MANUAL OF UROLOGIC SURGERY

Jackson E. Fowler, Jr., M.D.

Clarence C. Saelhof Professor of Urology and Chief of Urology,
University of Illinois College of Medicine, Chicago

ILLUSTRATED BY
Rong-Zeng Li

LITTLE, BROWN AND COMPANY
BOSTON/TORONTO/LONDON

MANUAL OF
UROLOGIC SURGERY

Contents

Preface

There are a number of basic urologic texts for medical students, house officers, and allied personnel. Well-illustrated descriptions of surgical procedures, however, are not commonly found in these works. This book is devoted to operative urology. It is extensively illustrated so that readers with little insight into the subject matter can appreciate the descriptive text. The book was produced initially by the University of Illinois Office of Publications Services, entitled *Methods of Urologic Surgery,* and supported by a grant from Mr. James Vance of the Van-Tec Corporation, Spencer, Indiana. The demand for the book exceeded our most optimistic expectations and prompted its republication in the current form.

The title of the original work has been changed to more accurately reflect the nature of its contents, and the format and text have been improved. The figures, however, are unchanged.

The first chapter addresses general considerations unique to urologic surgery. For brevity, the principles developed in this introductory section are not repeated in subsequent discussions of specific operative procedures to which they may apply. Most of the remaining chapters concern surgery of a specific component of the genitourinary system. The relevant anatomy and function are summarized in the introduction to each chapter. This is followed by a description of operations that may be used for a variety of disorders, or of operations for the treatment of a single disorder. When appropriate, postoperative management and complications are addressed after detailing the operative techniques.

Discussions of the pathophysiology, presentation, and evaluation of conditions that may require surgical intervention are brief, and the book is not referenced. Readers who wish to pursue specific topics in greater detail are encouraged to consult primary urologic texts. Categoric recommendations about the indications for operative intervention in general, and the optimal surgical approaches to individual disorders, have been omitted intentionally. These issues are subject to varying opinions based in large part on the training, experience, and philosophy of the surgeon, rather than on objective criteria.

The text was prepared with contributions from Drs. Jens Eldrup-Jorgensen and D. Preston Flanigan of the Peripheral Vascular Service at the University of Illinois Hospital and from Dr. Raymond Pollak of the Transplantation Service at the University of Illinois Hospital. While Rong-Zeng Li drew all the illustrations, many are adapted from the work of other artists whose perspectives and detail are difficult to surpass.

J. E. F., Jr.

Acknowledgments

The author wishes to thank James Vance, whose generosity made production of *Methods of Urologic Surgery* possible; Christopher Davis, formerly of Little, Brown and Company; and Susan Pioli, of Little, Brown and Company, whose enthusiasm and support made its republication in the current format possible. James Lau and Craig Smith, Residents in Urology, Clare Matz, Michele Mariano, and Catherine Judge helped in the preparation and review of the text.

CHAPTER 1

General Considerations

The primary ingredients for an optimal treatment outcome in any field of surgery include sound operative technique, attention to detail (both in and out of the operating room), and concern for the well-being of the patient. There are several considerations, however, that deserve particular attention in the management of urologic patients.

RENAL FUNCTION

A large number of urologic disorders have an adverse impact on renal function. Extirpative renal surgery also reduces overall renal function. Kidney function and functional changes associated with renal disease are most conveniently estimated by measuring the serum creatinine level or the creatinine clearance. The latter, which is a measure of the glomerular filtration rate (GFR), is determined by the formula $(U \times V)/P$, where U equals the concentration of urinary creatinine in milligrams per deciliters, V equals the volume of urinary excretion in milliliters per minute, and P equals the concentration of serum creatinine in milligrams per deciliter. Serial serum creatinine determinations are generally used to follow a patient's renal function over time. Because the creatinine clearance is inversely related to the serum creatinine level, it follows that a doubling of the serum creatinine represents a 50 percent decrease in GFR. This relationship is of clinical importance because a 1- to 2-mg/dl increase in the serum creatinine level and a 4- to 8-mg/dl increase both represent a 50 percent decrease of the preexisting renal function.

In a healthy person only about 20 percent of normal renal function, as measured by the GFR, is necessary for survival without dialysis or renal transplantation. Thus, the removal of one kidney is not associated with renal insufficiency over the long term when the serum creatinine level and the radiographic appearance of the contralateral kidney are normal. Nephrectomy may therefore be performed without hesitation for the treatment of a potentially lethal disorder or if the anticipated morbidity resulting from reparative surgery of a kidney or ureter is judged excessive. This consideration is particularly relevant if the affected kidney functions poorly.

In other circumstances, however, preservation of a diseased kidney may be advisable even when the contralateral kidney is normal. This is especially so when the disorder responsible for the diseased kidney may affect the remaining kidney at a later date. Urolithiasis, renal vascular disease, and infectious and inflammatory processes are examples of such conditions. At the other end of the spectrum, removal of both kidneys or of a functionally solitary kidney may be justified if the threat of the disorder is thought to be so great that survival with dialysis would be of a better quality and of longer duration than survival without nephrectomy. Sound clinical judgment and consultation with the patient must necessarily form the basis for therapeutic decision making in these situations.

The effects of aberrant renal function also impact on patient management and surgical risk. When overall renal function is less than 50 percent of normal, compensatory responses to fluid and electrolyte imbalance are impaired, and the risk of further renal deterioration from the stresses of surgery or infection is amplified. Severe renal insufficiency is associated also with a constellation of systemic disorders, including anemia, gastrointestinal and cardiovascular diseases, and impaired wound healing. The metabolism of many drugs, including most antibiotics, is abnormal. Urologic surgeons must optimize the general medical condition of patients with renal insufficiency before surgery and be prepared to deal with the complications arising from associated systemic diseases in the postoperative period.

ANTIMICROBIAL THERAPY

Susceptibility to urinary tract infection is often increased in patients with disorders of the urinary system. Culture documentation of a sterile urine is mandatory before operating on the urinary tract. If the urine is found to be infected before elective surgery, appropriate antimicrobial therapy is instituted and the operation is delayed until the urine is sterile. In conditions where rapidly recurring or persistent infection of the urinary tract is the rule, such as vesicointestinal fistulas or infected renal calculi, a sterile urine is almost always achievable with the administration of parenteral antibiotics just before surgery.

The value of perioperative prophylactic antimicrobial therapy in surgical procedures where bacterial contamination is unlikely remains controversial. For operations involving the kidney or urinary conduits, however, the rationale for preventative treatment is compelling. The urine has no natural antibacterial properties and is an excellent medium for the growth of gram-negative bacilli. Bacterial inoculation during surgery is possible and is inevitable in the postoperative period if exteriorized catheters are used for urinary drainage. The resultant bacteriuria impairs healing and the integrity of some suture materials. Leakage of infected urine before healing is complete predisposes to soft-tissue infections and abscesses. In addition, postoperative obstruction of urinary outflow potentiates the risks of acute bacterial nephritis and bacteremia; and acute bacterial prostatitis and epididymitis are recognized complications of urinary tract infection in men.

The potential efficacy of antibiotics for the prevention of postoperative bacteriuria is supported by three considerations. First, bacteria that usually infect the urine are limited to gram-negative enteric bacilli and enterococci. Most urinary tract infections, therefore, can be prevented or eradicated with well-defined antimicrobial regimens. Second, most antibiotics that are active against these bacteria are concentrated in the urine, reaching levels 50 to 100 times greater than those in the serum. This antibiotic concentration in the urine allows for increased activity against most organisms in the target fluid. Third, if antibiotics are not administered to patients with exteriorized catheters, bacteriuria develops within 8 days in about 50 percent of cases. The onset of infection, however, can be delayed with antimicrobial therapy. This provides a considerable therapeutic advantage because watertight healing of the urinary system usually occurs within 4 to 5 days of surgery, and drainage catheters are generally removed by the seventh postoperative day.

Urinary tract infection is almost inevitable if exteriorized catheters are required for more than 2 to 3 weeks. Unless the patient is at risk of serious morbidity from bacteriuria, prophylactic antibiotics should be administered for 5 to 7 days only after surgery. More prolonged treatment encourages infection with highly resistant organisms.

Regardless of the surgeon's approach to prophylactic therapy, the urine is always cultured, and isolates are tested for antimicrobial susceptibilities before exteriorized catheters are removed. If bacteriuria is suspected, one dose of an aminoglycoside is administered and a 7-day course of oral antibiotics is instituted. The agent chosen for oral therapy may have to be changed if susceptibility testing shows little activity against an infecting organism.

Categorical recommendations for the use of antibiotics are not warranted, and the guidelines summarized here are generalizations only. Nonetheless, we believe that prophylactic antimicrobial therapy and strict attention to urinary bacteriology will decrease the infectious complications of urologic surgery.

SUTURE MATERIALS

Foreign bodies within the urinary system promote stone formation. For this reason, naturally degradable suture materials are preferred for surgery of the urinary conduits. Absorbable sutures are also advisable for wound closure because some degree of urinary extravasation is inevitable in the postoperative period and bacteriuria may not be preventable. Suture abscesses are potentiated by nonabsorbable materials. Absorbable material is also useful for closing the skin of the scrotum and penis, as suture removal at these sites is difficult, and scars that are promoted by an inflammatory response are of no cosmetic importance.

The composition and proprietary name of natural and synthetic absorbable sutures are shown in Table 1.1. Gut sutures are derived from the intestinal submucosa of sheep and pigs whereas collagen sutures come from the tendons of cattle. The sutures are formed from twisted piles of the material and then polished. Plain gut or collagen is treated with an aldehyde solution to increase strength and resistance to degradation. Chromic gut or collagen is treated with chromium trioxide, which cross-links with the natural substance and further increases resistance to absorption.

Coated polyglactin 910 is a braided synthetic suture made from filaments of polymerized glycolide and lactide. It is coated with calcium stearate and a copolymer of lactic acid and glycolic acid. Polyglycolic acid sutures are made of braided strands of polymerized glycolide. Coated polyglycolic acid sutures are composed of the same material as the uncoated variety, but 188 poloxamer is applied to the surface as a lubricant.

Polyglyconate and polydioxanone monofilament synthetic sutures are made from polytrimethylene carbonate and from the polymerization of dioxanone, respectively.

Gut and collagen sutures are absorbed by enzymatic degradation and incite a pronounced inflammatory response. The rate of absorption is less predictable than that of synthetic absorbable suture material. It is en-

Table 1.1
ABSORBABLE SUTURES

Composition	Trade Name
Natural	
Plain gut	Plain Gut
Chromic gut	Chromic Gut
Reconstituted plain collagen	Plain Collagen
Reconstituted chromic collagen	Chromic Collagen
Synthetic	
Coated polyglactin 910 (braided)	Vicryl
Uncoated polyglycolic acid (braided)	Dexon S
Coated polyglycolic acid (braided)	Dexon Plus
Polyglyconate (monofilament)	Maxon
Polydioxanone (monofilament)	PDS

hanced by contact with urine, but is not altered by infection. Monofilament synthetic absorbable materials are more resistant to degradation than braided synthetic materials, and calculus formation is less likely when the latter are used to close the urinary tract.

Categoric recommendations concerning the optimal absorbable suture material for surgery of the urinary tract are also not warranted. Most urologists, however, prefer chromic gut or braided synthetic sutures for closure of the urinary conduits and monofilament synthetic sutures for wound closure.

DRAINS AND CATHETERS

In contrast to other hollow viscera, the components of the urinary system have a unique propensity for spontaneous healing. Watertight closures of the renal pelvis and ureter, which may be difficult or impossible, are not essential. Moreover, some degree of urinary extravasation is inevitable even when a thick-walled structure like the bladder is closed in three layers. It is generally advisable to position drains adjacent to suture lines in order to exteriorize urinary leakage. We prefer Penrose drains as opposed to suction drains. As a rule, the drains are left in situ until drainage has ceased. In situations where healing is compromised or the risks associated with premature drain removal are great, contrast studies to document the absence of urinary extravasation are done before the drain is manipulated.

The diversion of urine from the intrarenal collecting system or bladder lumen using an exteriorized catheter and stenting of the ureter or urethra with a catheter are fundamental components of urologic surgery. However, opinions vary concerning the desirability and technique of catheter drainage or stenting after specific operations. Drains and stents promote healing by decreasing urinary leakage and reducing tension on suture lines. Decompression of the urinary system also reduces the risks of acute renal infection. On the other hand, exteriorized catheters increase the likelihood of bacteriuria, and inflammation caused by a stent may encourage fibrosis and subsequent stricture formation. In addition, transient urinary extravasation routed to the skin via a drain does not usually result in postoperative complications.

Most urologists would agree that a conservative approach to catheter drainage or stenting is rarely regretted when the patient's overall medical condition is suboptimal, the prospects for prompt healing are uncertain, or the renal function is impaired.

Surgical Approaches

This chapter addresses the surgical approaches to the abdomen, retroperitoneum, and pelvis. Incisions for perineal and inguinal operations, and for surgery of the penis and scrotal contents, are summarized in the appropriate chapters. The muscular and fascial anatomy of the trunk is described in the introductory section to facilitate an understanding of the operative techniques.

Anatomy of the Abdominal Wall

The paired rectus muscles extend from the xiphoid and cartilage of the fifth, sixth, and seventh ribs to the symphysis pubis (Figures 2.1 and 2.2). They are separated in the midline by the linea alba, a decussation of the anterior and posterior rectus sheaths.

The anterior rectus sheath is formed from the aponeurosis of the external oblique muscle above the costal margin and for 8 cm below the xiphoid. Between the costal margin and the arcuate line it is derived from the aponeuroses of the external and internal oblique muscles; between the arcuate line and the symphysis pubis it is formed from the aponeuroses of the external oblique, internal oblique, and transversus muscles.

Above the costal margin the rectus muscle lies on the costal cartilage. For 8 cm below the xiphoid the posterior rectus sheath is derived from the aponeuro-

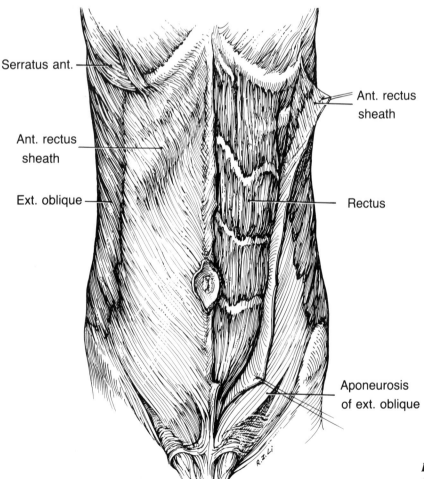

Serratus ant.

Ant. rectus sheath

Ext. oblique

Ant. rectus sheath

Rectus

Aponeurosis of ext. oblique

FIGURE 2.1
Superficial anterior abdominal musculature

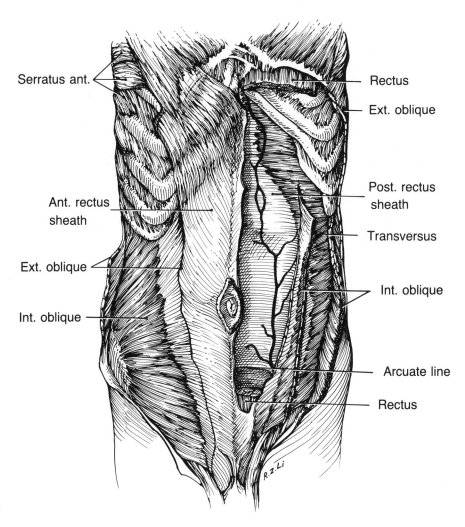

Serratus ant.

Rectus

Ext. oblique

Ant. rectus
sheath

Post. rectus
sheath

Transversus

Ext. oblique

Int. oblique

Int. oblique

Arcuate line

Rectus

R.Z.Li

FIGURE 2.2
Deep anterior abdominal musculature

sis of the transversus muscle only. From this level to the arcuate line it is formed from the aponeuroses of the internal oblique and transversus muscles. There is no true posterior sheath below the arcuate line. Only the areolar transversalis fascia and extraperitoneal fat lie between the rectus muscles and the peritoneum.

The external oblique muscle arises from the lower eight ribs, where there are interdigitations with the serratus anterior and latissimus dorsi muscles (Figures 2.3 to 2.5). The fibers course in an anteroinferior direction. The upper half of the external oblique muscle contributes to the anterior rectus sheath and decussates in the linea alba. The lower portion attaches to the iliac crest and forms the inguinal ligament between the anterior superior iliac spine and the pubic tubercle. The posterior border has no well-defined attachments.

The internal oblique muscle arises from the iliac crest and lateral inguinal ligament. The fibers course in an anterosuperior direction. Posterior fibers attach to the cartilage of the lower four ribs, and anterior fibers

contribute to the anterior and posterior rectus sheaths and decussate in the linea alba.

The transversus abdominis muscle arises from the iliac crest and lateral inguinal ligament, the transverse processes of the lumbar vertebrae, and the undersurface of the costal cartilage of the lower six ribs. The fibers course transversely to decussate in the linea alba. They pass posterior to the rectus muscle above the arcuate line and anterior to the rectus muscle below the arcuate line. In the posterolateral trunk the transversus muscle is aponeurotic and forms the lumbodorsal fascia.

The psoas muscle arises from the bodies of the twelfth thoracic and lumbar vertebrae and extends inferolaterally to insert in the lesser trochanter of the femur (Figure 2.6). The quadratus lumborum muscle arises from the posterior iliac crest and extends superomedially to the posterior segment of the lowest rib. The posterior border attaches to the transverse processes of the lumbar vertebrae.

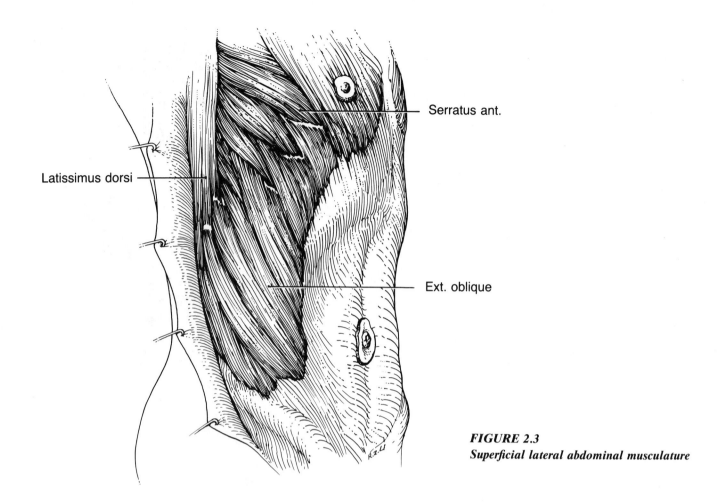

FIGURE 2.3
Superficial lateral abdominal musculature

Serratus ant.

Latissimus dorsi

Ext. oblique

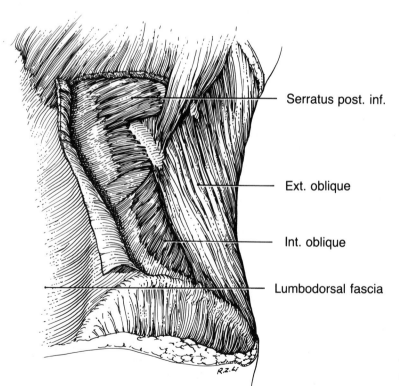

Serratus post. inf.

Ext. oblique

Int. oblique

Lumbodorsal fascia

FIGURE 2.4
Superficial posterolateral abdominal musculature

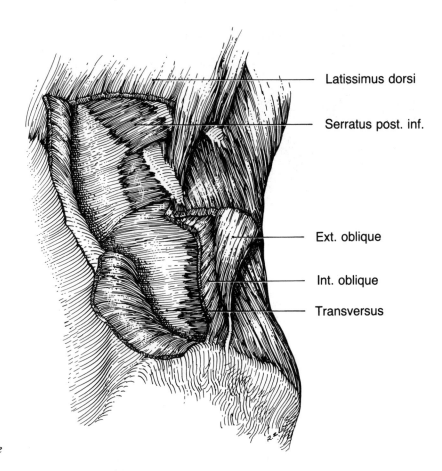

— Latissimus dorsi

— Serratus post. inf.

— Ext. oblique

— Int. oblique

— Transversus

FIGURE 2.5
Deep posterolateral abdominal musculature

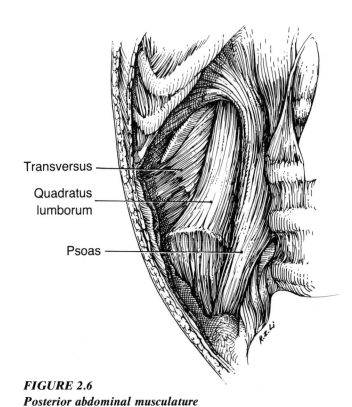

Transversus —

Quadratus
lumborum —

Psoas —

FIGURE 2.6
Posterior abdominal musculature

The sacrospinalis muscle (Figure 2.7) arises from the spines of the lower thoracic, lumbar, and sacral vertebrae and passes between the spines and the transverse processes of these vertebrae to insert in the posterior ribs and the thoracic and cervical vertebral spines.

The posterior abdominal musculature is compartmentalized by extensions of the lumbodorsal fascia. The superficial component (or posterior lamina) of the lumbodorsal fascia overlies the sacrospinalis muscle. The medial lamina courses between the sacrospinalis and quadratus lumborum muscles, and the anterior lamina passes deep to the quadratus lumborum. An appreciation of this anatomy is critical for the identification of muscular landmarks encountered during the lumbar approach to the retroperitoneum.

The serratus posterior inferior muscle (Figure 2.4) attaches to the spines of the lower thoracic and upper lumbar vertebrae and extends superolaterally to the lower ribs. This muscle is observed in the lateral aspect of flank incisions and may require transection to facilitate exposure.

The latissimus dorsi muscle (Figures 2.3 and 2.5) arises from the proximal humerus and fans out to

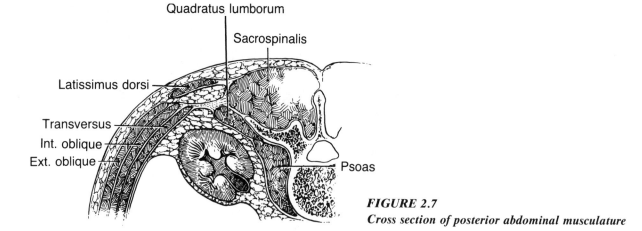

FIGURE 2.7
Cross section of posterior abdominal musculature

attach to the spines of the lower six thoracic, lumbar, and sacral vertebrae and to the posterior margin of the iliac crest. It is also attached to the lower three ribs, where there are interdigitations with the external oblique and serratus anterior muscles.

Incisions

A variety of operative approaches to the peritoneal cavity, retroperitoneum, and pelvis are available to the urologist. The most important criterion for choosing one incision over another is exposure of the operative field. Difficulties in identifying and exposing vital structures tax the surgeon and increase the risks of intraoperative complications.

FLANK INCISIONS

Flank incisions provide direct extraperitoneal access to the kidney and mid- and upper ureter. They are not well tolerated by patients with compromised cardiac or respiratory function because of the necessary lateral positioning. Exposure of the renal vessels without prior mobilization of the kidney is not possible through a standard flank incision. An injured kidney or large renal neoplasms, therefore, should be approached through a more anteriorly located transperitoneal incision.

The most appropriate level of the incision is dictated by the position of the kidney (or structure of surgical interest) and is best estimated by drawing — on the intravenous pyelogram — a horizontal line that crosses the midpoint of the anticipated area of dissection. The incision is made over the rib that is traversed by the line at the most lateral thorax. Uncertainty about the anticipated quality of exposure should always prompt an incision over the next highest rib.

The patient is placed on his or her side with the site of incision situated over the break of the table. The back is positioned near the table edge. The lower arm is extended on a board and a small pillow is positioned under the axilla. The upper arm is secured in a sling with the elbow flexed 90°. The lower leg is flexed 30° at the hip and 90° at the knee, and the upper leg is extended on a pillow. The hips and legs are strapped with heavy tape. While monitoring the blood pressure, the table is slowly flexed to spread the ribs and the musculature of the flank.

Unsuspected pleural injury is a potential complication of all flank incisions. A chest x-ray is routinely obtained in the recovery room to rule out a pneumothorax.

Subcostal Incision

The subcostal incision is usually adequate for exposure of a low-lying kidney or of the upper ureter. It is made 2 cm below the twelfth rib and extends from the sacrospinalis muscle to the rectus sheath (Figure 2.8). The investing fascia of the latissimus dorsi and external oblique muscles are exposed, and a plane is developed below the body of the muscles with a large clamp. The fibers between the open blades of the clamp or between the fingers are incised using electrocautery. The internal oblique muscle is divided in the same manner and the underlying subcostal neurovascular bundle is isolated and retracted superiorly or inferiorly to avoid injury. The lumbodorsal fascia is then opened bluntly in the direction of its transverse fibers. With a sponge-on-ring forceps the paranephric fat and peritoneum are swept from the undersurface of the lumbodorsal fascia and transversus abdominis muscle medially. Paranephric fat is then freed from the lumbo-

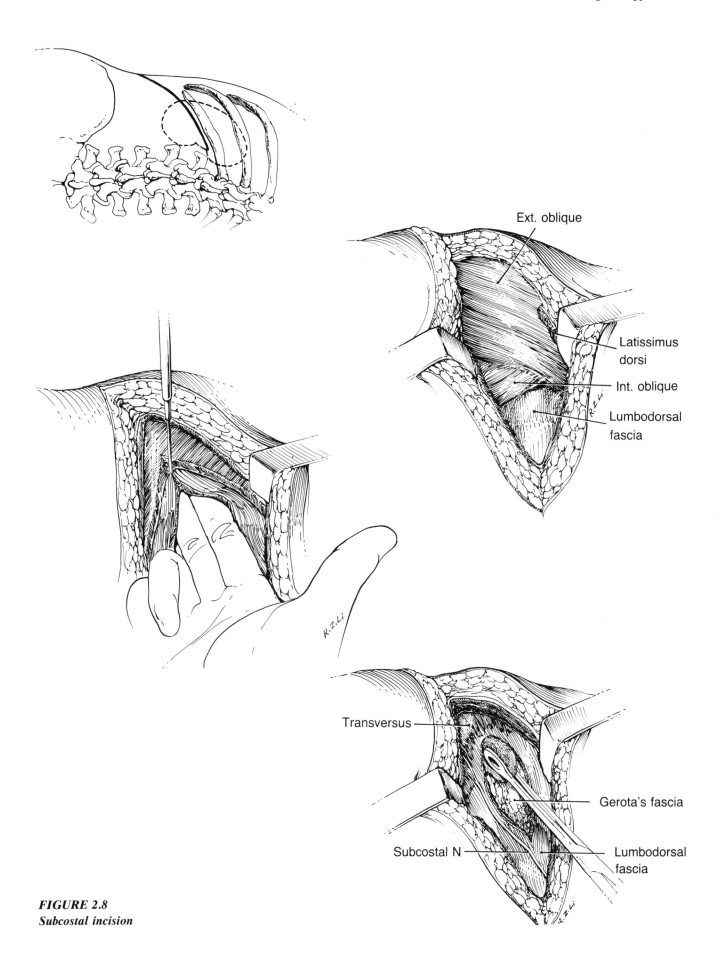

Ext. oblique

Latissimus dorsi

Int. oblique

Lumbodorsal fascia

Transversus

Gerota's fascia

Subcostal N

Lumbodorsal fascia

FIGURE 2.8
Subcostal incision

dorsal fascia inferiorly and superiorly and from the quadratus lumborum posteriorly. This permits wide separation of the wound with a self-retaining retractor. The fibers of the transversus abdominis muscle are bluntly separated along the length of the wound, moist pads are placed on the muscle edge, and a Finochietto or Balfour retractor is positioned to maintain exposure.

At the completion of the operation, drains and catheters are brought out through separate stab wounds below the incision. The muscle layers are systematically closed with interrupted figure-of-eight sutures that encompass the investing fascia but not the body of the muscle. Care must be taken to align each muscle layer properly because the oblique nature of the incision tends to shift the muscle edges. Flattening the table before closure eliminates undue tension as the sutures are tied. The subcutaneous tissue is approxi-

mated with interrupted or continuous absorbable sutures, and the skin is closed with staples or interrupted mattress sutures. Infiltration of the eleventh and twelfth intercostal nerves with 20 to 30 ml of bupivacaine significantly reduces postoperative discomfort.

Transcostal and Intercostal Incisions

A flank incision located at or above the twelfth rib is generally required to expose the entire kidney. The transcostal approach is made through a rib bed, whereas the intercostal approach is made between two ribs. Resection of the anterior portion of a rib does not lead to increased postoperative morbidity and may improve exposure. Wound closure is also facilitated because the rib bed provides abundant fibrous tissue for the placement of sutures.

The transcostal incision starts at the posterior axillary line, extends medially over the palpable rib, and

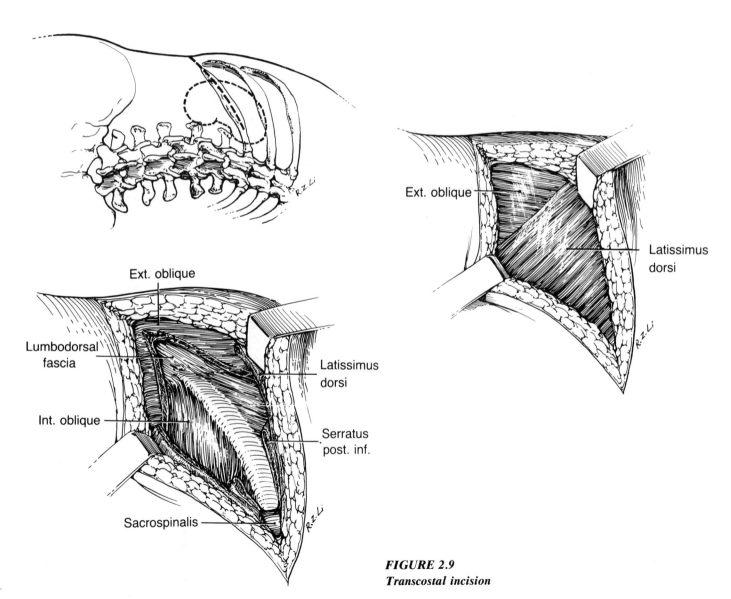

FIGURE 2.9
Transcostal incision

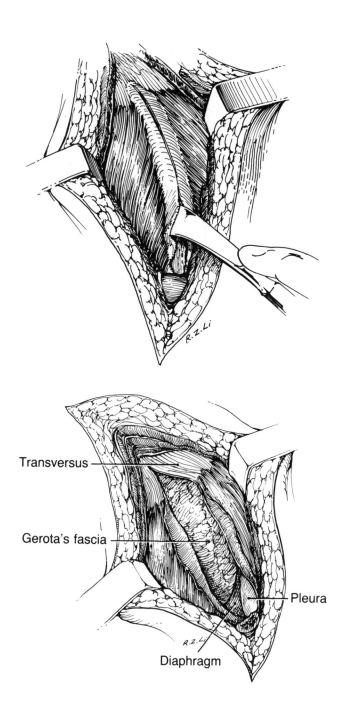

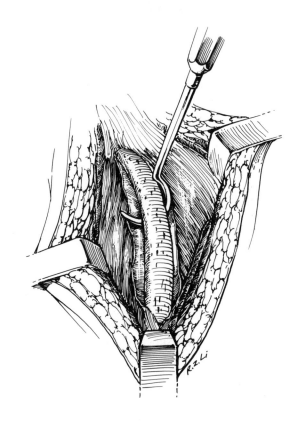

FIGURE 2.9
Transcostal incision (continued)

ends at the lateral margin of the rectus sheath (Figure 2.9). The latissimus dorsi, serratus posterior inferior, and external oblique muscles overlying the rib are divided with electrocautery. A finger is positioned over the upper and lower intercostal spaces to guide the incision. The external oblique and internal oblique muscles medial to the rib are then separated and individually transected with electrocautery.

The periosteum of the rib is scored with a scalpel and dissected from the anterior surface using a periosteal elevator. The intercostal muscles and fascia course obliquely in an anterior direction. They are sep-

arated from the rib by advancing the periosteal elevator downward on the upper rib edge and upward on the lower rib edge. The undersurface of the rib is freed from the periosteum with a flat or Doyen periosteal elevator. The lateral aspect of the incision is then retracted with a small Richardson retractor, and the rib is divided as far posteriorly as possible. The rib is grasped with a Kocher clamp, the cartilaginous tip is dissected sharply from fibrous tissues at the costal margin, and the segment is removed.

The rib bed is incised with a scalpel to expose the pleural reflection. The pleura is freed from its attachments to the diaphragm and reflected superiorly; the diaphragmatic fibers are transected. Paranephric fat and peritoneum are swept from the undersurface of the lumbodorsal fascia and transversus muscle medially. Paranephric fat is freed from the diaphragm and lumbodorsal fascia superiorly, the quadratus lumborum posteriorly, and the lumbodorsal fascia inferiorly. The lumbodorsal fascia and transversus muscle are then divided bluntly in the direction of their fibers to the medial aspect of the incision. The neurovascular bundle of the more superior rib is encountered above the transversus muscle and is isolated and retracted. Moist pads are placed over the margins of the rib bed and a Finochietto retractor is positioned to spread the wound.

Before closure of the wound, the lung is hyperexpanded to expose the pleura clearly. Tears in the pleura are managed by inserting a soft catheter into the thoracic cavity and approximating the edges of the defect with a continuous absorbable suture. A pursestring suture is placed in the pleura surrounding the catheter, and the end of the catheter is immersed in a basin of water. The lungs are expanded to evacuate the pleural space, and the pursestring suture is tightened as the catheter is removed.

The rib bed is closed in two discrete layers with interrupted sutures. The lumbodorsal fascia and muscle layers are systematically approximated as described for the subcostal incision. Infiltration of intercostal nerves above and below the incision with 20 to 30 ml of bupivacaine reduces postoperative discomfort.

The transcostal flank incision can also be done without rib resection. The rib is freed from the anterior, superior, and posterior periosteum using the techniques described above and retracted downward. The rib bed is incised, and the procedure is continued as with the transcostal incision with rib resection.

The incision for the intercostal approach is placed between rather than over the ribs. After transection of the latissimus dorsi and external and internal oblique muscles, the intercostal muscle is divided at the upper edge of the lower rib to avoid injury to the intercostal neurovascular bundle. The pleura is mobilized superiorly, and the diaphragmatic fibers are transected to expose the paranephric fat. The remainder of the incision is identical to that described for the transcostal approach.

Closure of the intercostal incision deviates from that of the transcostal incision because there is insufficient tissue for direct approximation of the intercostal muscle. We prefer to suture the intercostal muscle to the periosteum of the lower rib. To increase the strength of the closure, heavy absorbable sutures are passed around the upper and lower ribs at three or four points along the incision. These encircling sutures should hug the periosteum of the ribs to avoid injury to the intercostal vessels and nerve.

Muscle-Splitting Flank Incision

The muscle-splitting flank incision is an attractive option when exposure of a well-defined portion of the midureter only is required. If extensive ureteral surgery is contemplated, a vertical midline or paramedial incision is more appropriate.

The patient is placed in the supine position and the ipsilateral shoulder and buttock are elevated 30° with sandbags. A transverse incision is begun several centimeters below the tip of the twelfth rib and carried to the rectus sheath (Figure 2.10). The external oblique, internal oblique, and transversus muscles are sequentially separated in the direction of their fibers and retracted. Division of muscle is not necessary. The peritoneum is then swept off the psoas muscle to expose the ureter. The wound is closed by approximating the fascia that invests each muscle layer.

LUMBAR INCISION

The lumbar incision provides direct and rapid access to the kidney and upper ureter and is remarkably easy to close. Postoperative pain is minimal because only fascia is transected, and the natural interposition of muscle between the fascial closures prevents the development of incisional hernias. However, exposure is limited and intraoperative complications or unexpected anatomic variations may be troublesome. The approach can be used for upper ureterolithotomy, pyelolithotomy, pyeloplasty, renal biopsy, and removal of small kidneys. Bilateral incisions with the patient in the prone position are well suited for the removal of two small kidneys in patients with end-stage renal disease.

For the unilateral approach the patient may be placed in either the lateral or the prone position. With lateral positioning the midpoint between the iliac crest and lower rib is situated over the break of the table, and the back is positioned at the edge of the table. The arms and legs are positioned as described for a standard flank incision. The table is flexed to spread the muscle and fascia of the posterolateral trunk. With prone positioning the table is flexed to spread the muscle and fascia of the posterior trunk.

The incision is begun below the twelfth rib over the easily palpable sacrospinalis muscle and extended to a point just lateral to the most superior aspect of the iliac crest (Figure 2.11). The posterior lamina of the lumbar fascia is incised 2 cm medial to the edge of the sacro-

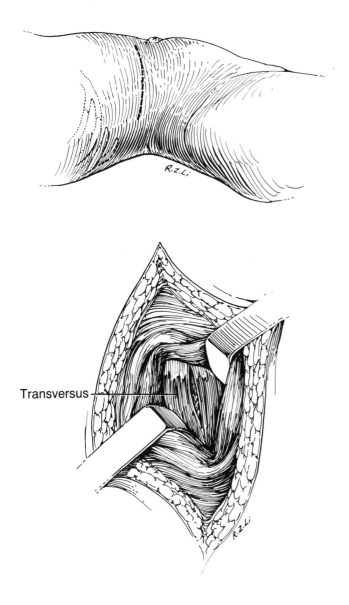

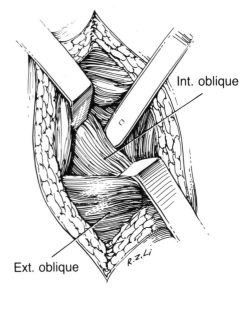

Int. oblique

Ext. oblique

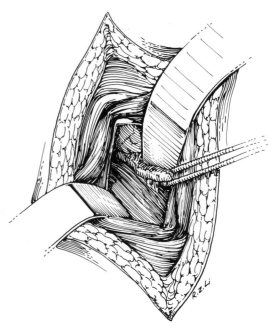

Transversus

FIGURE 2.10
Muscle-splitting flank incision

spinalis muscle. The lateral margin of the sacrospinalis is freed from its fascial investment and retracted medially; the middle lamina of the lumbar fascia is incised 2 cm medial to the edge of the quadratus lumborum muscle. The quadratus lumborum is also retracted medially, and the anterior lamina is incised to expose the paranephric fat. Care must be taken to avoid injury to the iliohypogastric nerve, which runs deep to the lumbodorsal fascia lateral to the incision, and to the ilioinguinal nerve at the inferior aspect of the incision. The wound is separated with a Finochietto retractor with protective pads under the blades.

Some urologists prefer to incise the lumbar fascia adjacent to the edge of the sacrospinalis and quadratus lumborum muscles. However, this approach does not permit insinuation of muscle between the fascial closures.

Exposure can be enhanced superiorly by division of the costovertebral ligament and upward retraction of the twelfth rib. Care is taken to avoid injury to the neurovascular bundle. Transection of the sacrospinalis muscle medial to the costovertebral ligament also improves exposure.

Before closing the wound, drains and catheters are brought out through separate stab wounds lateral to the incision. The three fascial divisions are closed separately with heavy interrupted absorbable sutures. The superior and inferior portions of each fascial closure should be completed before the middle portion is approximated.

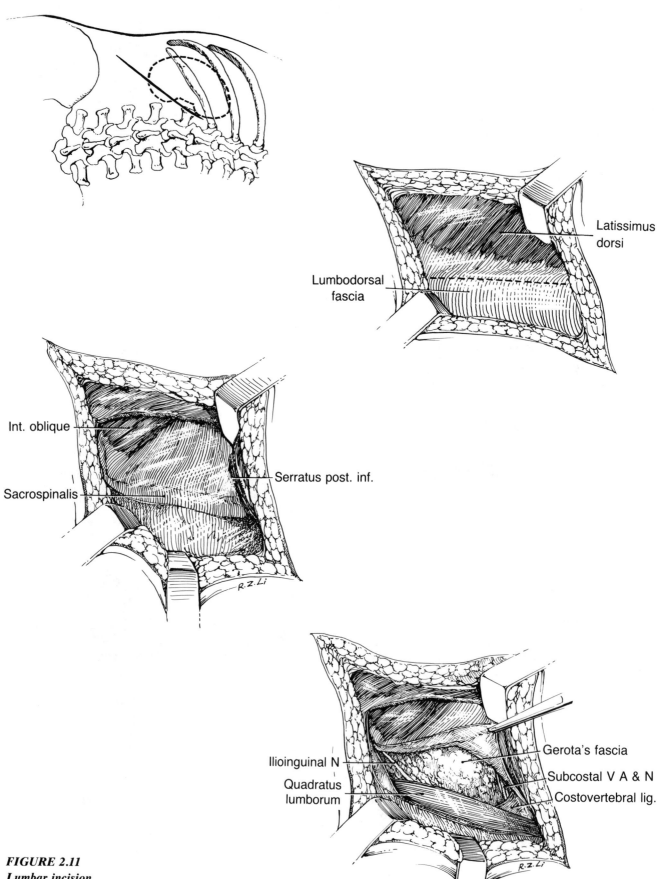

FIGURE 2.11
Lumbar incision

UPPER ABDOMINAL INCISIONS

Upper abdominal incisions are usually transperitoneal. An extraperitoneal dissection may be feasible in some circumstances, but the benefits rarely justify the efforts. A transperitoneal approach to retroperitoneal surgery is required when careful inspection of the intra-abdominal viscera is warranted, or if access to the renal vessels is desired before manipulation of the kidney.

Vertical Midline Incision

The vertical midline incision can be executed quickly and provides access to the entire peritoneal cavity and to the retroperitoneal space on each side. Exposure of the retroperitoneum above the renal vessels is satisfactory if the xiphoid is high.

The patient is placed in the supine position. The incision is initiated at the xiphoid and terminated above or below the umbilicus, as needed. The decussating fibers of the linea alba are divided along the length of the incision with the beveled edge of the scalpel. The rectus muscles are not seen if the incision is positioned properly and does not extend below the arcuate line. At the umbilicus the skin and fascial incisions should curve to the left. The abdominal cavity is preferentially entered in the upper aspect of the incision overlying the liver. The peritoneum is cleared of fat, grasped and tented with two hemostats, and incised with scissors or a scalpel. It is then divided along the length of the incision, taking care to identify and mobilize bowel or omentum that may be adherent at the incision line.

Before the wound is closed, the omentum is draped over the intestines, and a wide malleable retractor is positioned beneath the fascia to prevent the protrusion of bowel. The peritoneum may be closed separately with a continuous absorbable suture or encompassed in the fascial closure. The linea alba is approximated with interrupted heavy sutures. Retention sutures help to strengthen the closure and are used if the prospects for prompt healing are uncertain, or if intestinal distension creates tension on the suture lines. The sutures are placed through the rectus sheath but outside the peritoneal space before closing the linea alba and are tied over bolsters after the skin is approximated. Care is taken throughout the closure to avoid suture entrapment of bowel or omentum. Intermittent palpation of the undersurface of the suture line will identify unsuspected entrapments.

Paramedian Incision

The paramedian incision is made about 3 cm lateral to the midline (Figure 2.12). In contrast to the vertical

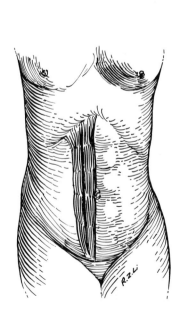

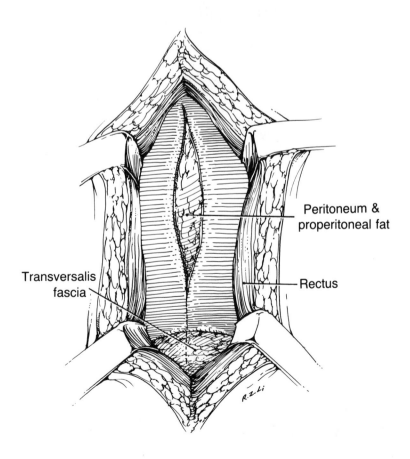

Transversalis fascia

Peritoneum & properitoneal fat

Rectus

FIGURE 2.12
Paramedian incision

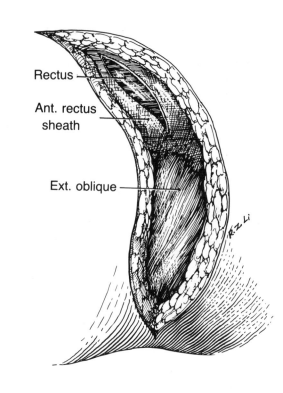

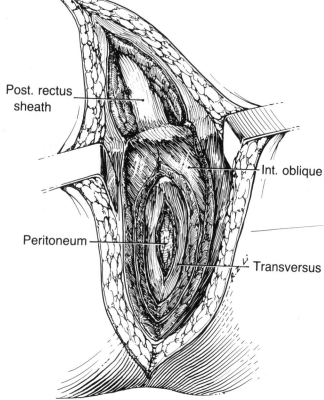

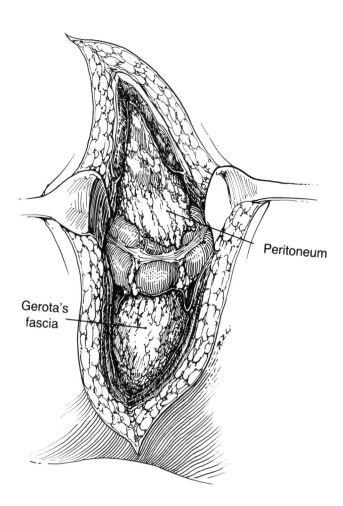

FIGURE 2.13
Anterior subcostal incision

midline incision, there are two fascial closures separated by the rectus muscle. This reduces the risks of incisional hernias.

The anterior rectus fascia is cut along the length of the skin incision, and the medial border of the rectus muscle is dissected from the rectus sheath. The muscle is retracted laterally, and the posterior rectus sheath and peritoneum are opened 3 cm lateral to the midline. The peritoneum and posterior rectus sheath and the anterior rectus sheath are closed separately with heavy interrupted sutures.

Anterior Subcostal and Chevron Incisions

The anterior subcostal incision provides exposure to the upper abdominal cavity and retroperitoneal space on one side, whereas the chevron incision permits exposure of both sides. Each necessitates the division of a rather large muscle mass. The patient is placed in a supine position with the ipsilateral flank elevated for the subcostal incision, and in the standard supine position for the chevron incision.

The anterior subcostal incision is begun in the midline several centimeters below the xiphoid and extends inferolaterally below the costal margin to the midaxillary line (Figure 2.13). The anterior rectus sheath and external oblique muscles are incised, and the rectus muscle is divided with cautery. Care is taken to ligate the superior epigastric vessels that lie

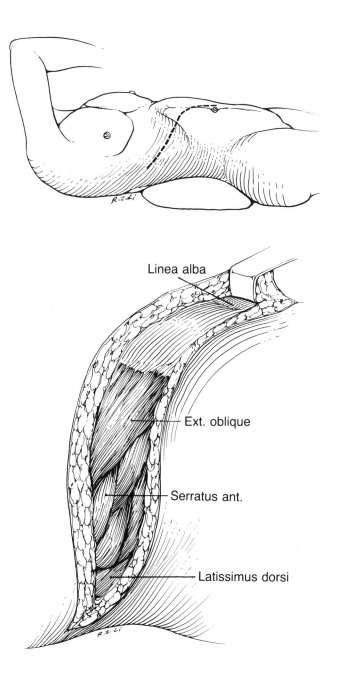

Linea alba

Ext. oblique

Serratus ant.

Latissimus dorsi

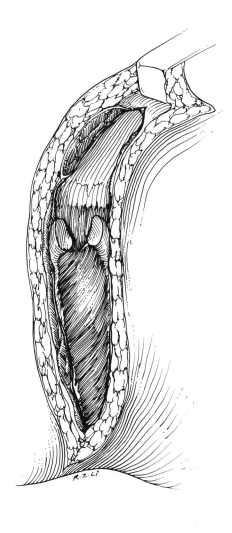

FIGURE 2.14
Thoracoabdominal incision

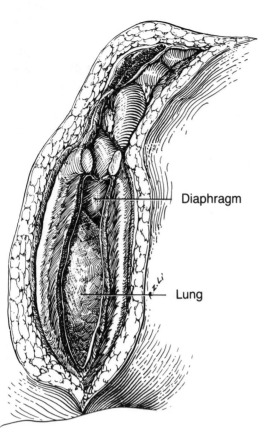
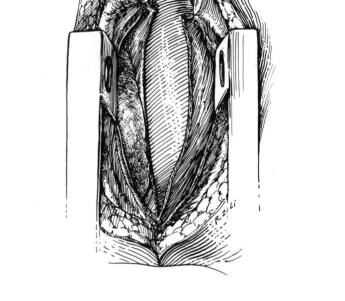

FIGURE 2.14
Thoracoabdominal incision (continued)

between the rectus muscle and the posterior sheath. The internal oblique and transversus muscles are then incised lateral to the rectus muscle, and the underlying peritoneum is opened. The incision is completed by dividing the posterior rectus sheath and adherent peritoneum. The wound is closed by systematic approximation of the fascial margins with interrupted heavy sutures.

The chevron incision is an anterior subcostal incision that is extended to the contralateral side by dividing the muscle and fascia in the same manner as the ipsilateral side. The falciform ligament must be transected to permit wide separation of the wound margins.

THORACOABDOMINAL INCISION

The thoracoabdominal incision traverses the pleural space and diaphragm and provides unparalleled exposure to the upper retroperitoneum and upper abdominal cavity. It is recommended for the removal of large renal, suprarenal, or retroperitoneal masses. The incision may be extended to the midline and directed infe-

riorly to the symphysis pubis when pelvic surgery is also anticipated.

The patient is initially placed in the supine position with the break of the table under the lower ribs. For midline masses we prefer a left-sided approach to obviate extensive retraction of the liver. The trunk is torqued by elevating the buttock 15° and the chest 30° with sandbags. The arms and legs are positioned as described for the flank incisions.

The incision may overlie the seventh to eleventh rib. However, unless an extrapleural dissection is planned, there is little reason to risk inadequate exposure by excising the ninth or tenth rib as opposed to the seventh or eighth. The incision begins at the midaxillary line and extends over the rib and costal margin to the rectus sheath (Figure 2.14). For more generous exposure it is carried to the midline and directed downward to the umbilicus or symphysis pubis. The latissimus dorsi and external oblique muscles are transected, and the underlying rib is removed using the techniques described for the transcostal flank incision. The cartilaginous costal margin of the seventh to tenth rib is usually intact, and a segment adjacent to the end of the rib is

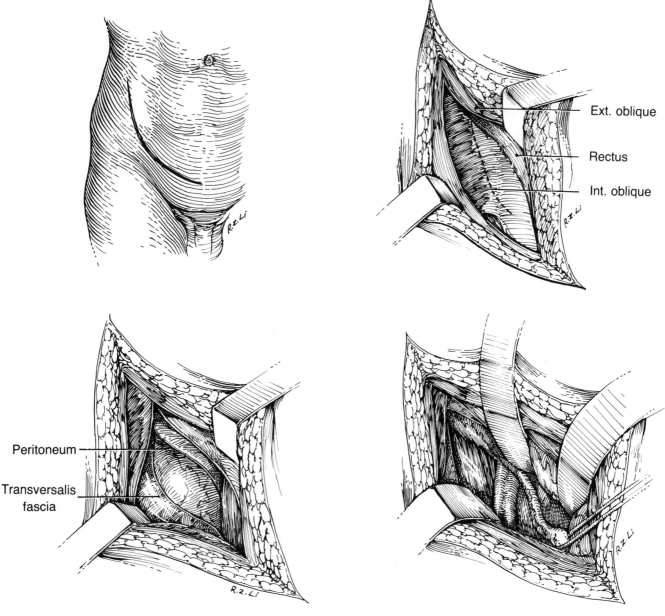

Ext. oblique

Rectus

Int. oblique

Peritoneum

Transversalis fascia

FIGURE 2.15
Gibson incision

removed to facilitate approximation of the rib bed during wound closure. The abdominal component of the incision is completed by dividing the internal oblique and transversus muscles and opening the peritoneum.

The pleural cavity is entered along the length of the rib bed. The tidal volume of respiration is then reduced to improve exposure of the diaphragm. The hand is placed on the undersurface of the diaphragm to protect the intra-abdominal viscera; with scissors the diaphragm and investing parietal pleura and peritoneum is incised directly under the thoracic wound. Several large vessels usually require suture ligation. A Fino-

chietto retractor is positioned so that the blades encompass the thoracic and diaphragmatic incision. If the incision is extended down the midline, a second self-retaining retractor is placed inferiorly.

The thoracic component of the incision is closed before the abdominal component. The diaphragm is approximated with through-and-through heavy absorbable figure-of-eight sutures. The knots are tied outside the pleural space. The parietal pleura may be sealed with an additional fine continuous suture. An 18 F Silastic chest tube is introduced at the midaxillary line through an inferior intercostal space. It is positioned posterior to the lung so as not to lie on the diaphragmatic suture line. To reduce tension during closure of the rib bed, the table is flattened and the rib approximator instrument is applied to the upper and lower ribs. The bed is approximated in two layers with interrupted heavy absorbable sutures. The knots of these sutures are also tied outside the pleural space. The costal margin is stabilized with a figure-of-eight suture of 28-gauge wire. When the diaphragmatic incision is extensive, it is advisable to close the lateral rib bed before closing the medial diaphragm. This reduces tension on the diaphragmatic suture line.

The remainder of the thoracic and abdominal wound closure is identical to that described for the transcostal flank and midline abdominal incisions.

LOWER ABDOMINAL INCISIONS

Lower abdominal incisions can be used for transperitoneal exposure of the pelvic viscera and extraperitoneal exposure of the bladder, prostate, and pelvic side wall.

Gibson Incision
The Gibson incision is particularly well suited for surgery of the lower ureter when extensive pelvic dissection is not anticipated. A curved incision is begun medial to the anterosuperior iliac spine and extended to a point two fingerbreadths above the symphysis pubis (Figure 2.15). The external oblique muscle and anterior rectus sheath are incised and the rectus muscle is retracted medially. The internal oblique muscle and transversalis fascia are then divided, and the peritoneum is swept medially from the psoas muscle to expose the iliac vessels and the ureter. Additional exposure can be achieved by transecting the rectus muscle just above the symphysis pubis. Care is taken to ligate the inferior epigastric artery and vein lying posterior to the rectus muscle.

The wound is closed by systematic approximation of the investing fascia of the internal and external oblique muscles and of the anterior rectus fascia.

Lower Midline Incision
The vertical lower midline incision provides exposure to the deep pelvis on each side and is always used when superior extension of a lower abdominal incision is contemplated. The incision begins above or below the umbilicus and is extended to a point slightly below the superior margin of the symphysis pubis. The linea alba is incised, the pyramidalis muscle is divided in the midline, and the transversalis fascia and peritoneum are opened along the length of the wound.

For extraperitoneal dissections it is critical to incise the filmy transversalis fascia and preperitoneal fat to develop a proper plane between the peritoneum and the pelvic side wall. In addition, the peritoneum should be freed from the undersurface of the posterior rectus sheath before dividing the linea alba above the arcuate line. This reduces the risk of inadvertent entry of the peritoneal cavity.

The wound is closed by approximation of the linea alba with heavy interrupted sutures.

Transverse Incision
The transverse lower abdominal incision, or Pfannenstiel incision, has an advantage over the vertical midline incision in that muscle is situated between the peritoneal cavity and the fascial closure, and the scar is located below the beltline.

The incision is made 4 cm above the symphysis pubis and extends in a gentle upward curve beyond the lateral border of the rectus muscle on each side. The anterior rectus sheath is divided along the length of the incision and freed from the rectus muscles inferiorly and superiorly (Figure 2.16). The rectus and pyramidalis muscles are then separated in the midline and pulled apart. For transperitoneal approaches, the transversalis fascia and peritoneum are incised, and exposure is maintained with a self-retaining retractor.

For extraperitoneal surgery the transversalis fascia is incised, and the peritoneum is swept from the undersurface of the fascia and pelvic side walls. This permits

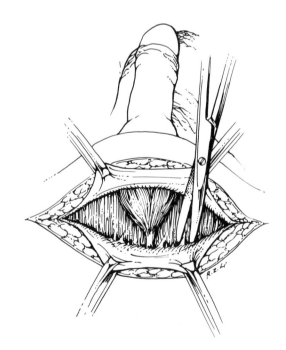

FIGURE 2.16
Transverse lower abdominal incision

wide separation of the rectus muscles with a self-retaining retractor. If drainage of the pelvis is planned, a midline stab wound of the skin and anterior rectus sheath is made several centimeters below the incision. A large Penrose drain is introduced through the defect and pulled inferiorly to facilitate exposure. Division of the rectus muscles just above the symphysis pubis also enhances exposure of the deep pelvis.

The wound is closed by approximating the rectus muscles with several loose interrupted sutures and closing the anterior rectus sheath with heavy interrupted sutures.

Surgery of the Kidney

The kidneys are situated in the upper retroperitoneum at the level of the twelfth thoracic vertebra to the third lumbar vertebra. The upper portion of the kidney is protected by the lower ribs. Posterior to the kidney and the encompassing fascia and fat are the psoas and quadratus lumborum muscles. Relationships between the kidneys and adjacent viscera are shown in Figure 3.1. Overlying the right kidney are the right liver lobe, the descending duodenum, and the hepatic flexure of the colon. Overlying the left kidney are the stomach, spleen, splenic flexure of the colon, pancreas, and jejunum.

Each kidney and adrenal gland is surrounded by Gerota's fascia, which is closed superiorly, laterally,

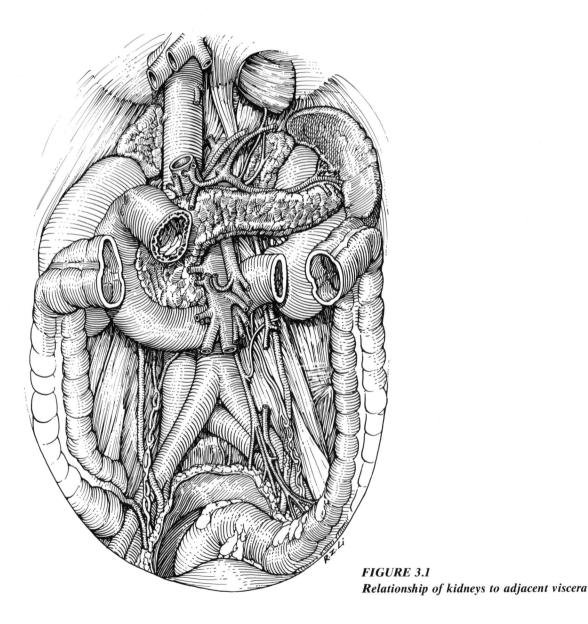

FIGURE 3.1
Relationship of kidneys to adjacent viscera

and (to a variable extent) medially before it crosses the midline anterior and posterior to the great vessels. Gerota's fascia encompasses the upper one third of the ureter but is not fused at the most dependent portion. Fluid collections within Gerota's fascia, therefore, extend inferiorly into the retroperitoneal space. Gerota's fascia is surrounded by pararenal fat and separated from the renal capsule by perirenal fat.

The kidney is 10 to 12 cm long and weighs approximately 150 g. Its fibrous capsule extends from the margins of the calyces surrounding the renal pyramids (Figure 3.2) and is easily stripped from the parenchyma. The renal parenchyma is divided into an outer cortex and an inner medulla. The glomeruli and most of the renal tubules lie in the cortex. The medulla is composed of 10 to 20 conical pyramids and intervening cortical tissue. The pyramids contain the loops of Henle and collecting ducts, and their bases demarcate the medulla from the cortex.

The apex of each pyramid is surrounded by a minor calyx, the most proximal component of the urinary collecting system. The minor calyces are muscular conduits lined by transitional epithelium. Major calyces are derived from the merger of two or more minor calyces and drain through infundibula into the renal pelvis. Although there is great variability of the intrarenal collecting system, the configuration of the collecting systems of companion kidneys is usually similar. The renal pelvis is situated behind the renal

vessels and may be surrounded largely by renal parenchyma (an intrarenal pelvis) or protrude from the renal hilus (an extrarenal pelvis).

About 75 percent of kidneys are supplied by only one renal artery, which branches from the aorta below the superior mesenteric artery. The inferior adrenal artery and small arteries to the renal pelvis, capsule, and upper ureter branch from the renal artery proximal to the hilus. The right renal artery courses behind the inferior vena cava and right renal vein, and the left renal artery is situated behind the left renal vein. The renal artery branches into an anterior and posterior division as it enters the renal hilus. The posterior branch passes behind the renal pelvis and supplies the posterior segment of the kidney (see Figure 3.17). The anterior branch courses between the renal pelvis and the renal vein and branches to supply the superior, inferior, and anterior segments of the kidney. There are no significant communications between the segmental renal arteries, and occlusion usually results in infarction of the perfused segment.

The intra- and extrarenal courses of the renal veins parallel those of the renal arteries, but there are numerous anastomotic connections. The renal veins converge into one or more major renal veins situated anterior to the renal artery. The right renal vein is substantially shorter than the left and has few or no extrarenal connections. The left renal vein usually lies anterior to the aorta, but anomalies are not infrequent. The entire venous drainage of the left kidney or one of several renal veins may pass posterior to the aorta. The inferior phrenic and adrenal veins drain into the superior aspect of the left renal vein, the gonadal vein drains into the inferior aspect, and a lumbar vein may drain into the posterior aspect.

The lymphatics of the right kidney course from the renal hilus to the nodal chains lateral to the inferior vena cava and between the vena cava and aorta both above and below the renal vessels. On the left the lymphatics drain to the nodal chain lateral to the aorta above and below the renal vessels. The innervation of the kidney is of no surgical importance.

PERCUTANEOUS NEPHROSTOMY

Percutaneous nephrostomy is the procedure of choice for temporary or emergent renal drainage when retrograde catheterization is not possible. In addition, advances in instrumentation permit the removal of calculi and visual inspection of the collecting system through the nephrostomy tract. Bleeding diatheses, a solitary kidney, or the absence of a safe access route are relative contraindications to percutaneous nephrostomy.

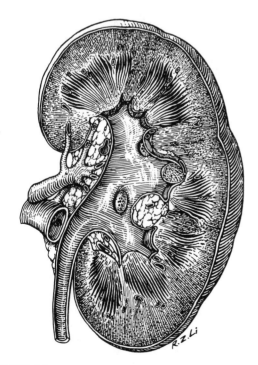

FIGURE 3.2
Renal parenchyma and collecting system

OPERATIVE TECHNIQUE Percutaneous nephrostomy is performed usually with sedation and local anesthesia only. The patient is placed in the prone position with the ipsilateral flank elevated 30° so that the posterior calyces have a vertical orientation (Figure 3.3). Fluoroscopy is used to visualize the collecting system, which is opacified by the administration of intravenous contrast medium. If the kidney functions poorly, contrast medium can be introduced via a ureteral catheter. Ultrasonography may be used as an alternative means for visualizing the collecting system.

A number of percutaneous nephrostomy kits containing all materials necessary for the procedure are available. A 10- to 15-cm, 22-gauge needle is inserted below the twelfth rib and into a posterior calyx. Urine is aspirated to confirm puncture of the collecting system, and contrast material is injected if opacification by alternative means is not possible. Extravasation of contrast material makes fluoroscopic visualization of the collecting system difficult and should be avoided.

A small stab wound is made in the skin and an 18-gauge flexible needle with a hollow internal obturator is advanced alongside the first needle. The first needle and the obturator of the flexible needle are withdrawn, and a guide wire is introduced into the collecting system and maneuvered into the upper ureter. The flexible needle is removed, and with the guide wire taut, the tract is dilated to an appropriate size for the drainage catheter. A coiled drainage catheter is then passed over the wire and positioned in the collecting system. The wire is removed and the nephrostomy tube is sutured to the skin and connected to a drainage system.

POSTOPERATIVE CARE AND COMPLICATIONS Hematuria for 12 to 24 hours is not uncommon, but perirenal

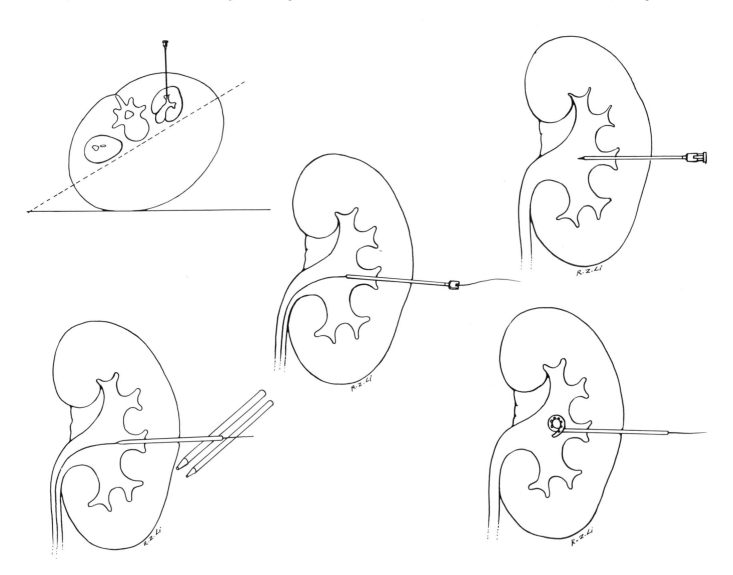

FIGURE 3.3
Percutaneous nephrostomy

bleeding is unusual. Dislodgment of the nephrostomy tube within several days after insertion predisposes to hemorrhage because the tube acts to tamponade the nephrostomy tract.

PERCUTANEOUS INTRARENAL MANIPULATIONS

Inspection of the renal collecting system (nephroscopy) and removal of renal stones (nephrostolithotomy) may be performed at the time of percutaneous nephrostomy or several days after the nephrostomy tract is established. Before nephrostolithotomy the precise location of the stone and the anatomy of the collecting system are delineated with anteroposterior and oblique x-rays of the kidney. Renal pelvic and upper calyceal stones are approached through a lower calyx, and lower or midrenal calyceal stones are approached through the involved calyx. Puncture of a middle calyx is desirable for stones in the upper ureter.

Most of the techniques and instruments used for nephroscopy and nephrostolithotomy are unique, and substantial practice is required before the procedures can be done with any degree of excellence. The following descriptions are intended as a brief overview.

OPERATIVE TECHNIQUE Catheterization of the bladder is advisable to evacuate irrigant that drains from the renal pelvis. The guide wire is positioned in the upper ureter, and the nephrostomy tract is enlarged by passing dilators of increasing size over the wire, or by balloon dilation. The goal is to create a tract that is 4 F larger than the instrument used for the procedure. Before dilatation beyond 8 to 10 F, a second guide wire is introduced into the renal pelvis and the first guide wire is sutured to the skin. The latter serves as a safety wire should the second wire become dislodged during subsequent dilatations and manipulations.

Nephroscopy is performed with a rigid or flexible nephroscope. A forceps or electrode inserted through the working channel of the instrument is used for biopsy or fulguration of mucosal lesions. Small calculi may be grasped and extracted with a forceps.

Stones larger than 2 cm require fragmentation with an electrohydraulic or ultrasonic lithotripter. It is advisable to insert a ureteral catheter before the procedure to prevent the migration of stone particles into the ureter. With electrohydraulic lithotripsy a shock wave is created by an electrical discharge and adjacent stones are pulverized. The probe of the electrohydraulic lithotripter is flexible and does not need to be in contact with the stone. With ultrasonic lithotripsy the energy is delivered through a solid probe that must be in direct contact with the stone. Fragmented stones are flushed from the collecting system or grasped and removed.

POSTOPERATIVE CARE AND COMPLICATIONS A nephrostomy tube is reinserted after the procedure to tamponade bleeding in the tract and to encourage healing of perforations in the collecting system. After 1 to 2 weeks an antegrade pyelogram is performed, and the tube is removed if there is no obstruction, extravasation, or residual stone material. An intravenous pyelogram or renal sonogram is generally obtained after 3 to 6 months to rule out delayed ureteral obstruction.

Early complications include perirenal hematomas, retroperitoneal fluid collections, bleeding from the nephrostomy tract, and accidental tube dislodgment. Most respond to conservative, nonoperative management. Stricture of the ureter or collecting system and residual calculi are the principal late complications.

OPEN NEPHROSTOMY

Open surgical procedures done solely for placement of a nephrostomy tube have been supplanted by percutaneous nephrostomy techniques and by the development of ureteral stents suitable for prolonged internal drainage. However, nephrostomies are commonly used for drainage of the collecting system after open renal surgery.

OPERATIVE TECHNIQUE The kidney is approached through an extraperitoneal flank incision. Gerota's fascia is incised, and perinephric fat is dissected from the upper ureter, renal pelvis, and lower pole of the kidney. A small pyelotomy is made between stay sutures, and a Randall stone forceps (or the equivalent) is positioned in the lower-pole calyx with the thinnest overlying parenchyma. The forceps is then thrust through the renal parenchyma and capsule (Figure 3.4). The tip of a 24 to 28 F Malecot catheter with one or two of the four wings removed is grasped and brought into the renal pelvis. Proper positioning is ensured by visualizing the catheter tip through the pyelotomy. Bleeding from the renal parenchyma is usually tamponaded by the catheter, but a heavy absorbable pursestring suture that encompasses the renal capsule only should also be placed around the puncture site. The suture is wrapped around the catheter and tied again to stabilize the tube.

The pyelotomy is closed with a continuous fine absorbable suture, and the nephrostomy is irrigated to remove clot and to document patency. A stab wound is made below the flank incision and immediately adjacent to the nephrotomy to create a short, straight, and dependent tract for the catheter. The catheter is pulled through the defect and secured to the skin with a heavy nonabsorbable suture. Fixation of the renal

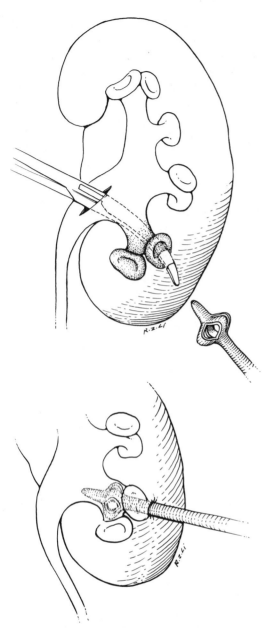

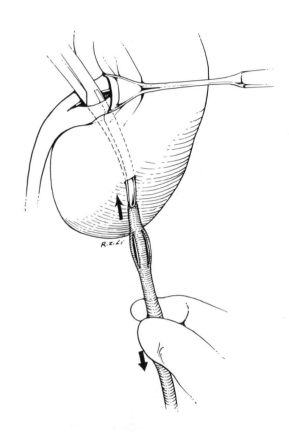

FIGURE 3.4
Open nephrostomy

capsule to adjacent abdominal musculature also helps to maintain a short nephrostomy tract. A Penrose drain is positioned next to the pyelotomy and brought out through a second stab wound.

A U-tube nephrostomy exiting through two calyces is favored by some urologists (Figure 3.5). Accidental dislodgment is difficult. However, the drainage inlets of the catheter may slide into the nephrostomy tract if the position of the catheter changes.

POSTOPERATIVE CARE AND COMPLICATIONS   Complete accidental dislodgment of the nephrostomy tube or displacement of the drainage ports into the renal parenchyma are not uncommon. In the immediate postoperative period the tract may be reestablished with flexible guide wires or small catheters using fluoroscopic guidance. Reinsertion of the catheter is less difficult when the tract has matured. However, obstruction at the level of the renal capsule is often encountered when the interval between removal and reinsertion is longer than 6 hours.

Encrustation and blockage of the catheter lumen is inevitable if a nephrostomy tube is not electively

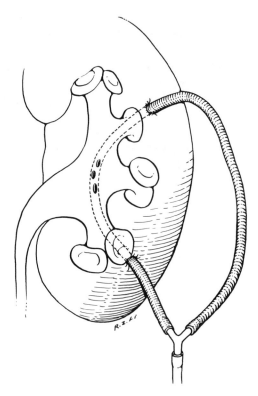

FIGURE 3.5
U-tube nephrostomy

changed every 6 to 8 weeks. Intermittent irrigation with a 10 percent hemiacidrin solution (Renacidin) helps to dissolve small crystalline deposits.

OPEN RENAL BIOPSY

A renal biopsy is generally performed to determine the etiology of parenchymal disorders that produce renal insufficiency. Although renal biopsies are often done by percutaneous techniques, an open biopsy may be requested if a needle biopsy is unsuccessful, or if such conditions as severe hypertension or coagulopathies make the percutaneous approach dangerous. An open biopsy may be advisable also in cases of a solitary kidney.

OPERATIVE TECHNIQUE Tissue fixatives for immunologic and electron microscopic investigations must be available before the operation is begun. Biopsy requires exposure of the lower pole of the kidney only, and a subcostal flank incision or lumbar incision is usually adequate. Gerota's fascia is incised and perinephric fat is freed from the lower pole. An elliptical segment of the renal cortex is then excised with the scalpel (Figure 3.6). Care should be taken to avoid crushing of the specimen during removal.

The defect in the renal parenchyma is closed with several simple absorbable sutures that encompass the renal capsule and superficial cortex. Brisk bleeding is not common because the perfusion of diseased kidneys is usually reduced. A Penrose drain is positioned next to the biopsy site, and Gerota's fascia is approximated over the lower pole. As renal insufficiency impairs the healing process, the wound is closed meticulously with interrupted sutures of heavy nonabsorbable material, and the skin sutures are not removed for 10 to 14 days. The Penrose drain is removed on the first postoperative day unless drainage is excessive.

PARTIAL NEPHRECTOMY

Subtotal excision of the renal parenchyma is by and large limited to the upper and lower poles. The

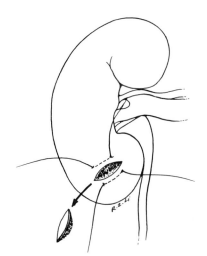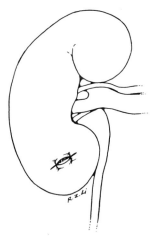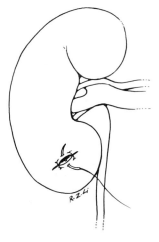

FIGURE 3.6
Open renal biopsy

vascular supply to these segments is well defined, and defects in the collecting system can be repaired without difficulty. Small renal cell carcinomas, calculi in upper- or lower-pole calyces that are associated with parenchymal atrophy, obstructed duplicated renal segments, and traumatic renal injuries may be managed by partial nephrectomy. Less common indications include symptomatic arteriovenous fistulas that are not amenable to embolization and ischemic segments that cause hypertension.

OPERATIVE TECHNIQUE   An extraperitoneal flank incision is generally used for the procedure. The exposure should always be sufficiently generous to permit isolation and control of the renal artery. When the operation is done for a benign disorder, the kidney is completely mobilized from the perinephric fat, and the renal artery is isolated. The capsule of the upper or lower pole is then incised and stripped from the parenchyma to the level of anticipated amputation (Figure 3.7). When removing a tumor, one does not disturb the fat and fascia surrounding the involved renal segment, and the renal capsule is incised at the level of anticipated amputation.

The margins of the superior or inferior renal segment are delineated by isolation and occlusion of the appropriate segmental artery. The main renal artery is then secured with a bulldog clamp, and the renal parenchyma is divided in a medial-to-lateral direction. This allows early identification and ligation of large intrarenal vessels. Transected calyces or infundibula are oversewn with a continuous fine absorbable suture, and residual bleeders are ligated after the arterial

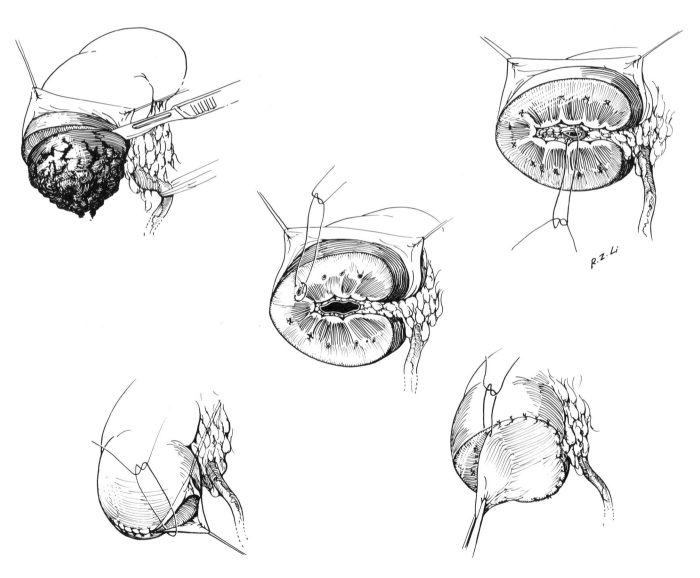

FIGURE 3.7
Partial nephrectomy

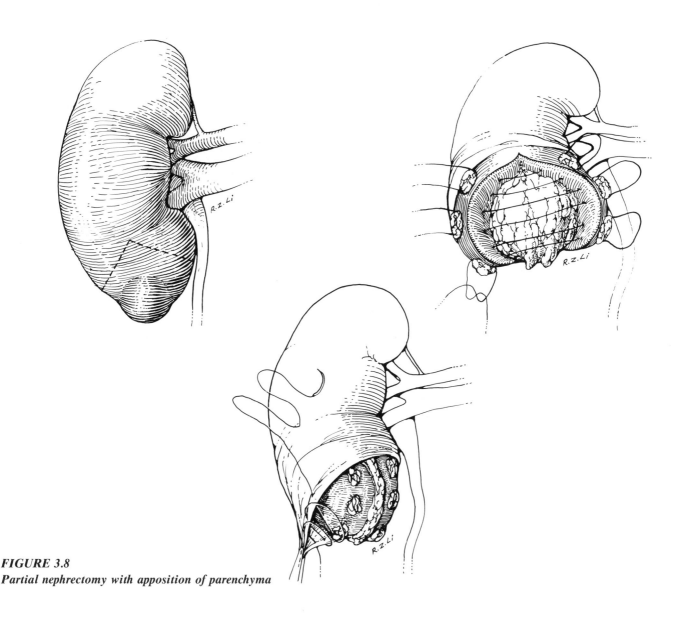

FIGURE 3.8
Partial nephrectomy with apposition of parenchyma

clamp is released. The parenchyma is covered with the redundant renal capsule or a patch of peritoneum.

If a wedge-shaped segment is removed, omentum or fat is positioned in the defect. The parenchyma is approximated with heavy absorbable mattress sutures that encompass the capsule and superficial cortex and are buttressed with fat or Gelfoam (Figure 3.8). Nephrostomy drainage is prudent if there is concern about the integrity of the closure of the collecting system. A Penrose drain is positioned adjacent to the renal closure, and Gerota's fascia is replaced around the kidney and secured with absorbable sutures.

If a partial nephrectomy is performed on a functionally solitary kidney or if prolonged arterial occlusion is anticipated, renal cooling as described in the section on anatrophic nephrolithotomy is advisable.

SIMPLE NEPHRECTOMY

Simple nephrectomy is the excision of a kidney without removal of the adrenal gland or of the surrounding fat or fascia. Indications for the procedure are benign kidney disorders causing nonfunction, such as chronic obstruction, vascular compromise, and granulomatous processes. Renovascular hypertension that is not amenable to alternative treatment is also an indication for the procedure.

In situations where extensive fibrosis obliterates the plane between the renal capsule and the perinephric fat, a radical nephrectomy may be technically easier than a simple nephrectomy. A subcapsular nephrectomy performed by separating the renal parenchyma from the capsule should be considered if dissection outside Gerota's fascia is also difficult.

OPERATIVE TECHNIQUE The optimal surgical approach is based primarily on the reason for the nephrectomy. An extraperitoneal flank incision is usually suitable, but a transperitoneal approach is preferred if control of the renal vessels before nephrectomy is desirable. The lumbar approach can be used when the kidney is small and low lying.

Gerota's fascia is incised on the lateral border of the kidney, and perinephric fat is dissected from the lower pole. The ureter is isolated, doubly ligated, and transected; perinephric fat is cleared from the renal capsule working toward the upper pole. An extension of Gerota's fascia separates the adrenal gland and its vasculature from the perinephric fat, and injury to these structures is unusual if the dissection is confined to the renal capsule. The kidney is then retracted laterally, and the renal artery and vein are isolated just medial to the renal hilus. The artery is secured with two nonabsorbable sutures placed as far from the hilus as possible, and the vein is secured with one or two nonabsorbable sutures. Both vessels are then transected distal to the ties. Residual medial attachments from the renal hilus are then divided and the specimen is removed. Isolation of the renal vessels may not be feasible when there is extensive fibrosis around the hilus. In these circumstances the entire vascular pedicle is secured with ligatures placed as far medially as possible and transected distal to the ties.

Drainage of the renal fossa is advisable when the nephrectomy is performed for an infectious process or hemostasis is less than optimal.

RADICAL NEPHRECTOMY

Radical nephrectomy refers to en bloc excision of the kidney, adrenal gland, perirenal fat, upper ureter, and surrounding Gerota's fascia. It is the procedure of choice for renal cell carcinoma or transitional cell carcinoma of the renal pelvis, because the likelihood of complete tumor removal is enhanced if there is extension beyond the renal capsule. The operation may be appropriate for benign disorders when dissection outside Gerota's fascia is technically easier than dissection next to a scarred or fibrotic renal capsule. A regional lymphadenectomy in conjunction with radical nephrectomy for tumor is recommended by some authorities.

The arterial anatomy of the kidney is often established before surgery by diagnostic angiography (Figure 3.9). Inferior vena cavography is advisable if a suspected tumor is large or located near the renal hilus. In these cases tumor extension into the renal vein or inferior vena cava is not uncommon (Figure 3.10) and should be documented before surgery. Computed

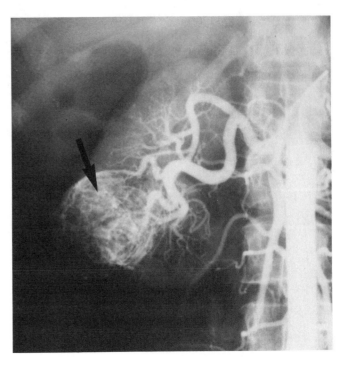

FIGURE 3.9
Renal arteriogram demonstrating renal cell carcinoma (arrow)

tomography or magnetic resonance imaging can also demonstrate venous involvement.

Preoperative embolization of the renal artery with coils or Gelfoam may be advisable if the tumor is extremely large or extends into the vena cava. Embolization permits transection of the renal vein or removal of a caval thrombus before isolation of the less accessible renal artery.

OPERATIVE TECHNIQUE Transperitoneal exposure is recommended. We routinely use a thoracoabdominal incision if there is a large renal tumor. The intra-abdominal contents are inspected for undetected visceral metastases, and the tumor is carefully palpated to assess resectability. The renal vessels are approached through an incision in the posterior peritoneum medial to the inferior mesenteric vein (Figure 3.11). The duodenum is then reflected laterally to expose the renal veins.

For a left radical nephrectomy all branches of the left renal vein are ligated and transected, and the vein is retracted superiorly or inferiorly. A 2-cm length of the artery is isolated and secured with two heavy nonabsorbable sutures applied flush with the aorta and $\frac{1}{2}$ cm distal to the aorta. A third tie is placed about 2 cm distal to the aorta, and the vessel is transected with a knife between the second and third ligatures. For a right radical nephrectomy the artery may be approached between the aorta and the vena cava after

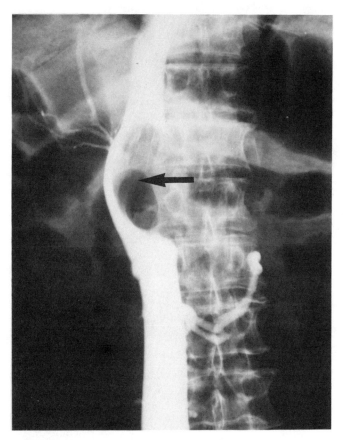

FIGURE 3.10
Inferior venacavogram demonstrating tumor thrombus (arrow)

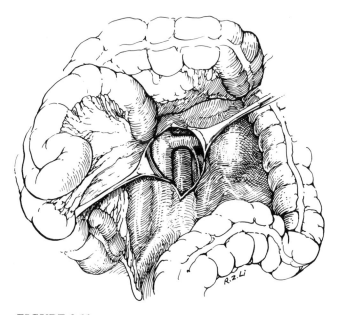

FIGURE 3.11
Exposure of renal vessels for radical nephrectomy

isolating and retracting the left renal vein. Alternatively, it can be exposed just lateral to the vena cava after mobilization and retraction of the right renal vein.

The renal vein or veins are ligated flush with the vena cava and 1 to 2 cm distal to the vena cava and transected with a knife between the ties. The stumps of the renal artery and vein can be further secured with suture ligatures.

The renal vessels can also be approached after incising the paracolic gutter and mobilizing the colonic mesentery from Gerota's fascia. However, the more direct approach to the renal vessels should always be used if any difficulty is encountered during this dissection.

We prefer to isolate the inferior, inferomedial, and posterior aspects of Gerota's fascia before approaching the superior and superomedial margins. Troublesome bleeding from the adrenal vessels is more easily identified and controlled after the specimen has been removed. If it has not already been done, the colon is reflected medially to expose the anterior surface of Gerota's fascia (Figure 3.12). The ureter and gonadal vessels are isolated at the pelvic brim, individually ligated with nonabsorbable sutures, and transected. The Gerota's fascia that envelopes the ureter is freed to the lower pole of the kidney, and the plane of dissection is extended superiorly behind the kidney. The ureter and surrounding fascia are pulled laterally, and the medial ramifications of Gerota's fascia are divided adjacent to the aorta or vena cava to the level of the previously transected renal vessels.

The specimen is retracted downward with the hand, and the superior margins of Gerota's fascia above the adrenal gland are freed from the posteroinferior diaphragmatic fibers. Exposure may be limited if the tumor is large, but care must be taken to avoid splenic or hepatic laceration from overzealous retraction. The superior aspect of the specimen is then retracted laterally with the hand, and the adrenal arteries and veins are secured with ligatures or hemostatic clips. The medial extensions of Gerota's fascia above the renal vessels are divided next to the aorta or vena cava and the specimen is removed.

The renal fossa is liberally irrigated with sterile water, and residual bleeders are ligated or fulgurated. The posterior peritoneal and paracolic incisions are closed with interrupted sutures. Drainage of the renal fossa is usually not necessary.

If nephrectomy is performed for transitional cell carcinoma of the renal pelvis or ureter, the ureter is removed in its entirety using the techniques described in Chapter 7.

A regional lymphadenectomy, if performed, is begun after removal of the kidney. This component of

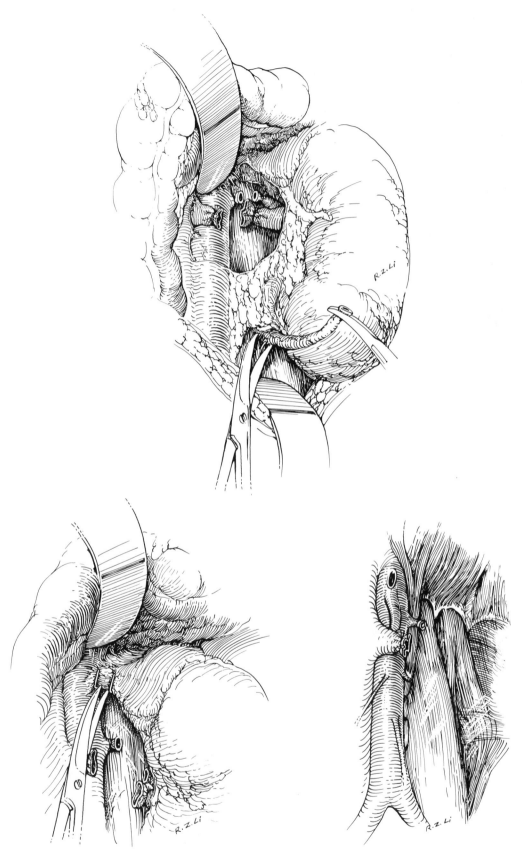

FIGURE 3.12
Radical nephrectomy

the operation is accomplished using the techniques described in the section on retroperitoneal lymphadenectomy in Chapter 17. We excise all lymphatic tissue from the level of the inferior mesenteric artery to the takeoff of the superior mesenteric artery. For right-sided tumors, tissue lateral to the vena cava and between the vena cava and the aorta is removed. For left-sided tumors, tissue lateral to the aorta and between the aorta and vena cava is removed. The appropriate anatomic constraints of the lymphadenectomy, however, are poorly defined.

Tumor extension into only the main renal vein does not necessitate substantial alteration of the foregoing surgical approach. A large Satinsky clamp is applied to the lateral aspect of the vena cava adjacent to the renal vein, and a cuff of vena cava is excised with the renal vein to assure that the entire thrombus is removed. The cavotomy is closed with a continuous suture of 5-0 polypropylene.

Vena caval thrombi that do not extend above the hepatic veins may be managed without undue blood loss if vascular control is satisfactory. Exposure of the suprarenal vena cava is enhanced by division of the triangular ligament of the liver and lateral retraction of the left lobe. Vessel loops are passed around the vena cava below or between the hepatic veins and around the contralateral renal vein and infrarenal vena cava (Figure 3.13). Lumbar veins between the vessel loops are tied and transected if feasible. The vessel loops are tightened using Rommel tourniquets immediately before opening the vena cava. A cavotomy is made just above the thrombus and extended into the involved renal vein. The thrombus rarely invades the intima of the vena cava but may be adherent and require delicate dissection. Excessive bleeding from intact lumbar veins is controlled by suture ligation of the orifices through the cavotomy. The renal vein is then transected flush with the vena cava, and the cavotomy and stump of the vein are closed with a single continuous suture of 5-0 polypropylene.

Profound hypotension may occur after occlusion of the vena cava, and the surgeon and assistants must be prepared to work expeditiously in a coordinated manner. After removal of the thrombus, the cavotomy can be temporarily closed by the application of one or more large Satinsky clamps. The edges of the cavotomy are grasped with Allis clamps to prevent slippage from the blades of the Satinsky clamp. The vessel loops are then released to restore venous blood flow.

Tumor extension above the hepatic veins usually necessitates exposure through a median sternotomy and is best managed in conjunction with a cardiovascular surgeon. Cardiopulmonary bypass may be required if the thrombus extends to or into the right atrium.

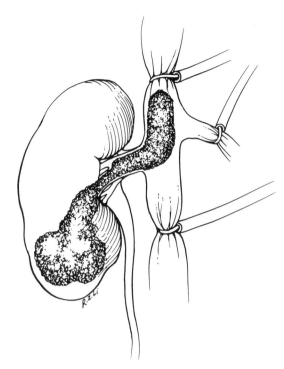

FIGURE 3.13
Control of vena cava for removal of tumor thrombus

OPERATIONS FOR RENAL STONES

Open surgery for the removal of renal calculi is performed infrequently because of the availability of percutaneous nephrostolithotomy and extracorporeal shock-wave lithotripsy. Indeed, contemporary indications for surgery are based primarily on factors that might contraindicate or complicate these procedures.

Renal stones that are accompanied by recurring bacteriuria due to an organism that synthesizes urease are usually composed of struvite. The bacteria colonize the interstices of the stone and usually cannot be eradicated with antibiotics. However, in most cases a sterile urine can be maintained in the perioperative period with parenteral antimicrobial therapy that is selected on the basis of susceptibility testing.

Pyelolithotomy
With the exception of branched renal calculi involving multiple calyces, or stones in calyces with narrow infundibula, most renal calculi can be removed through an incision in the renal pelvis.

OPERATIVE TECHNIQUE   An extraperitoneal subcostal or transcostal flank incision usually provides adequate exposure. The lumbar approach is superb if the kidney is not situated too high and a difficult dissection is not anticipated.

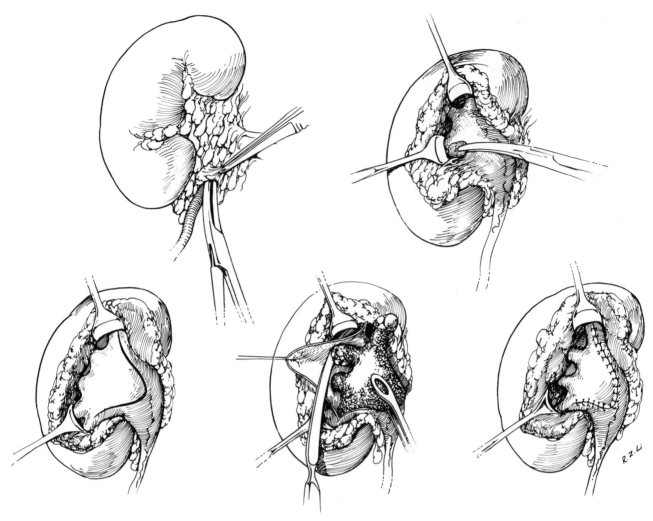

FIGURE 3.14
Pyelolithotomy

The posterolateral aspect of Gerota's fascia is opened adjacent to the lower pole of the kidney, and the upper ureter is isolated and secured with a vessel loop. Areolar tissue and fat are then freed from the adventitia of the ureter and posterior renal pelvis (Figure 3.14). Retraction of renal parenchyma overlying the pelvis with a vein or renal sinus retractor is often necessary for satisfactory exposure of an intrarenal pelvis. The edge of the retractor is positioned between the renal capsule and the pelvis to prevent parenchymal laceration.

Small renal calculi are extracted through a transverse pyelotomy made between stay sutures. Extension of the pyelotomy into the upper and lower infundibula is recommended for the removal of large renal pelvic stones or calculi that involve the intrarenal collecting system. In most cases the posterior surface of major infundibula can be exposed with impunity if the plane of dissection is confined to the adventitia. A parenchymal incision between the posterior and infe-

rior renal segments facilitates access to the lower collecting system without risk of vascular injury (Figure 3.15). Under direct vision the stone or stones are grasped with forceps and removed. Impacted stones or stones occupying the entire renal pelvis must usually be teased from the urothelium.

All calyces are flushed with saline using a malleable irrigator. Retained stone material should be suspected if the configuration of the retrieved calculi does not correspond with that seen on preoperative x-rays. Intraoperative x-rays, nephroscopy, or ultrasonography help to localize residual fragments.

A coagulum prepared from cryoprecipitate plasma, thrombin, and calcium chloride is a useful adjunct for the recovery of multiple renal calculi or calyceal stones that are smaller than the associated infundibulum. The maneuver is generally performed before making the pyelotomy. The proximal ureter is occluded with a vessel loop, and the approximate volume of the collecting system is determined by injection and

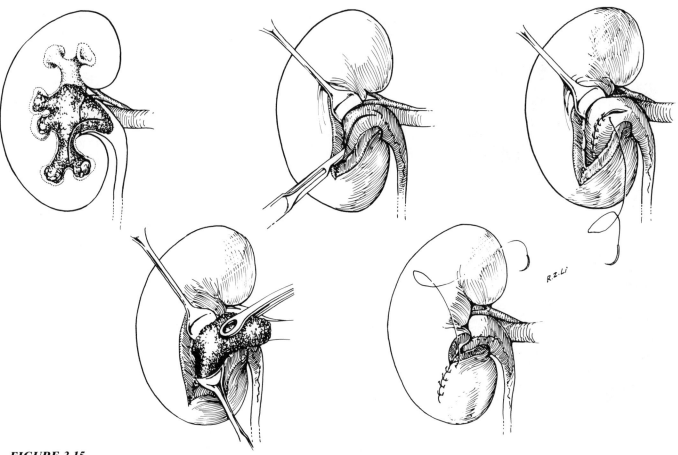

FIGURE 3.15
Pyelolithotomy with parenchymal incision

aspiration of saline. Volume determination is important because overdistention with the cryoprecipitate may lead to extravasation and venous thrombosis. The collecting system is then filled with cryoprecipitate plasma using a needle and syringe. The plasma solidifies about 10 minutes after injection of thrombin and calcium chloride. The coagulum and embedded stones are removed through a pyelotomy.

After the calculus has been removed, a catheter is advanced to the bladder to ensure ureteric patency, and the pyelotomy is closed with a continuous absorbable suture. Heroic efforts to approximate the apical aspects of infundibular incisions are not warranted. Renal parenchyma overlies these sites and promotes prompt healing. If the renal parenchyma has been incised, the capsule is approximated with a continuous absorbable suture. When a stone is composed of struvite, some authorities recommend routine postoperative irrigation of the collecting system to dissolve retained fragments. If this is planned, a large Hemovac drain is brought through the parenchyma overlying a lower-pole calyx and is positioned in an upper-pole calyx to serve as an inlet for the irrigation. In other situations nephrostomy drainage or placement of a

double-coiled ureteral stent is indicated only when the prospects for prompt healing of the pyelotomy are remote. A Penrose drain is positioned adjacent to the renal pelvis, and Gerota's fascia is approximated over the kidney.

Simple Nephrolithotomy

Stones that are not amenable to pyelolithotomy are retrieved through incisions of the renal parenchyma. Such stones are almost always located in calyces and may accompany large calculi that occupy the renal pelvis. When the renal parenchyma is attenuated, the stone is often palpable, and injury to intrarenal vessels and difficult-to-control hemorrhage during the nephrotomy are uncommon. However, entry into the proper calyx can be problematic when the parenchyma is of normal or near-normal thickness, and brisk bleeding or segmental infarction due to transection of intrarenal arteries are potential complications.

OPERATIVE TECHNIQUE Extraperitoneal exposure that permits access to the renal vessels is recommended. The precise location of nonpalpable calyceal stones is established by intraoperative x-ray or ultrasonography. Posterior calyces are entered through the

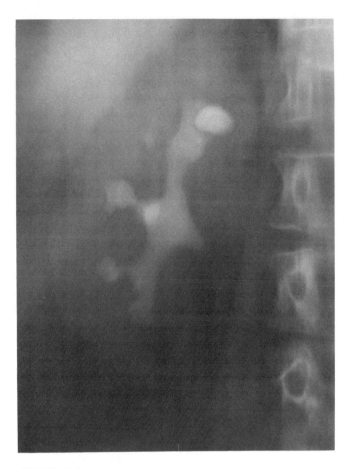

FIGURE 3.16
Branched renal calculus removed by anatrophic nephrolithotomy

avascular plane separating ramifications of the posterior and anterior renal arteries. Anterior calyces and calyces in the upper or lower poles are entered through radial nephrotomies that parallel the course of the intrarenal arteries. Control of the main renal artery is advisable even if only one nephrotomy is anticipated. This allows prompt occlusion should arterial injury lead to troublesome bleeding and facilitates localization and ligation of the lacerated vessel. Renal artery occlusion and renal cooling are recommended when complete stone removal requires numerous nephrotomies. The collecting system is closed with interrupted fine absorbable sutures, and the renal capsule is approximated with a continuous absorbable suture.

Anatrophic Nephrolithotomy

Anatrophic nephrolithotomy exposes the entire intrarenal collecting system and is the procedure of choice for complete removal of large branched calculi (Figure 3.16). The parenchyma is divided in the avascular plane between the posterior and anterior renal segments. The peripheral margin of this plane is located about 2 cm posterior to the lateral border of the kidney (Figure 3.17) and may be demonstrated intraoperatively by temporary occlusion of the posterior branch of the renal artery.

OPERATIVE TECHNIQUE   Sterile iced slush must be available for renal cooling. A generous extraperitoneal flank incision that is adequate for exposure and mobilization of the entire kidney is required. The lateral margin of Gerota's fascia is incised, and the upper ureter is isolated and secured with a vessel loop. Perinephric fat is then cleared from the entire renal capsule. A surgical tape or opened sponge is draped around the kidney for retraction into the wound.

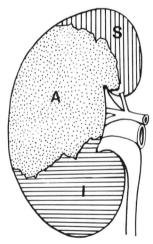
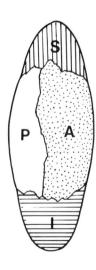
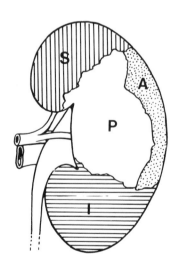

FIGURE 3.17
Segmental arterial supply to kidney

The renal artery is located by palpation, freed from the renal vein and hilar fat, and secured with a vessel loop. A plastic sheet is draped around the renal pedicle to hold the iced slush. We prefer to use a Lahey intestinal bag that is opened on the bottom and secured around the pedicle by tightening of the straps on the top. The proximal ureter is occluded with the vessel loop to prevent distal migration of stone particles, the renal artery is occluded with a bulldog clamp, and the plastic drape is filled with slush. Cooling of the kidney reduces metabolic requirements, and acute tubular necrosis is uncommon despite $\frac{1}{2}$ to 1 hour of total ischemia.

The renal capsule is incised over the avascular line, and the parenchyma is separated by blunt dissection with the knife handle. The direction of the incision is shown in Figure 3.18 and should lead to the anterior surface of the posterior calyces and infundibula. The renal pelvis is opened with a scissors, and the incision is extended as required to include the anterior border of the posterior calyces and the posterior border of the anterior calyces (Figure 3.19). The stone is exposed as completely as possible, teased from the urothelium, and removed with a stone forceps or the equivalent. Most branched calculi are composed of struvite and may crumble or fracture with manipulation.

It is advisable to compare the configuration of retrieved stone material with that on the preoperative x-rays to identify missing portions. Intraoperative x-rays of the kidney, however, are always done to demonstrate residual fragments and to document complete stone removal. Nephroscopy or ultrasonography also help to locate retained stone material. Calyceal stones can be extracted with a forceps that is introduced through the infundibulum or through a small nephrotomy. However, when the collecting system is complex or not dilated, these maneuvers can be extremely difficult.

The intrarenal collecting system is vigorously irrigated. The occluding loop around the upper ureter is removed, and a catheter is passed to the bladder to document ureteric patency. Even if the x-rays reveal complete stone removal, we routinely use a large Hemovac drain as a nephrostomy tube and inlet for postoperative irrigation.

The necessity for reconstruction of the collecting system is controversial. At a minimum, the renal pelvis and large infundibula and calyces should be closed with interrupted fine absorbable sutures, making no effort to change the preexisting anatomy. Alternatively, two or more calyces and infundibula may be combined to promote renal drainage and, possibly, to reduce the risks of recurrent stone formation. This is accomplished by approximating the free edges of adjacent calyces and infundibula (Figure 3.20). Some calyces may not be amenable to this procedure because of intervening renal parenchyma.

The occlusive clamp on the renal artery is released but not removed. If the parenchymal incision was properly positioned, troublesome bleeding is unusual. Manual compression of the kidney for 15 to 30 seconds reduces oozing from the parenchyma and permits identification of larger vessels. Bleeders are secured with fine absorbable suture ligatures that encompass the vessel but minimal renal tissue. If excessive hemorrhage is encountered, the renal artery is reoccluded with the bulldog clamp, and the responsible vessels are ligated. The renal capsule is closed with a continuous absorbable suture.

A Penrose drain is positioned adjacent to the nephrotomy, and the drain and nephrostomy are brought out through separate stab wounds below the incision. Perinephric fat and Gerota's fascia lying adjacent to the renal hilus are draped over the kidney and approximated with absorbable sutures.

POSTOPERATIVE CARE AND COMPLICATIONS

An antegrade pyelogram is performed 5 to 7 days after surgery. If there is no extravasation and the ureter is patent, the Penrose drains are removed, and plain-film tomograms of the kidney are obtained the following day. When the stone is composed of struvite, irrigation of the collecting system for 24 to 48 hours with a 10 percent hemiacidrin solution (Renacidin) is recommended if no residual fragments are seen. This effectively dissolves clinically inapparent stone debris, which can lead to persistent bacteriuria and

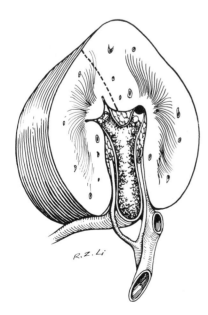

FIGURE 3.18
Parenchymal incision for anatrophic nephrolithotomy

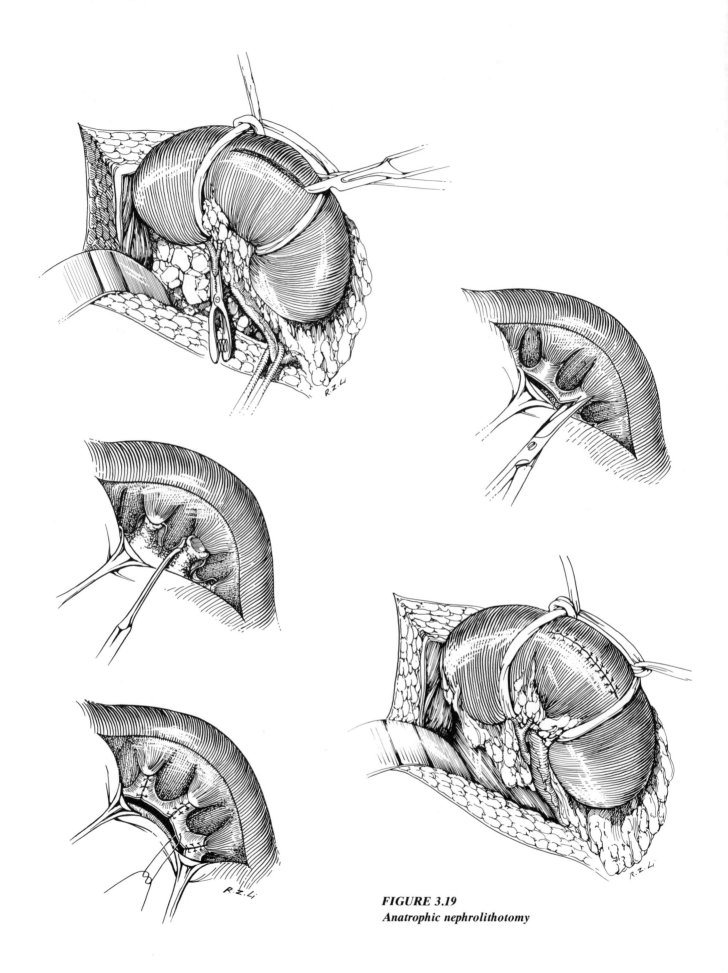

FIGURE 3.19
Anatrophic nephrolithotomy

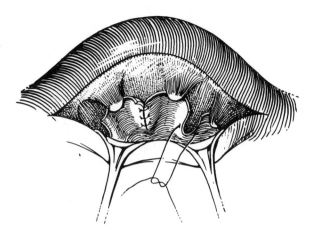 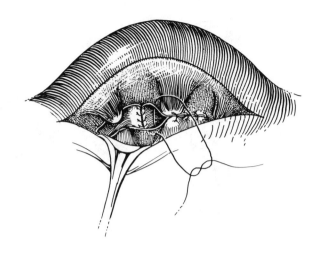

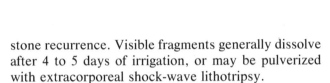

FIGURE 3.20
Calyceal and infundibular reconstruction

stone recurrence. Visible fragments generally dissolve after 4 to 5 days of irrigation, or may be pulverized with extracorporeal shock-wave lithotripsy.

Postoperative hematuria usually subsides within 1 to 2 days. Arteriovenous fistulas may cause severe bleeding but can be occluded by selective embolization of the responsible artery. Urinary leakage from the collecting system is managed by extended nephrostomy drainage or placement of a double-coiled ureteral stent. Persistent bacteriuria following the complete removal of infected struvite calculi is treated with long-term suppressive antimicrobial therapy. Renal artery thrombosis is unusual, and hypertension due to scarring of the parenchyma is infrequent.

OPERATIONS FOR RENAL CYSTS

Renal cysts are the most common space-occupying lesions of the renal parenchyma. They do not communicate with the collecting system, are frequently multiple, and may become quite large. Most are simple cysts that are lined with epithelium and filled with a straw-colored fluid. Multilocular cysts contain fibrous septa but are uncommon.

The vast majority of cystic lesions are asymptomatic and are discovered incidentally with intravenous pyelography or renal imaging. Differentiation between cystic and solid lesions is usually not difficult with ultrasonography, computed tomography, or magnetic resonance imaging. If uncertainty remains after these tests, arteriography may be of diagnostic benefit. In addition, cysts can be punctured to obtain fluid for cytologic examination and for the injection of contrast medium to define the contour of the cyst cavity. In rare cases surgical exploration is advisable to elimi-

nate the possibility of malignancy with complete certainty.

Hemorrhage into a cyst or obstruction of the intrarenal collecting system by a cyst can produce pain. Infected cysts are unusual but may be refractory to conventional antimicrobial therapy. Surgical intervention is at times advisable for the management of these complications.

OPERATIVE TECHNIQUE The kidney is exposed through an extraperitoneal approach, and the cyst is localized after opening Gerota's fascia. Most cysts are found in the periphery of the parenchyma (Figure 3.21). The superficial cyst wall is easily excised and is sent for frozen section examination. A biopsy of cyst cavity irregularities is done for frozen-section examination, or the irregularities are scraped with a scalpel for cytologic examination. The margin of the cyst is oversewn with a continuous absorbable suture, a Penrose drain is placed in the cavity, and Gerota's fascia is closed.

Cysts in the deep cortex can be localized with intraoperative ultrasonography or needle aspiration. Control of the renal artery before incising the parenchyma is advisable. In addition, temporary occlusion of the artery softens the renal parenchyma and may facilitate location of the mass by palpation. Cysts adjacent to the renal hilus must be exposed carefully to avoid injury to the major renal vessels.

OPERATIONS FOR CONGENITAL ANOMALIES

Duplication anomalies and anomalies of position and fusion are often asymptomatic and associated with normal renal function. Duplication of the renal

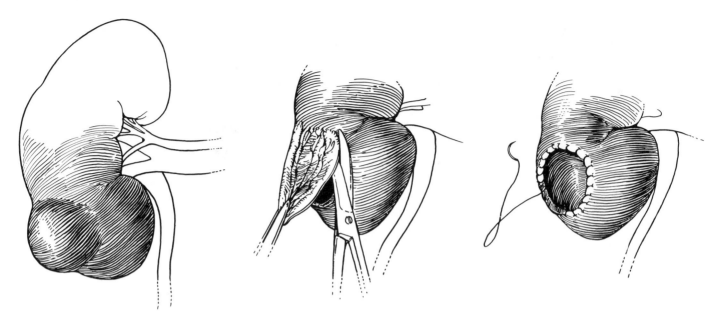

FIGURE 3.21
Marsupialization of renal cyst

collecting system and ureter, however, may be complicated by obstruction of the ureteropelvic junction, vesicoureteral reflux, or ureteroceles. Ectopic kidneys, which are usually located in the pelvis, are also vulnerable to ureteropelvic junction obstruction. Techniques for the repair of these conditions are addressed in Chapters 6 and 8.

The horseshoe kidney (Figure 3.22) is the most common anomaly of fusion. The lower poles of the horseshoe kidney are fused by an isthmus of varying thickness lying anterior to the aorta. The ureteropelvic junctions are located anterior to the isthmus and are susceptible to obstruction. If clinically indicated, the obstruction can be repaired with a flap or dismembered pyeloplasty. Division of the isthmus and lateral rotation of the lower poles, however, may be necessary to create a funneled anastomosis that drains dependently.

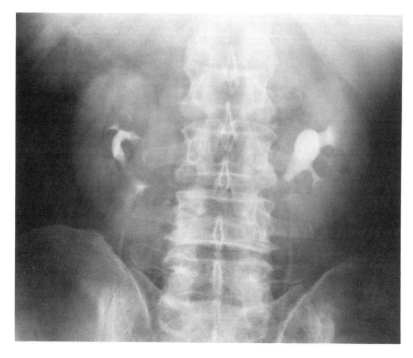

FIGURE 3.22
Intravenous pyelogram demonstrating horseshoe kidney

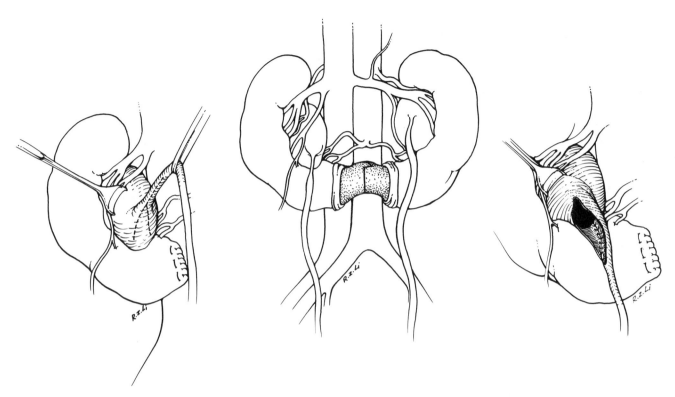

FIGURE 3.23
Division of isthmus of horseshoe kidney and repair of ureteropelvic junction obstruction

The surgical principles of symphysiotomy parallel those of partial nephrectomy. However, the arterial supply of the horseshoe kidney is unpredictable, and arteriography is recommended before surgery.

OPERATIVE TECHNIQUE   A flank incision that is extended medially provides adequate exposure to one side of a horseshoe kidney, but an anterior transperitoneal approach is usually advisable when symphysiotomy is anticipated. The isthmus is exposed by incising the posterior peritoneum. The ileum and cecum are reflected upward as needed.

The capsule of the isthmus is incised circumferentially and stripped laterally (Figure 3.23). Temporary occlusion of the artery that perfuses one side of the isthmus helps to delineate an avascular parenchymal plane. A thick isthmus is separated with the handle of a knife, but thin, fibrous connections can be transected with scissors. Entries into the collecting system are oversewn with a continuous absorbable suture, and bleeding vessels are secured with ligatures. The renal capsule is then drawn over the exposed parenchyma and approximated with a continuous absorbable suture. Lateral rotation of the lower poles is accomplished by anchoring the renal capsule to the posterior abdominal musculature or by placement of a nephrostomy.

OPERATIONS FOR RENAL ABSCESSES

Abscesses that involve the kidney may be intrarenal (confined to the renal parenchyma), perirenal (contained within Gerota's fascia), or pararenal (extending beyond Gerota's fascia) (Figure 3.24). Most are caused by gram-negative bacilli and are preceded by acute or chronic renal infections. Ureteral obstruction, infected renal stones, and diabetes mellitus are important predisposing factors.

Abscesses are typically manifested by fever, chills, and flank discomfort of several weeks' duration. Flank or abdominal tenderness is common, and a mass may be palpable. Pyuria, bacteriuria, and leukocytosis are characteristic laboratory findings. Obliteration of the psoas shadow and mottled gas overlying or adjacent to the kidney are often seen on the abdominal x-ray. Elevation of the ipsilateral diaphragm, pleural effusion, or empyema may be seen on the chest x-ray.

Abnormalities seen on the intravenous pyelogram include a mass lesion with distortion of the collecting system or impaired excretion of contrast material. On the sonogram abscesses appear as irregular sonolucent masses with internal echoes. Computed tomography (CT) is the most useful diagnostic study. The abscess appears on the CT scan as a mass lesion with low

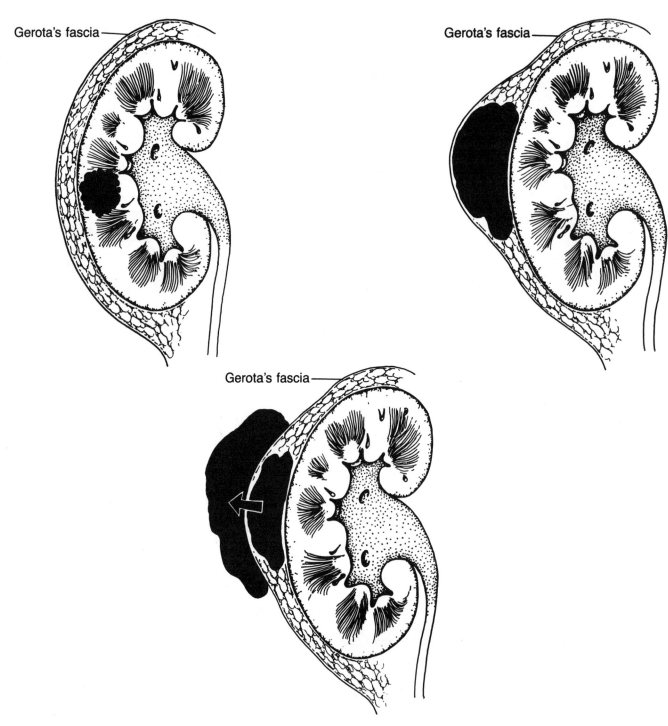

FIGURE 3.24
Renal, perirenal, and pararenal abscesses

attenuation surrounded by a rim of increased enhancement. Irregularity and accentuation of the perinephric fat and extrarenal fluid collections suggest extension of the infectious process into the perirenal or pararenal space (Figure 3.25).

Renal and perirenal abscesses can be drained by per-cutaneous techniques. However, the collections of pus are often loculated, and open drainage is required for satisfactory evacuation. Parenteral antibiotics are always administered in the perioperative period. We prefer the combination of an aminoglycoside and am-picillin to cover infections caused by gram-negative

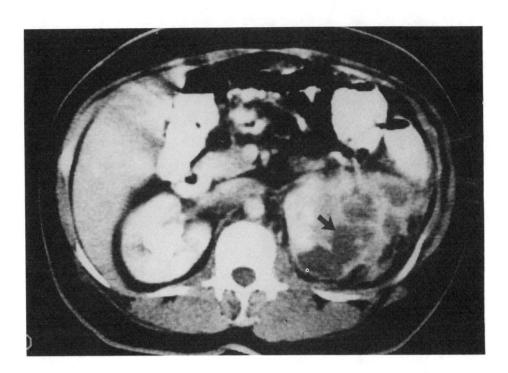

FIGURE 3.25
A CT scan demonstrating perirenal abscess (arrow)

bacilli and enterococci. Coexisting obstructive processes are managed initially by percutaneous or open nephrostomy or with a ureteral stent.

OPERATIVE TECHNIQUE A subcostal flank incision is recommended to avoid entry of the peritoneal and pleural cavities. The abscess is usually palpable and is entered with blunt dissection. All loculations are broken to drain the entire collection of pus. Intrarenal abscesses usually accompany pararenal or perirenal abscesses and should also be identified and drained.

Multiple Penrose drains are placed in the abscess cavity and the wound is closed. The subcutaneous tissue and skin are preferentially approximated with large nylon sutures spaced 2 cm apart. Some surgeons prefer to leave the subcutaneous tissue and skin open to prevent wound infection.

Nephrectomy at the time of abscess drainage may be hazardous. On the other hand, if the kidney is nonfunctional or functions poorly, a secondary nephrectomy may be necessary to eliminate a focus of persistent infection. This procedure is often complicated by dense perirenal fibrosis, and a subcapsular nephrectomy should be considered to reduce the risks of injury to adherent and difficult-to-identify viscera.

POSTOPERATIVE CARE AND COMPLICATIONS The Penrose drains are slowly removed after 5 to 7 days if the patient's condition is stable and the drainage is minimal. Oral antibiotics are generally administered for 2 to 4 weeks after hospital discharge.

Renal stones or obstructive processes are treated with conventional methods if the kidney is salvageable. These interventions or secondary nephrectomy are not performed until the infection and inflammation have resolved. This typically requires 1 to 2 months.

OPERATIONS FOR RENAL TRAUMA

The primary objective in the management of a traumatized patient with a renal injury is to prevent death. Preservation of renal function is an important but secondary objective. Extrarenal injuries are usually the most lethal, and decisions concerning overall surgical management must be deferred to the trauma team. Penetrating renal trauma generally results from gunshot wounds and stab wounds, and injury of other viscera is the rule. Blunt renal injuries result usually from motor-vehicle accidents. Associated extrarenal injuries are not uncommon, and their incidence correlates roughly with the magnitude of the renal injury.

The advisability of surgical intervention for the sole purpose of treating an injured kidney is determined by estimating the extent of injury with radiographic and imaging studies. Most patients with isolated renal trauma do not require an emergency operation, and thorough investigation is generally feasible.

A high-dose infusion intravenous pyelogram helps to delineate the nature of an injury and documents the presence and status of the contralateral kidney. Rib or vertebral fractures, which may accompany blunt renal injuries, and absence of the psoas shadow are often seen on the preliminary x-ray. Extravasation or impaired excretion of the contrast medium or complete absence of a nephrogram is not uncommon. The depth

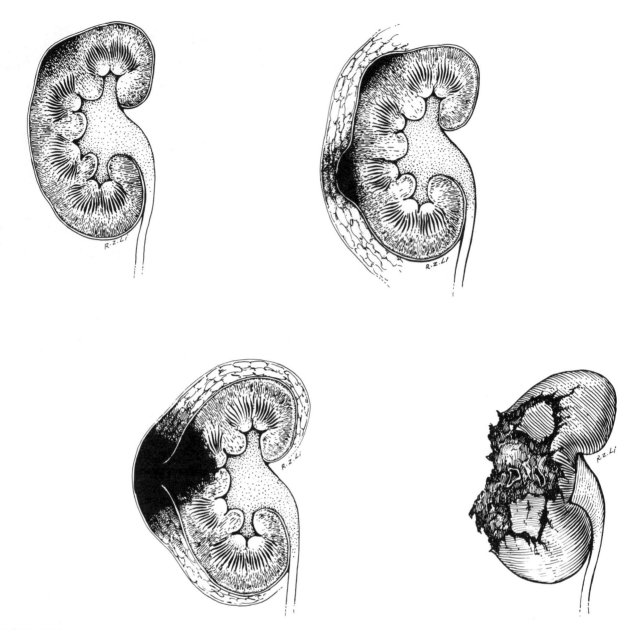

FIGURE 3.26
Renal contusion and shallow lacerations (top); major laceration and shattered kidney (bottom)

and multiplicity of parenchymal disruptions are defined best with renal arteriography or computed tomography. The former is always advisable to rule out injury to the renal artery when there is complete nonvisualization of the affected kidney.

Renal contusions or superficial lacerations are reasonably categorized as minor injuries (Figure 3.26). Major lacerations denote one or several disruptions through the corticomedullary junction that often extend into the collecting system (Figure 3.27). Severe injuries include multiple deep lacerations (the shattered kidney) or injury to the main renal artery or vein. Approximately 70 percent of renal injuries are minor,

15 percent are major lacerations, and 15 percent are severe injuries.

There is general agreement that minor injuries can be managed conservatively with bedrest, intermittent physical examination, and serial hematocrit determinations. Patients with severe injuries should undergo an exploratory procedure and, in most cases, nephrectomy. The optimal management of major lacerations is not established and should be individualized. Deep lacerations may heal spontaneously. However, nonoperative management presents a risk of delayed bleeding or abscess; and exploration several days after the injury is more difficult and associated with a higher

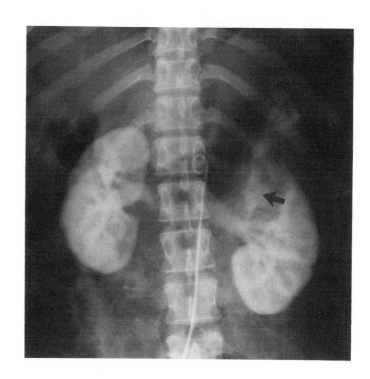

FIGURE 3.27
Arteriogram demonstrating major renal laceration with extravasation of contrast medium (arrow)

rate of nephrectomy than is immediate intervention. Further, patients who are managed conservatively generally remain in the hospital longer than those who undergo surgical treatment.

OPERATIVE TECHNIQUE Broad-spectrum antibiotics are administered before surgery. A vertical midline incision is recommended for speed and generous exposure. Arterial control of the affected kidney is achieved immediately unless extrarenal injuries require initial attention. The small bowel is reflected superiorly, and the posterior peritoneum is incised medial to the inferior mesenteric vein. The left renal vein is isolated, and its branches are ligated and transected. Superior retraction of the vein exposes the takeoffs of the right and left renal arteries, and a bulldog clamp is applied to the artery that supplies the injured kidney (Figure 3.28).

The paracolic peritoneum is incised and the colon is reflected medially. Gerota's fascia is opened, hematomas are evacuated, and perinephric fat is dissected from the renal capsule to expose the injury. Renal cooling is advisable if the anticipated time required for reparative procedures is greater than 30 minutes.

Minor lacerations and most major lacerations are amenable to debridement. Care is taken to identify and ligate all bleeding vessels and to oversew tears of the collecting system (Figure 3.29). A partial nephrectomy may be advisable if there are major lacerations of the superior or inferior poles. Primary closure of the renal capsule is rarely feasible, and the denuded renal

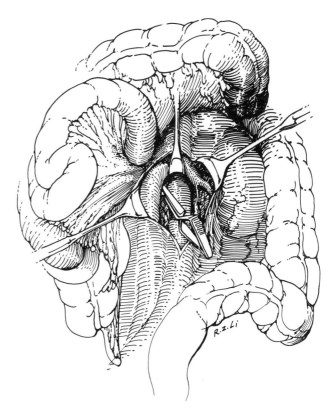

FIGURE 3.28
Approach to renal arteries before exploration of traumatized kidney

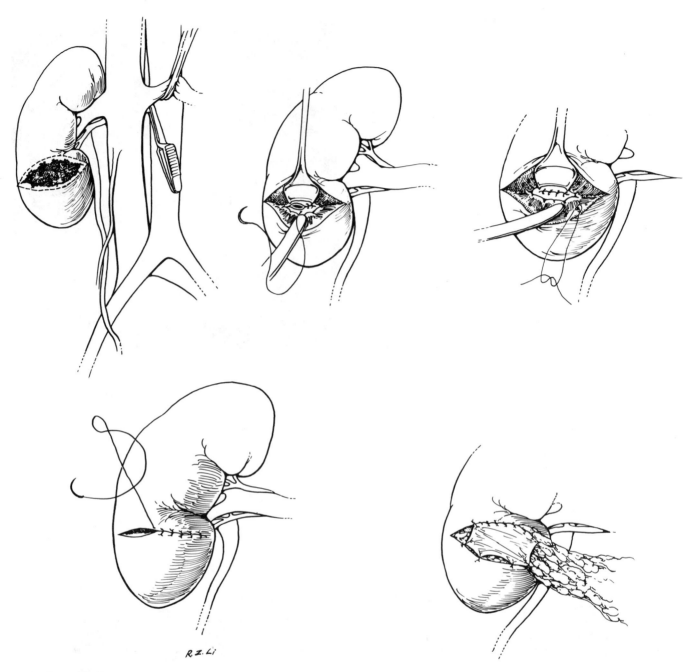

FIGURE 3.29
Repair of major renal laceration

parenchyma must be covered with perinephric fat or omentum and a patch of peritoneum. Nephrostomy drainage is generally not necessary. Several Penrose drains are positioned next to the repair, and Gerota's fascia is approximated over the kidney.

Shattered kidneys are removed because the likelihood of preserving meaningful renal function is small, and the risk of postoperative complications is large. Tears of the renal vein can usually be closed primarily, or the vein can be ligated. Reported experiences con-

cerning the repair of major arterial injuries are not abundant. Unless the surgeon is adept at vascular reconstructions and the injury is clearly amenable to repair, nephrectomy is probably the procedure of choice.

POSTOPERATIVE CARE AND COMPLICATIONS Abscesses and urinary extravasation are the primary complications of reparative renal surgery. Persistent urinary leakage often responds to the placement of a double-coiled ureteral stent.

CHAPTER 4

Renal Transplantation

Raymond Pollak, M.B., F.R.C.S. (Edin.)

Kidney transplantation is one of several forms of therapy for chronic end-stage renal disease. Because of the associated morbidity and mortality of dialytic treatment and because of improved results with transplantation, renal transplantation is now frequently recommended before dialysis is even required. The 1-year graft survival with a cadaveric kidney is 80 to 85 percent, whereas that with living donors is about 90 percent.

Candidates for renal transplantation must be able to tolerate a major operative procedure and should be free of chronic infectious or malignant diseases that might be exacerbated by immunosuppressive therapy. Noncompliance with postoperative immunosuppressive treatment is a cause of graft rejection; psychosocial stability is therefore a prerequisite. Bilateral nephrectomy before transplantation may be advisable if the native kidneys are susceptible to infection.

Patients judged suitable for transplantation are placed on a waiting list if a cadaveric kidney is to be implanted. If procurement of a graft from a living related donor is feasible, evaluation of potential donors is initiated.

Donor Operations

CADAVERIC DONOR NEPHRECTOMY

Cadaveric donors are the major source of kidneys for transplantation. Patients who have been declared brain dead but who have normal cardiovascular function are acceptable donors if they do not have a transmissible infectious disease, an underlying renal disease, or a recent history of malignancy.

OPERATIVE TECHNIQUE A bilateral nephrectomy is performed through a generous vertical midline incision. Exposure of the retroperitoneum is achieved by incising the posterior peritoneum from the cecum to the ligament of Treitz, dividing the right paracolic gutter, and reflecting the cecum and ascending colon upward. The ureters and periureteral tissues are mobilized to the level of the common iliac arteries and transected. The kidneys and a segment of the aorta and vena cava are removed en bloc without isolating the renal vasculature. Cold Collins solution is infused through the aorta to flush the kidneys in situ, or after removal to a basin containing ice-cold saline slush. The renal vessels are then separated from the aorta and vena cava, taking care to preserve the entire length of the right renal vein. The kidneys are preserved using one of a number of methods, including simple cold storage. The spleen and mesenteric lymph nodes are also removed to facilitate tissue typing and cross-match studies.

After suitable cross-matching with recipient serum, the kidneys are distributed to the appropriate centers for implantation.

LIVING RELATED DONOR NEPHRECTOMY

Siblings, parents, or close relatives of the recipient are potential candidates for kidney donation. A donor's overall health, and cardiovascular and respiratory function, must be satisfactory. Psychosocial stability and a commitment to the proposed procedure are key ingredients for a smooth postoperative course. Blood group and tissue compatibility between the prospective donor and the recipient are assessed to determine the risks of rejection.

The final evaluation of a suitable donor involves transfemoral aortography to delineate the anatomy of the renal vasculature. The left kidney is preferred for transplantation because of the greater length of the renal vein. Multiple renal arteries are a relative contraindication to donor nephrectomy.

OPERATIVE TECHNIQUE Procurement of a kidney from a living donor deviates from a standard simple nephrectomy in the following respects. The ureter is mobilized as distally as possible, but is not divided until the operative field of the recipient is prepared for the transplant. Care is taken to preserve a generous

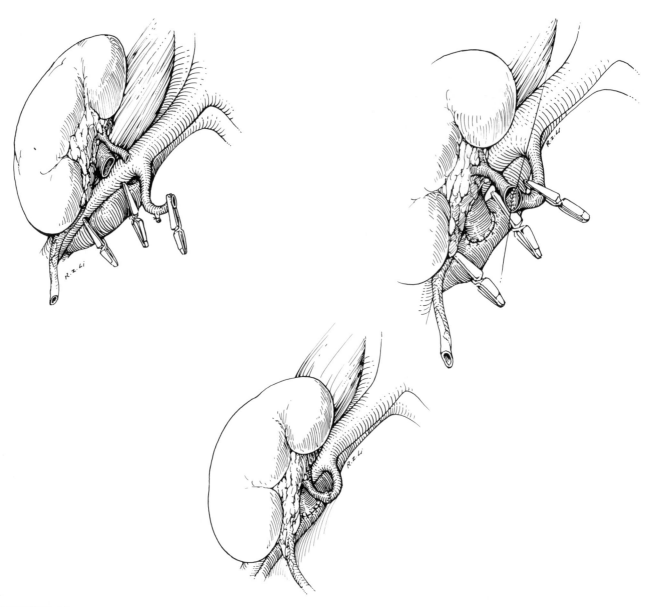

FIGURE 4.1
Recipient operation in the adult

amount of periureteral tissue. The renal vein is mobilized to the vena cava, and the adventitia of the artery is freed from investing tissues. An appropriate dose of heparin is administered, the ureter is divided, and about 3 minutes later the artery and vein are clamped and transected. The kidney is then handed to the team that is managing the recipient procedure. They cannulate the artery and infuse a cold (4° C) Collins solution until the effluent from the renal vein is clear.

The renal artery is doubly ligated with heavy nonabsorbable sutures, and the renal vein is oversewn with fine cardiovascular polypropylene. An appropriate dose of protamine is administered to inactivate the heparin, and the wound is closed in a conventional manner.

Postoperative care and complications parallel those of simple nephrectomy. It is customary to obtain serum creatinine and creatinine clearance determinations before hospital discharge and at 6 weeks, 6 months, and 1 year after the operation.

Recipient Operations

ADULT

The recipient of a transplant undergoes dialysis before surgery to ensure optimal fluid and electrolyte balance. In adults the graft is preferentially placed in the right pelvis.

OPERATIVE TECHNIQUE   The right lower quadrant is approached through a low Gibson incision. The peritoneum is reflected medially to expose the psoas muscle and the common, external, and internal iliac vessels. The spermatic cord is mobilized posterior to the cecum.

Our preference is to use the internal iliac artery whenever possible for anastomosis with the renal artery. The artery is isolated from the bifurcation to a point above the takeoff of the superior vesical artery. Branching vessels are secured with nonabsorbable ligatures. The proximal artery is occluded with a curved coarctation vascular clamp and the distal aspect is ligated and divided. The lumen is then inspected to ensure that an endarterectomy is not warranted. If the internal iliac artery is unsuitable for anastomosis, the adventitia of the external iliac artery is exposed for 3 to 4 cm to create an alternative anastomotic site. Care is taken to ligate the adjacent lymphatics. The adventitia of the external iliac vein is exposed for about 6 cm between the bifurcation and circumflex iliac vein. Lymphatic tissue is again secured with suture ligatures.

The arterial anastomosis is done first. Interrupted 6-0 polypropylene sutures are used for construction of an end-to-end anastomosis (Figure 4.1). For an end-to-side anastomosis, an arteriotomy is made in the external iliac artery between occlusive vascular clamps. The anastomosis is performed with a continuous suture of 6-0 polypropylene using the triangular technique. A venotomy is then made in the external iliac vein between occlusive vascular clamps, and an end-to-side anastomosis is performed with a continuous 5-0 polypropylene suture.

After removal of the arterial and venous clamps, the kidney typically increases in turgor and develops a pink color. Capsular vessels are secured with sutures or small hemostatic clips. When the period of cold storage has been relatively brief, urine can be seen emanating from the ureter shortly after the start of renal perfusion. The central venous pressure is maintained at 10 cm H_2O, and intravenous mannitol (1 g/kg) is infused to maximize the urinary output.

The ureter is positioned behind the spermatic cord, and the ureteroneocystostomy is performed with the Lich technique (see Chapter 8). This eliminates the need for a cystotomy and reduces the risks of postoperative urinary leakage. The bladder is decompressed with a urethral catheter but drains are not used.

CHILDREN

In children the graft is placed in the midretroperitoneum, and the vascular anastomoses are made with the aorta and the inferior vena cava.

OPERATIVE TECHNIQUE   The retroperitoneum is approached through a generous midline incision. The small intestine is packed superiorly, and the right colon is reflected medially to expose the distal aorta, vena cava, and common iliac vessels. Fibroareolar tissue is dissected from the adventitia of the infrarenal aorta and vena cava, and proximal and distal vascular control is obtained with vessel loops. End-to-side anastomoses between the renal artery and aorta and the renal vein and vena cava are performed with continuous 6-0 polypropylene sutures (Figure 4.2). Bicarbonate is administered before release of the vascular loops to prevent acute acidosis and cardiac irritability. Mannitol is infused after the initiation of renal perfusion to promote a diuresis.

The ureteroneocystostomy is then performed as in adults. The mesentery of the right colon is replaced over the graft, and the paracolic gutter is closed with interrupted sutures.

POSTOPERATIVE CARE AND COMPLICATIONS

After surgery the recipient is monitored in a specialized organ transplant unit. Immunosuppressive therapy is begun using one of a variety of standardized protocols. Intravenous fluids are administered judiciously, based on the patient's weight and urine output. The urethral catheter is removed usually on the second or third postoperative day. A renal sonogram is obtained to identify hydronephrosis or fluid collections adjacent to the graft and to serve as a control for

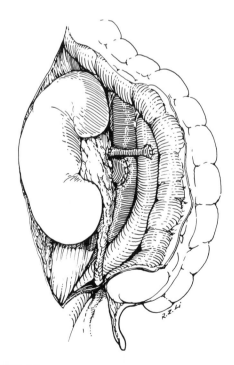

FIGURE 4.2
Recipient operation in the child

subsequent studies. A baseline renal scan is also performed to assess graft perfusion and patency of the renal artery. After hospital discharge the patient is seen twice a week to allow prompt detection of graft rejection or other complications.

General postoperative complications include wound infection in 1 to 2 percent of patients, peritransplant hematoma or lymphocele in 5 to 10 percent, and urinary extravasation at the ureteroneocystostomy in 10 to 15 percent. Urinary extravasation necessitates immediate surgical intervention and, in most cases, reconstruction of the ureteroneocystostomy.

Acute tubular necrosis develops in about 60 percent of patients when transplantation is performed after more than 24 hours of cold storage. Fluid restriction and dialysis are generally required for 10 to 14 days. Hyperacute rejection is usually evident at the time of surgery and is rarely reversible. The risks of early acute rejection have been greatly reduced with improved immunosuppressive therapies. Accelerated rejection, however, is seen in 10 to 20 percent of patients but often responds to treatment with antilymphocyte globulin or monoclonal OKT3 antibody.

Graft rejection, hypertension, excessive weight gain, drug toxicity, steroid-induced diabetes mellitus, and opportunistic infections are the primary late complications of transplantation. Obstruction of the ureter, which may result from extrinsic compression by fluid collections or ureteral stenosis, must always be ruled out in the patient with deteriorating renal function. The risks of lymphoreticular malignancies and epithelial neoplasms of the skin and cervix are substantially increased because of immunosuppression.

CHAPTER 5

Renovascular Surgery

J. Eldrup-Jorgensen and D. P. Flanigan

Operations on the renal arteries are performed primarily for the treatment of renovascular hypertension. Traumatic injury and aneurysms are also indications for renovascular surgery. About 5 to 10 percent of all hypertensive patients, and about 20 to 30 percent with severe or malignant hypertension, are thought to have renovascular hypertension. The disorder more often affects the young and the elderly; it is unusual in blacks. Renovascular hypertension should be suspected if the hypertension is recent in onset and poorly controlled with medication, there is no family history, or an abdominal bruit can be auscultated. The absence of these characteristics, however, does not exclude a renovascular etiology for increased blood pressure.

Renal artery stenosis is the cause of renovascular hypertension and results usually from atherosclerotic lesions or fibromuscular hyperplasia. A hemodynamically significant stenosis produces a drop in the perfusion pressure to the kidney and the release of renin by the juxtaglomerular cells of the afferent arterioles. Renin is an enzyme that converts angiotensinogen to angiotensin I. In the pulmonary circulation a second enzyme cleaves off part of angiotensin I, forming angiotensin II. Angiotensin II is a potent vasoconstrictor that acts on the smooth muscle of arteries. It also stimulates aldosterone secretion, and the retention of salt and water may contribute to hypertension.

There are no screening tests for renovascular hypertension that are sufficiently sensitive and specific for routine clinical use. Further, the indications for evaluating hypertensive patients for renovascular disease and the optimal sequence of available investigations are not well defined. The study of patients who are candidates for an operation and have a diastolic blood pressure greater than 105 mm Hg, however, is generally warranted.

Quantitation of the peripheral plasma renin activity is the most simple test for renovascular hypertension.

The results are expressed as a function of sodium excretion and are meaningful only if the patient discontinued all antihypertensive medications for 2 weeks, restricted sodium intake for 2 weeks, and was recumbent for 12 hours before blood collection. Despite strict adherence to these recommended guidelines, test findings are normal in as great as 50 percent of patients with renovascular hypertension.

An intravenous pyelogram is done primary to rule out other renal diseases. Findings suggestive of renovascular hypertension on a rapid sequence study include delayed opacification of the collecting system, hyperconcentration of contrast medium in the calyces, and a 1.5-cm or greater disparity in renal size. Ureteral notching due to increased collateral circulation is seen occasionally. Arterial lesions, however, are often bilateral and false-negative studies are common. Renal artery stenosis may produce delayed perfusion and excretion on radionuclide scans, but the test has generally proved unreliable.

Arteriography is the only available study that clearly defines stenotic lesions of the renal arteries. An aortic flush, as well as selective renal artery injections viewed in anterior and oblique projections, is desirable. Intravenous digital subtraction angiography is an alternative to arteriography but is associated with a high incidence of false-positive interpretations. Deep abdominal duplex ultrasonography is a promising but new diagnostic modality.

When arteriography demonstrates narrowing of the renal artery, the functional significance of the abnormality is determined by renal vein renin assays. The preparation for this study parallels that described for peripheral renin assays. Catheters must be accurately placed in each main renal vein, and the blood specimens are collected simultaneously. A 1.5 or greater ratio of the renal vein renin activity in blood from the affected kidney as compared with the contralateral

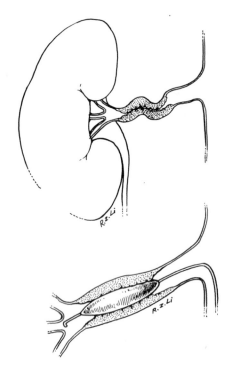

FIGURE 5.1
Percutaneous angioplasty of renal artery stenosis due to fibromuscular dysplasia

kidney is suggestive of a hemodynamically significant lesion. However, renal vein renin ratios may not be diagnostic in patients with bilateral arterial disease. For this reason, some authorities prefer to compare the renal vein renin activity with the systemic venous renin activity.

Compared with medical management, operative treatment of renovascular hypertension usually results in improved blood pressure control, decreased mortality, and better preservation of renal function. Percutaneous transluminal angioplasty (Figure 5.1) has been introduced recently as an alternative to open surgical interventions. When performed by experienced angiographers, the procedure is safe and has an initial success rate of greater than 90 percent in selected patients. Recurrence of renal artery stenosis, however, is common among patients with atherosclerotic lesions. Ostial stenoses are associated with a particularly low initial success rate. In patients with fibromuscular hyperplasia, however, the response to angioplasty is usually quite durable.

BYPASS GRAFTS

Endarterectomy or bypass grafting is the principal technique for in situ repair of renal artery stenoses. Ex

vivo arterial reconstruction has been used for stenoses of multiple branch vessels or for reoperations. Nephrectomy is reserved for patients with renal vessels that are not amenable to reconstruction and should be viewed as an option of last resort if there is meaningful renal function. Vascular disease may progress to involve the contralateral renal artery, and significant improvement in renal function is not uncommon after renal revascularization.

Before endarterectomy or bypass grafting is performed, antihypertensive medications are reduced to a minimum. Preoperative hydration is critical for patients whose drug regimen included diuretic medications. Parenteral broad-spectrum antibiotics are administered routinely, and perioperative monitoring with a Swann-Ganz catheter is advisable for patients with coronary artery disease or cardiac dysfunction.

OPERATIVE TECHNIQUE A generous transperitoneal midline incision is recommended. The left renal artery is approached by incision of the posterior peritoneum to the ligament of Treitz, transection of the tributaries to the left renal vein, and superior or inferior retraction of the vein. Alternatively, the left renal vasculature may be exposed by medial reflection of the descending colon. The right renal artery is approached by medial reflection of the ascending colon and duodenum. The right renal vein is isolated and retracted superiorly or inferiorly to expose the artery.

We prefer bypass grafting to endarterectomy unless there are bilateral atheromatous ostial stenoses. Autologous saphenous vein or hypogastric artery and synthetic grafts may be used for the bypass. We generally choose the greater saphenous vein, but synthetic grafts have comparable patency rates and must be used when autologous conduits are not available.

The proximal anastomosis is performed on the infrarenal aorta if technically feasible and is done first. Alternative in-flow sites include the suprarenal aorta, the iliac, hepatic or splenic artery, or an aortic graft. A side-biting clamp is applied to the lateral aspect of the aorta, and a full thickness ellipse of the arterial wall is removed (Figure 5.2). For procedures on the right side, the graft may be tunneled anterior or posterior to the inferior vena cava. This decision should be made before the proximal anastomosis is begun. The saphenous vein is anastomosed to the aortic defect with a continuous 6-0 polypropylene suture. The vascular clamp is then moved distal to the anastomosis, and the suture line is inspected for leaks. The distal anastomosis is usually constructed in an end-to-side manner. The renal artery is controlled with gentle microvascular clamps, and an anterior arteriotomy at least 1 cm in length is made between the clamps. This anastomosis is performed with the aid of Loupe magnification using a continuous 6-0 polypropylene suture. The postopera-

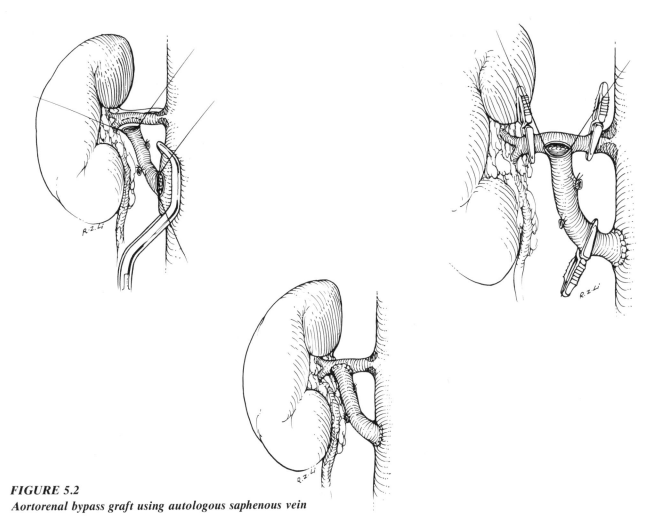

FIGURE 5.2
Aortorenal bypass graft using autologous saphenous vein

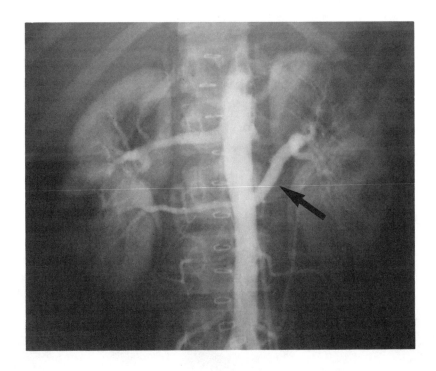

FIGURE 5.3
Arteriogram demonstrating left aortorenal bypass graft of saphenous vein (arrow)

tive arteriogram of a successful left renal artery bypass using saphenous vein is shown in Figure 5.3.

POSTOPERATIVE CARE AND COMPLICATIONS   The blood pressure is closely monitored in the immediate post-operative period, as hypotension following successful revascularization is common. An abrupt recurrence of hypertension suggests graft stenosis or thrombosis and should be investigated by arteriography. If convalescence is uneventful, a renal arteriogram is obtained before the patient leaves the hospital to confirm the technical adequacy of the reconstruction.

CHAPTER 6

Surgery of the Ureteropelvic Junction

The ureteropelvic junction is the site where the funneled renal pelvis joins with the upper ureter. Obstruction at the ureteropelvic junction is the primary disorder of surgical concern. Congenital obstruction is caused by segmental peristaltic dysfunction, intrinsic stricture, extrinsic compression by adhesions or segmental renal arteries, or insertion of the ureter into the upper aspect of the renal pelvis (Figure 6.1). Obstruction may also result from stone or tumor; treatment of these two conditions is addressed in other chapters but may involve the operative techniques described in this chapter.

Obstructions of the ureteropelvic junction result in dilatation of the renal pelvis and intrarenal collecting system and deterioration of renal function. Chronic or intermittent flank pain and hematuria following minor trauma are not uncommon. The site of obstruction is delineated by intravenous pyelography, but retrograde

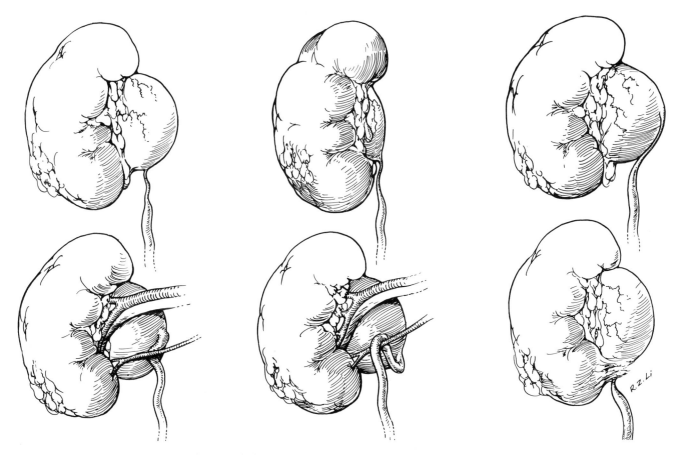

FIGURE 6.1
Causes of obstruction at the ureteropelvic junction: intrinsic stricture or peristaltic dysfunction with extrarenal and intrarenal pelvis, and high insertion of ureter (top), and compression by segmental renal artery, kinking by segmental renal artery, and fibrosis following unsuccessful pyeloplasty (bottom)

pyelography is often required to detail the nature and extent of the process and the status of the lower ureter.

In some instances the obstruction may be asymptomatic and of limited functional importance. Periodic observation only is warranted in this setting. Conversely, the loss of renal function with a chronic, high-grade obstruction may be so severe that nephrectomy rather than reparative surgery is advisable. On occasion the degree of functional obstruction and the advisability of operative intervention are impossible to determine by radiographic examination alone. The diuretic renogram is an excellent test to differentiate between a dilated but nonobstructed collecting system and a collecting system that is dilated because of obstruction. This study also provides a baseline for assessing the functional results of surgery.

PYELOPLASTY

Pyeloplasty is an operative procedure designed to correct obstruction of the ureteropelvic junction and is performed using one of two general techniques. Flap procedures enlarge the ureteropelvic junction by insinuation of tissue from the renal pelvis. Dismembered procedures involve excision of the ureteropelvic junction and anastomosis of the upper ureter with the renal pelvis. The optimal method of repair is dictated by the anatomy of the renal pelvis and ureter and by the cause of the obstruction. Regardless of the technique used, fibrosis at the site of repair may lead to recurrent obstruction. The risks of this complication can be reduced if the tissue is handled in an atraumatic manner, a tension-free anastomosis is created, and the blood vessels lying in the adventitia and periadventitial tissues of the ureter and renal pelvis are not disturbed.

An extraperitoneal flank incision that provides access to the upper ureter and renal pelvis is most commonly used for unilateral procedures. The lumbar approach is acceptable in selected instances. A transabdominal approach is preferred for simultaneous bilateral repairs.

To determine the optimal technique for pyeloplasty, and to remove a portion of the renal pelvis if needed, one exposes the entire renal pelvis and upper ureter. The posterior renal pelvis and the ureteropelvic junction are generally approached first. The lower pole of the kidney is then rotated laterally, and the renal vasculature is mobilized from the anterior renal pelvis. Before the pelvis is decompressed, stay sutures are applied to delineate critical margins of the proposed incision. With dismembered procedures it is helpful to mark the medial border of the transected ureter with a

stay suture for proper orientation of the lumen during the subsequent anastomosis.

Opinions concerning the value of double-coiled or exteriorized ureteral stents to support the anastomosis and the necessity for nephrostomy drainage are variable. Neither may be used if the patient is in good health, the contralateral kidney is normal, and the repair seems technically excellent. Under less favorable conditions it is advisable to use one or both of these adjuncts. Suture fixation of the kidney to the psoas muscle helps to prevent kinking or angulation of the anastomosis caused by normal renal mobility. A nephrostomy, if used, achieves the same goal.

Foley Y-Plasty
The Foley Y-plasty is the most straightforward technique of pyeloplasty but is best reserved for obstructions caused by high insertion of the ureter. The size of the renal pelvis is not reduced with this operation.

OPERATIVE TECHNIQUE The lateral aspect of the ureter is incised from the ureteropelvic junction to a point 1 cm below the obstruction (Figure 6.2). A wide-based, V-shaped flap of the dependent renal pelvis is developed by incising the anterior and posterior walls of the pelvis. Each incision begins at the apex of the ureterotomy and extends toward the renal hilus. The flap must be sufficiently long to reach the distal end of the ureterotomy when dropped inferiorly.

The apex of the flap is rounded to prevent ischemia and is fixed to the distal ureterotomy with a fine absorbable suture. The back wall of the repair is closed by approximating the margins of the renal pelvis and the flap with the edges of the ureter using a continuous fine absorbable suture. The closure begins superiorly and progresses inferiorly so that the flap can be trimmed if it is redundant. A stent or nephrostomy, if used, is positioned at this juncture. The anterior margins of the renal pelvis and flap are then joined with the edge of the ureter with a continuous fine absorbable suture. A Penrose drain is placed near the suture line, and Gerota's fascia is repositioned around the renal pelvis.

Spiral Flap and Vertical Flap Procedures
The spiral flap and vertical flap pyeloplasties can correct long obstructive segments of the ureteropelvic junction but are feasible only when the renal pelvis is dilated. To create a flap that lies conveniently next to the ureterotomy when rotated downward, the spiral technique is used when the angle between ureter and dependent renal pelvis is greater than 90°. The vertical technique is used when the angle is 90° or less. Obstructions that are caused by high ureteral insertions are not amenable to repair with either of the flap proce-

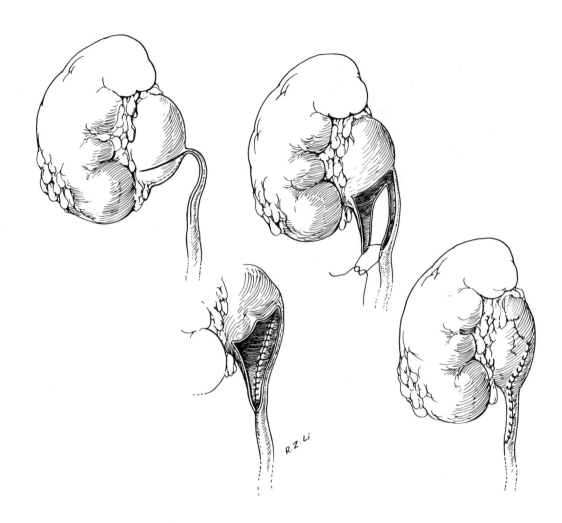

FIGURE 6.2
Foley Y-plasty

dures because the availability of renal pelvic tissue above the obstruction is limited.

OPERATIVE TECHNIQUE With both spiral flap (Figure 6.3) and vertical flap (Figure 6.4) pyeloplasties, the first incision is made in the inferomedial aspect of the posterior renal pelvis and extended through the ureteropelvic junction to a point 1 cm below the obstruction. A flap is then developed that is sufficiently long to reach the distal ureterotomy when swung downward. The spiral flap is derived from the posteromedial renal pelvis, whereas the vertical flap is derived from the posterior pelvis only. With both procedures the length of flap should be no greater than three times the width of the base to reduce the risks of ischemia.

The apex of the flap is fixed to the distal ureterotomy with a fine absorbable suture. The medial margin of the flap and the lateral margin of the ureterotomy are then anastomosed with a continuous fine absorbable suture. The closure begins superiorly to permit trimming of an excessively long flap. A stent or nephrostomy, if used, is positioned, and the repair is completed by joining the opposing edges of the renal pelvis and the more inferior opposing margins of the flap and ureter. A Penrose drain is positioned near the suture line, and Gerota's fascia is closed around the renal pelvis.

Dismembered Procedures
Dismembered procedures are ideal for the repair of most obstructions caused by high insertion of the ureter. However, these procedures are not suitable for long strictures unless normal ureter can be manipulated without tension to the midrenal pelvis, and they are technically difficult if the renal pelvis is small.

OPERATIVE TECHNIQUE The medial portion of a redundant renal pelvis and the diseased ureteropelvic junction are excised en bloc (Figure 6.5). The ureter is transected just below the site of obstruction. The dependent renal pelvis is then incised between the hilus and the ureteropelvic junction. The incision is extended into the anterior and posterior renal pelvis in the direction of the hilus. This creates a "tongue" of tissue for anastomosis with the spatulated ureter. Each incision is then directed superiorly to meet where the

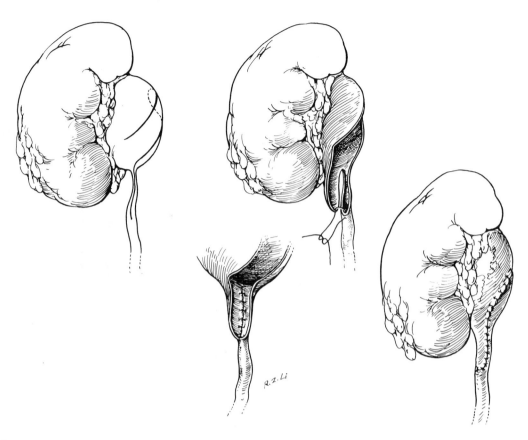

FIGURE 6.3
Spiral flap pyeloplasty

renal pelvis abuts against the parenchyma of the upper pole, and the surgical specimen is removed.

The lateral border of the ureter is spatulated for 1 cm, and the dependent tongue of renal pelvis is fixed to the lower angle of the ureterotomy with a fine absorbable suture. The back wall of the anastomosis is completed by joining the margins of the ureteral spatulation and one half of the luminal end of the ure-

ter with the opposing edge of the renal pelvis using a continuous absorbable suture. A stent or nephrostomy, if used, is positioned and the front wall of the anastomosis is closed in the same manner. The free edges of the renal pelvis above the anastomosis are then approximated with a continuous suture.

When reduction in the size of the renal pelvis is not necessary, a dismembered pyeloplasty can be per-

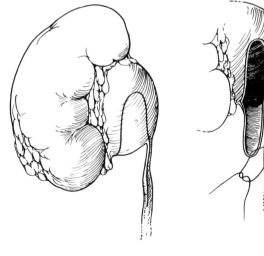

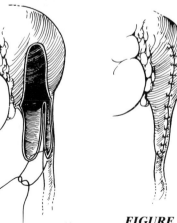

FIGURE 6.4
Vertical flap pyeloplasty

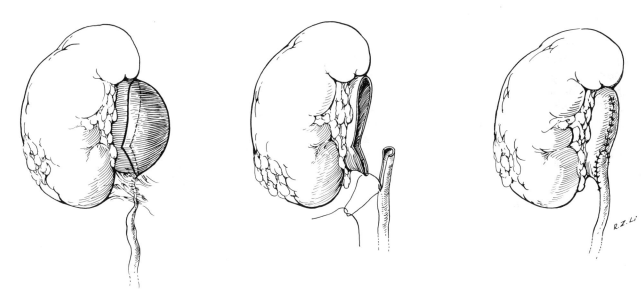

FIGURE 6.5
Dismembered pyeloplasty with excision of redundant renal pelvis and anastomosis of ureter to flap of dependent renal pelvis

formed by direct anastomosis of the spatulated ureter to the defect in the renal pelvis created by excision of the ureteropelvic junction (Figure 6.6). Alternatively, after excision of the ureteropelvic junction, one may create a V-shaped flap from the dependent renal pelvis (Figure 6.7). The flap resembles that developed in the Foley Y-plasty and is swung inferiorly and anastomosed with the spatulated ureter.

POSTOPERATIVE CARE AND COMPLICATIONS

All types of pyeloplasty have similar postoperative care and complications. Urinary drainage is often pro-

fuse for 1 to 2 days but then tapers rapidly. The Penrose drain is removed 24 hours after the drainage has ceased. If a stent or nephrostomy has not been used, an intravenous pyelogram is obtained before the patient leaves the hospital to assess patency of the anastomosis. Double-coiled ureteral stents are extracted during cystoscopy 14 days after surgery, and intravenous pyelography is performed 1 to 2 weeks later.

When the repair is protected with a nephrostomy and an exteriorized stent, an antegrade pyelogram is obtained between the fifth and seventh postoperative

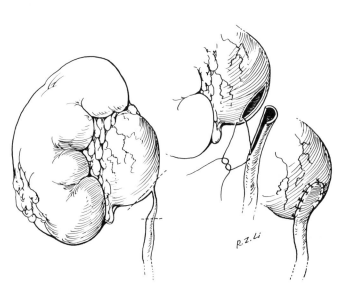

FIGURE 6.6
Dismembered pyeloplasty without excision of redundant renal pelvis

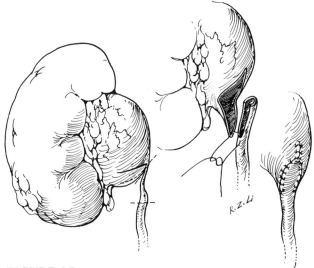

FIGURE 6.7
Dismembered pyeloplasty without excision of redundant renal pelvis and anastomosis of ureter to flap of dependent renal pelvis

day. If the anastomosis is watertight, the stent is removed and the nephrostomy is clamped for 24 hours. Antegrade pyelography is repeated the following day, and the tube is removed if there is no obstruction to the drainage of contrast material.

Variations on these management themes are favored by other surgeons. In addition, the duration of nephrostomy or stent drainage is usually extended if the prospect for promptly healing of the anastomosis is questionable.

Inadequate drainage of the operative field or unintentional removal of a nephrostomy or stent may lead to the collection of urine in the retroperitoneal space. A percutaneous nephrostomy or a ureteral stent that is gently introduced with fluoroscopic guidance usually corrects the problem. When the retroperitoneal collection is small, uninfected, and asymptomatic, drainage is generally not warranted.

An intravenous pyelogram is obtained 3 months after an uneventful recovery. Some degree of dilatation of the intrarenal collecting system is inevitable, but delayed excretion of contrast medium by the affected kidney suggests persistent obstruction. The diuretic renogram is the most sensitive test for documenting impaired drainage of the renal pelvis and should be obtained when this issue is of clinical concern. Some authorities recommend the diuretic renogram only as a means for assessing the results of surgery.

Anastomotic obstructions generally result from technical error or fibrosis. Obstructions may resolve with placement of a double-coiled ureteral stent for 1 to 2 months. Anastomotic strictures can also be managed by incision or balloon dilatation using percuta-

neous techniques. Operative intervention is recommended only when the foregoing maneuvers fail or are not feasible.

PYELOPYELOSTOMY

With partial or complete duplication of the renal pelvis and ureter, obstructions of the ureteropelvic junction usually involve the superior segment. Anastomosis of an obstructed renal pelvis to its unobstructed companion is an excellent alternative to pyeloplasty because the lumen is capacious and postoperative obstruction is unusual.

OPERATIVE TECHNIQUE The upper and lower renal pelves are exposed through an extraperitoneal approach. The opposing walls of the renal pelves are incised, and the adjacent margins are approximated with interrupted or continuous fine absorbable sutures (Figure 6.8). If there is reflux to the obstructed segment, the ureter is transected and ligated. Nephrostomy or stent drainage is usually not required. A Penrose drain is positioned at the anastomosis, and Gerota's fascia is replaced around the renal pelves.

URETEROPYELOSTOMY

In some cases of complete duplication the upper renal pelvis is dilated because of vesicoureteral reflux or obstruction below the ureteropelvic junction. In this setting the ureteropyelostomy is a reasonable alterna-

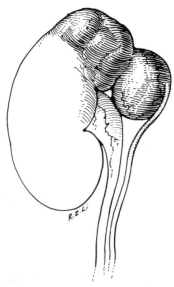
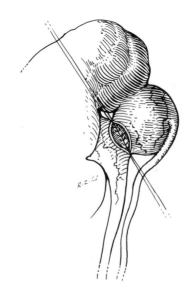
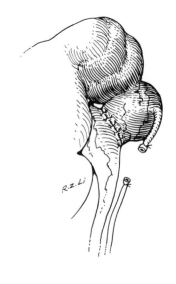
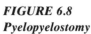

FIGURE 6.8
Pyelopyelostomy

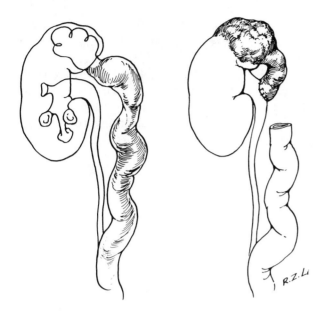

FIGURE 6.9
Ureteropyelostomy

tive to pyelopyelostomy when the renal pelves cannot be joined without undue tension.

OPERATIVE TECHNIQUE The upper and lower renal pelves and the dilated upper ureter are exposed through an extraperitoneal approach. The ureter is transected adjacent to the lower renal pelvis and ligated distally (Figure 6.9). The superomedial border of the lower renal pelvis is incised and anastomosed with the proximal ureter using a continuous fine absorbable suture. Stent or nephrostomy drainage is generally not necessary if the anastomotic lumen is large. A Penrose drain is positioned adjacent to the suture line, and Gerota's fascia is replaced around the renal pelves.

URETEROCALYCOSTOMY

Anastomosis of the ureter with an inferior calyx should be considered when a ureteropelvic junction obstruction cannot be corrected by pyeloplasty, the lower pole calyces are dilated, and preservation of renal function is of critical importance. The operation should not be performed unless the unobstructed

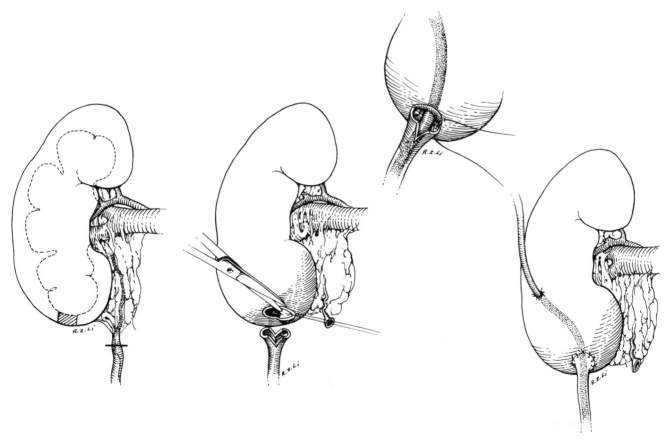

FIGURE 6.10
Ureterocalycostomy

ureter can be manipulated 1 to 2 cm above the lower pole of the kidney without tension.

OPERATIVE TECHNIQUE   The upper ureter and lower pole of the kidney are exposed in an extraperitoneal manner. The ureter is mobilized as distally as possible, taking care to prevent devascularization. It is then transected just distal to the obstruction and the proximal end is ligated (Figure 6.10). A disc of parenchyma overlying an inferior calyx is excised, and the spatulated ureter is anastomosed directly to the calyx with interrupted absorbable sutures. In some cases the kidney must be mobilized and displaced downward to create a tension-free anastomosis. Nephrostomy drainage and stenting of the anastomosis are advisable, as the procedure is rarely performed under favorable surgical conditions.

Surgery of the Ureter

The ureter is a retroperitoneal tubular conduit that conveys urine from the renal pelvis to the bladder by peristaltic contraction. The anatomic relationships of the ureter to the retroperitoneal vasculature are shown in Figure 7.1. The ureter courses lateral to the inferior vena cava or aorta, posterior to the gonadal vessels, and anterior to the common iliac vessels at the bifurcation. The common iliac vessels are a useful landmark for locating the ureter during pelvic surgery. The ureter passes behind the vas deferens in the male (see Figure 12.1) and behind the uterine vessels and broad ligament in the female (Figure 7.2).

The epithelium of the ureter is transitional, and the muscularis is a meshwork of fibers in an oblique orientation. The vascular supply is derived from branches of the aorta and the renal, gonadal, iliac, hypogastric, vesical, uterine, and hemorrhoidal arteries. These feeding vessels lie medial to the upper and midureter, and lateral to the pelvic ureter. A generous longitudinal communication of arteries and veins in the adventitia prevents ischemia despite extensive mobilization. Lymphatic drainage is diffuse and parallels the arterial supply. Neural innervation is similarly diffuse and of minimal surgical importance.

The primary indications for ureteral surgery are congenital or acquired obstructions that produce pain or deterioration of renal function, transitional cell carcinomas, and traumatic injury.

The following surgical principles facilitate prompt healing of reparative procedures and help to prevent the formation of strictures. The ureter is always handled gently and never grasped with crushing clamps or forceps. Extensive mobilization is discouraged, but all anastomoses must be tension-free. Ureteral defects are closed with through-and-through interrupted sutures using fine absorbable material on atraumatic needles. Some degree of urinary leakage, however, is inevitable, and drainage of the operative site is always prudent. Proximal urinary diversion with a nephrostomy should be considered after upper ureteral surgery if the prospects for prompt healing are in doubt, the patient is in poor general medical condition, or the overall renal function is impaired. A double-coiled stent introduced before closure of the ureter at any site reduces urinary leakage and promotes healing without the burden of an exteriorized catheter.

URETERECTOMY

Removal of the entire ureter is performed usually in conjunction with nephrectomy or, on occasion, as a secondary procedure after nephrectomy. En bloc nephroureterectomy that includes a cuff of bladder surrounding the ureteral orifice is the recommended treatment for transitional cell carcinomas of the renal

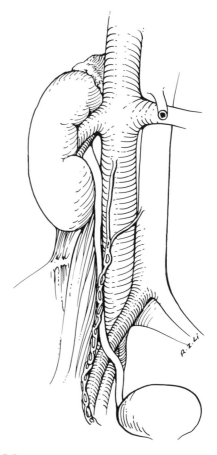

FIGURE 7.1
Relationship of ureter to retroperitoneal vasculature

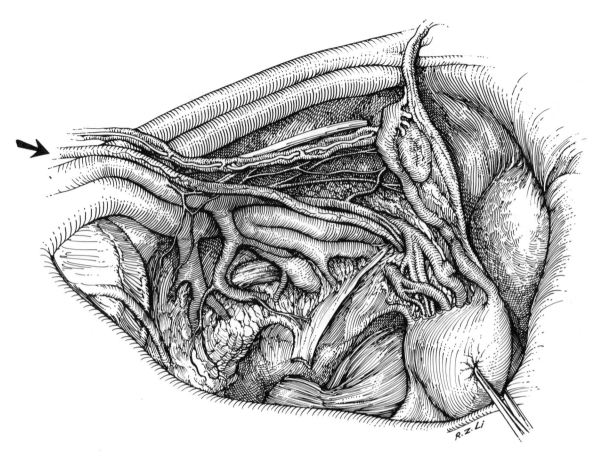

FIGURE 7.2
Relationship of ureter (arrow) to female pelvic viscera

pelvis or ureter. These malignancies have a propensity for recurrence on the side of initial involvement, and surveillance of the supravesical urinary system is difficult. Preservation of the kidney in selected cases of ureteral cancer may be possible by excision of the involved segment and ureteroureterostomy or ureteroneocystostomy. When tumors are managed in this fashion, periodic inspection of the ureter with ureteroscopy is advisable.

Poorly functioning, chronically infected kidneys associated with distal ureteral obstruction and tuberculosis of the kidney and ureter with minimal renal function are additional indications for nephroureterectomy.

Secondary ureterectomy after simple or radical nephrectomy is advisable if the original operation was performed for transitional cell carcinoma, or if there is chronic infection of the retained ureter.

OPERATIVE TECHNIQUE En bloc nephroureterectomy can be performed through a single incision that resembles an anterior flank incision that is extended inferiorly to connect with a Gibson incision. This approach is most appropriate for thin patients of short stature.

An anterior flank incision that provides sufficient exposure for the nephrectomy and mobilization of the upper ureter and a separate Gibson or lower midline incision to expose the distal ureter are also reasonable. With both of these approaches the thorax is rotated only 45° and repositioning of the patient is not necessary. However, some surgeons prefer to expose the kidney through a standard flank incision, and then reposition the patient for a lower abdominal incision after closing the initial wound.

We prefer to approach the kidney and distal ureter through two separate incisions that do not necessitate repositioning the patient. The nephrectomy is performed as described in Chapter 3, but the ureter is not transected. A radical nephrectomy is advisable if transitional cell carcinoma of the renal collecting system is the reason for surgery. The upper ureter is mobilized as distally as possible, and the kidney is positioned in the lower retroperitoneum. The wound is closed and the pelvis is exposed through a lower abdominal incision.

The pelvic ureter is isolated and freed in its entirety to the bladder. The ureter is ligated and transected

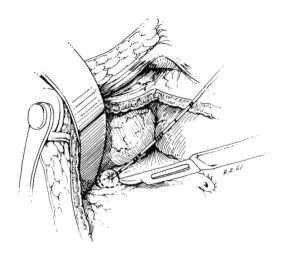

FIGURE 7.3
Excision of bladder cuff with ureterectomy

flush with the detrusor if the operation is performed for a benign condition. With transitional cell carcinoma, however, the intramural and submucosal ureter and a cuff of adjacent bladder mucosa are excised in continuity with the more proximal ureter. This is accomplished under direct vision through a cystotomy (Figure 7.3). The ureteral orifice is circumscribed to include a 1-cm margin of bladder mucosa, the ureter is dissected from the detrusor hiatus, and the surgical specimen is removed. The detrusor hiatus and cystotomy are closed in the usual manner, and Penrose drains are positioned at both sites. Transurethral rather than suprapubic catheter drainage is advisable to reduce the risk of tumor implantation in the catheter tract.

The distal ureter and bladder cuff may also be removed in an extravesical manner. This approach, although more expeditious, risks injury to the contralateral ureteral orifice. The ureter is grasped adjacent to the bladder, retracted, and circumscribed with a portion of the adjacent bladder wall. The defect is closed in two layers.

Secondary ureterectomy is performed through a lower abdominal incision. The ureter is mobilized proximally to the site of previous transection and distally to the bladder hiatus. The intramural and submucosal ureters are managed as described previously.

URETEROLITHOTOMY

The availability of ureteroscopy, intraureteral lithotripsy, and extracorporeal shock-wave lithotripsy have all contributed to a substantial decline in indications for ureterolithotomy. Nonetheless, ureteral cal-

culi are common, and all stones are not amenable to these treatment modalities.

OPERATIVE TECHNIQUE The level of the stone in the ureter, which is reconfirmed by an abdominal radiograph immediately before surgery, dictates the surgical approach. The upper ureter is exposed with a subcostal or lumbar incision. The lumbar incision, however, may be inadequate if the stone migrates into the distal ureter during surgery. The muscle-splitting flank incision is most appropriate for midureteral stones, and a Gibson incision or vertical or transverse lower abdominal incision are used to approach lower ureteral stones. In women, calculi in the most distal ureter that are palpable on bimanual examination may be removed through a transvaginal incision (Figure 7.4).

The ureter is approached extraperitoneally whenever feasible. The calculus or surrounding indurated tissue is palpated, and Babcock clamps or vessel loops are applied to the ureter above and below the stone to prevent migration. A longitudinal ureterotomy is then made directly over the stone, and the stone is extracted with forceps (Figure 7.5). Patency of the proximal and distal ureter is demonstrated by passage of a ureteral catheter. The ureterotomy is closed with loose, interrupted sutures, and a Penrose drain is positioned near the suture line.

On occasion the stone may migrate during the interval between the last x-ray and exposure of the ureter.

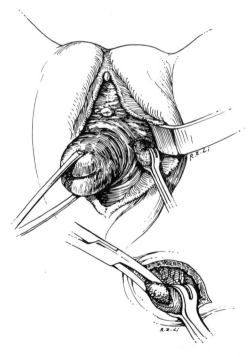

FIGURE 7.4
Transvaginal ureterolithotomy

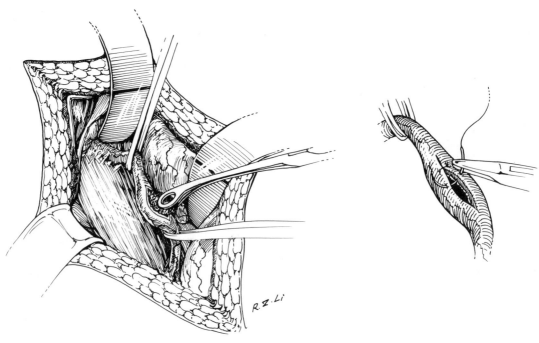

R.Z.Li

FIGURE 7.5
Ureterolithotomy

This frustrating intraoperative complication is managed by locating the position of the stone with intraoperative x-rays or with a flexible ureteroscope. It is usually possible to expose the site of stone migration by extending the incision, or to retrieve the stone with a basket. However, heroic efforts to extract distal ureteral stones that have migrated proximally are not warranted. In this situation a double-coiled stent is introduced through the ureterotomy, and the stone is pulverized at a later date with extracorporeal shockwave lithotripsy.

POSTOPERATIVE CARE AND COMPLICATIONS Persistent urinary leakage is the most common postoperative complication. An abundant drainage of urine for 1 to 2 days that rapidly decreases over the ensuing 12 to 24 hours is not unusual. Drainage for more than 5 to 7 days should be investigated with a retrograde pyelogram to rule out distal ureteral obstruction caused by unrecognized stone particles. Placement of a double-coiled ureteral stent is advisable when delayed healing is the cause of prolonged drainage.

Resolution of drainage accompanied by inordinate pain or fever should alert the surgeon to the possibility of a retroperitoneal urinoma. Large urinomas can be demonstrated easily with ultrasonography and require open or percutaneous drainage.

Stricture formation following ureterolithotomy is not common, but it is advisable to obtain an intravenous pyelogram 2 months after surgery to document the absence of obstruction.

URETEROURETEROSTOMY

End-to-end anastomosis of the ureter is performed after segmental excision for stricture or tumor and after traumatic disruption. Some degree of ureteral mobilization proximal and distal to the anastomosis is required for a tension-free closure. On occasion, mobilization and downward displacement of the kidney is also necessary. Alternatives to ureteroureterostomy, which are described in the following sections, should be considered when a satisfactory tension-free anastomosis is not feasible.

OPERATIVE TECHNIQUE The surgical approach is dictated by the location of the diseased ureter and parallels that described for ureterolithotomy. However, if the prospects for straightforward ureteroureterostomy are not great, exposure sufficient to perform alternative maneuvers is advisable.

The ureter is mobilized for 3 to 4 cm proximal and distal to the area of interest and the affected segment is excised. With traumatic disruption the free ends are debrided. If the ureter is not dilated, the ends are spatulated on opposing sides and anastomosed with interrupted fine absorbable sutures spaced at 2 to 3 mm intervals (Figure 7.6). The caliber of the anastomosis may be increased by a Z-plasty anastomosis (Figure 7.7). A stenting ureteral catheter is always advisable if the anastomosis is less than perfect. Drains are positioned near the suture line.

Postoperative care and early and late postoperative

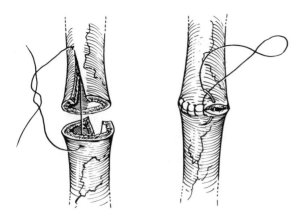

FIGURE 7.6
Ureteroureterostomy with spatulation of opposing sides of ureteral ends

complications are similar to those following ureterolithotomy. Because of the circumferential suture line, however, the risks of prolonged urinary leakage and stricture formation are probably greater.

When a tension-free ureteroureterostomy is not feasible, one can use various maneuvers to "bridge the gap." The applicability of alternatives to ureteroureterostomy is based, in large part, on the site and length of the defect. In the lower ureter, continuity of the urinary system can be restored with a psoas hitch or Boari flap and ureteroneocystostomy. Transureteroureterostomy is occasionally required when the defect is of sufficient length to preclude repair with the former approaches. The excision of extensive strictures of the midureter or upper ureter may be obviated by management with intubated ureterostomy. When most or all of the ureter is unsalvageable, ureteral substitution with ileum or renal autotransplantation is the only viable means for restoring continuity of the urinary system. The surgeon should be satisfied that both the need to preserve renal function and the functional potential of the ipsilateral kidney justify the potential morbidity of these two more extensive procedures.

PSOAS HITCH

The psoas hitch involves superlateral displacement of the bladder to permit tension-free ureteroneocystostomy. Fixation of the bladder to the psoas muscle prevents downward migration and anastomotic disruption or stricture. The operation is performed only when there is a compliant bladder of normal capacity.

OPERATIVE TECHNIQUE The pelvis is approached in an extraperitoneal or transperitoneal manner through a lower abdominal incision. The bladder is freed from the symphysis pubis, and the peritoneum and bladder are reflected medially from the pelvic side wall on both the ipsilateral and contralateral sides. The bladder is distended with saline and peritoneum is peeled from the dome. The affected ureter is transected above the diseased site, and the distal segment is either removed or secured with a ligature (Figure 7.8).

A transverse cystotomy is made between stay sutures, and the opened hand is inserted into the bladder to assess vesical mobility. Usually, the *contralateral* anterolateral vascular pedicle of the bladder must be divided to position the ipsilateral bladder over the external iliac vessels. The most superior margin of the bladder is then secured to the tendon or body of the

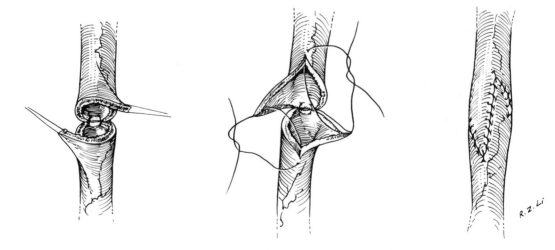

FIGURE 7.7
Ureteroureterostomy with angled spatulation of same side of ureteral ends and Z-plasty

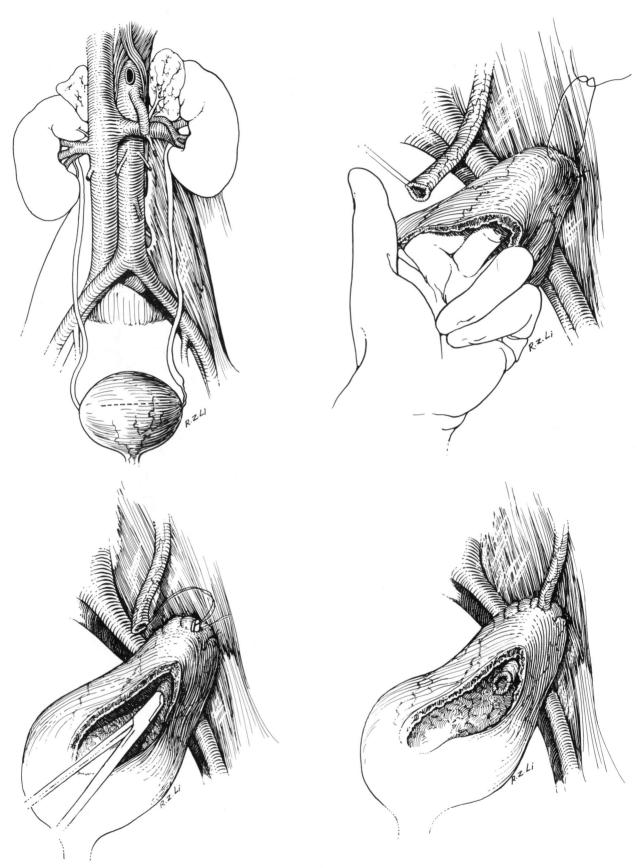

FIGURE 7.8
Psoas hitch with ureteroneocystostomy for distal left ureteral stricture

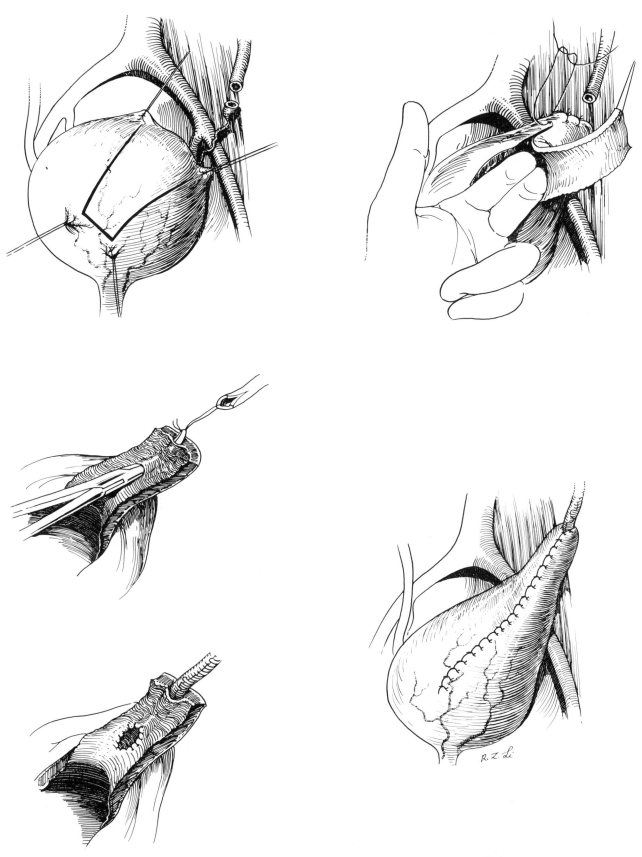

FIGURE 7.9
Boari flap with ureteroneocystostomy for distal left ureteral stricture

psoas muscle with heavy absorbable sutures. The sutures in the bladder should encompass the full thickness of the detrusor.

A stab wound for the ureteroneocystostomy is made at an appropriate site between the fixation sutures, and a tunneled ureteroneocystostomy is performed as described in Chapter 8. Care is taken to avoid angulation of the ureter as it traverses the detrusor. If the ureteral length is not sufficient for a tunneled anastomosis, an end-to-side anastomosis or a Boari flap procedure is performed.

The anastomosis is supported with a ureteral stent, and a suprapubic cystostomy is used for bladder drainage. The cystotomy is closed in the conventional manner, and drains are positioned adjacent to the bladder closure and the ureteroneocystostomy.

Ureteral obstruction and anastomotic leakage are uncommon, and voiding disturbances in the long term are unusual despite distortion of normal bladder anatomy.

BOARI FLAP

The Boari flap extends the psoas hitch about 5 to 10 cm upward and is recommended when a tension-free ureteroneocystostomy cannot be performed after bladder displacement alone.

OPERATIVE TECHNIQUE The bladder is mobilized and sutured to the psoas muscle as described for the psoas hitch procedure. The corners of a trapezoid flap with a 4-cm base and 3-cm apex are marked with stay sutures (Figure 7.9). The length should correspond to the defect requiring replacement. The sides and apex of the flap are incised, and the flap is reflected superiorly to the distal ureter. If feasible, a tunneled ureteroneocystostomy is performed. The defect in the fundus of the bladder is closed in the conventional manner, and the flap is tubularized by approximation of the lateral margins with two layers of absorbable sutures. The end of the tube is closed taking care to avoid strangulation of the ureter.

Edema of the tubularized bladder segment may lead to postoperative obstruction, and drainage with a double-coiled ureteral stent is prudent. A suprapubic cystostomy is used for bladder drainage. Drains are positioned next to the tubularized flap and the cystostomy.

TRANSURETEROURETEROSTOMY

Favorable experiences with the psoas hitch and Boari flap procedures have limited the indications for transureteroureterostomy. However, the procedure

should always be considered when satisfactory mobilization of the bladder is precluded by coexisting vesical disease. A proximal ureteral segment of inadequate length to cross the midline for a tension-free, end-to-side anastomosis with the contralateral ureter is an absolute contraindication. Relative contraindications include urinary stone disease, which may lead to bilateral ureteral obstruction if a calculus becomes lodged in the distal recipient ureter, and reflux of the recipient ureter. The advisability of salvaging a diseased kidney with an operation that has the potential for jeopardizing the function of a normal contralateral kidney must also be factored when contemplating a transureteroureterostomy.

OPERATIVE TECHNIQUE The pelvis is exposed with a transabdominal incision, and the mesenteric small bowel is displaced superiorly. The right ureter is isolated at the level of the common iliac artery. Mobilization of the cecum and ascending colon is required for satisfactory exposure of the upper ureter. The left ureter is approached by incision of the paracolic gutter and medial reflection of the sigmoid colon. The donor ureter is mobilized proximally and transected above the diseased segment (Figure 7.10). The distal segment is ligated or excised. A tunnel beneath the posterior peritoneum and mesentery of the sigmoid colon is created with blunt dissection either above or below the inferior mesenteric artery. The donor ureter is then drawn through the retroperitoneal space, taking care to avoid angulation or twisting.

The medial border of the recipient ureter is incised for 1 cm, and the donor ureter is spatulated. The superior and inferior angles of the anastomosis are secured with through-and-through fine absorbable sutures. The posterior wall of the anastomosis and then the anterior wall are approximated with interrupted absorbable sutures.

A small-caliber ureteral stent may be positioned in the donor ureter and distal recipient ureter, but obstruction of the recipient ureter at the anastomosis is a potential complication. If the distal recipient ureter is sufficiently capacious, a second stent may be introduced to obviate the problem. A Penrose drain is positioned at the anastomosis and tracted through the retroperitoneal space to a stab wound in the lower abdomen. The peritoneal incisions are closed with continuous absorbable sutures to prevent urinary leakage into the abdominal cavity.

POSTOPERATIVE CARE AND COMPLICATIONS Persistent urinary drainage is the most common postoperative complication. The gentle placement of a ureteral stent under fluoroscopic control or percutaneous nephrostomy, or both, usually reduces the magnitude of drainage and promotes healing of the anastomosis.

Late complications are confined primarily to anasto-

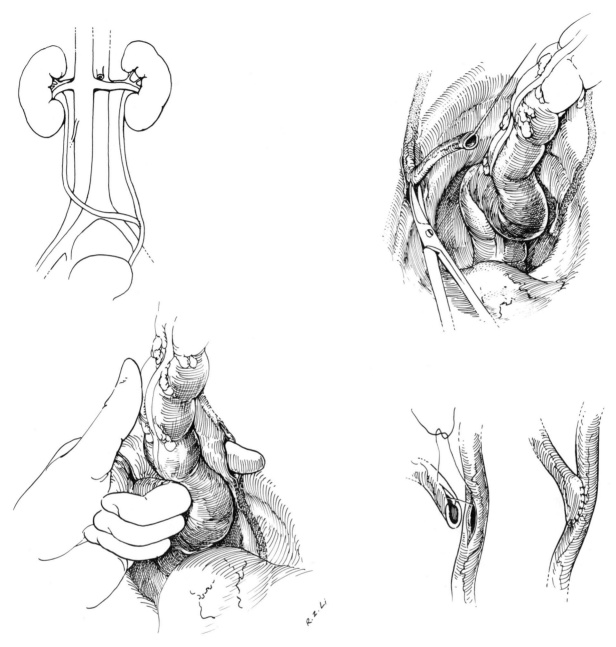

FIGURE 7.10
Transureteroureterostomy

motic stenosis, which may lead to obstruction of both ureters. Medial retraction and obstruction of the recipient ureter is inevitable if the donor ureter is of insufficient length for a tension-free anastomosis. These complications usually necessitate operative revision.

INTUBATED URETEROTOMY

Intubated ureterotomy is indicated for long strictures of the middle or upper ureter that are not amenable to simple excision. The procedure is straightforward and based on the ability of the ureter to heal over a stenting catheter.

OPERATIVE TECHNIQUE The ureter is exposed through an extraperitoneal approach. The diseased segment and 1 cm of normal ureter above and below the stricture are incised longitudinally on the lateral border (Figure 7.11). A snug-fitting, double-coiled stent, or a straight ureteral catheter exiting with a nephrostomy, is positioned in the ureter. The mucosal edges of the ureterotomy are then drawn toward one

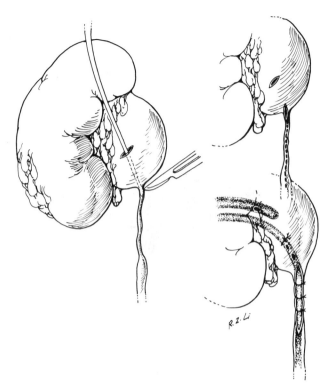

FIGURE 7.11
Intubated ureterotomy

another with fine absorbable bridging sutures. Nephrostomy drainage is advisable, and the ureterotomy is drained generously.

POSTOPERATIVE CARE AND COMPLICATIONS The drains are removed after 5 to 7 days; the ureteral stent is left indwelling for 6 to 8 weeks. Before removal of the stent, an antegrade pyelogram is obtained. If there is no extravasation, the stent is removed and ureteral integrity is reassessed with a second antegrade pyelogram. Extravasation seen with this study necessitates replacement of the ureteral stent.

ILEAL URETER

The isoperistaltic ileal segment is an effective replacement for the entire ureter or for a long segment of distal ureter. The technique is employed usually for bypassing an extensively strictured ureter when more conservative approaches have been exhausted. Ileal ureters have also been constructed to facilitate stone passage in patients with uncontrollable urolithiasis. Functional ureter proximal to a diseased segment may be anastomosed to the ileum. However, the entire distal ureter must be bypassed because mucus produced by the ileum does not easily traverse the lumen. It is important to delineate the normal and abnormal ureteral segments before surgical intervention with retrograde and, if necessary, antegrade pyelography.

Reflux into an ileal ureter is expected, and patients with hypertonic neurogenic bladder dysfunction are inappropriate candidates for the operation. As with all procedures involving transposition of bowel to the urinary tract, a hyperchloremic, metabolic acidosis that is accentuated by renal insufficiency is a recognized complication. An ileal ureter should not be constructed if the serum creatinine level is greater than 2.0 mg/dl.

OPERATIVE TECHNIQUE A generous transperitoneal approach is required for satisfactory exposure. For right ureteral substitution the cecum, ascending colon, and ileum are mobilized superomedially by incision of the lateral gutter and the posterior peritoneum from the cecum to the ligament of Treitz. For left ureteral substitution the paracolic gutter is incised and the descending and sigmoid colon are reflected medially. The ureter is isolated and the length required for substitution is measured. Functional proximal ureter may be preserved, but all distal ureter is bypassed or excised.

A segment of ileum somewhat longer than appears to be required is chosen so that the distal mesentery can be divided between the right colic and ileocolic arteries. The distal mesenteric incision should be 15 to 20 cm in length, but the proximal incision is shorter. The bowel is transected, and intestinal continuity is reestablished with an anastomosis performed anterior to the mesentery of the isolated segment. The ileal segment is positioned in the right retroperitoneum through a defect in the mesentery of the ascending colon or by rotation of the proximal end behind the cecum and ascending colon (Figure 7.12). The ileum is positioned in the left retroperitoneum through a defect in the mesentery of the descending colon. Care should be taken to avoid acute angulation or twisting of the vascular pedicle.

If the proximal ureter is dilated, an end-to-end ureteroileal anastomosis may be feasible. Otherwise, the proximal ileum is closed in two layers, and the spatulated ureter is anastomosed in an end-to-side manner. In the absence of usable proximal ureter, the renal pelvis is transected above the ureteropelvic junction, the ureter is ligated, and the ileal lumen and the renal pelvis are joined with an end-to-end anastomosis. Alternatively, one can leave the diseased ureter in situ and anastomose the ileum to the renal pelvis in an end-to-side fashion.

A cystotomy is performed and a disc of the bladder wall above the ipsilateral ureteral orifice is removed. The ileovesical anastomosis is then done in two layers with interrupted absorbable sutures. Alternatively, the

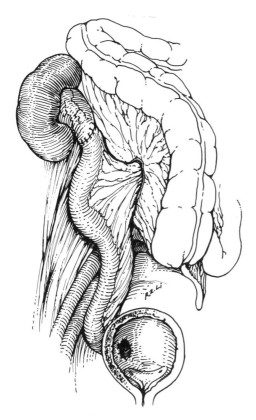

FIGURE 7.12
Ileal ureter

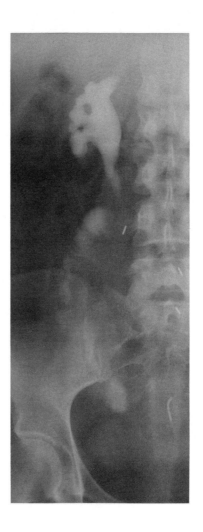

FIGURE 7.13
Intravenous pyelogram demonstrating right ileal ureter

distal ileal segment can be tapered and implanted into the bladder using the tunneling technique of ureteroneocystostomy. If desired, the ileovesical anastomosis can be stabilized with a psoas hitch procedure.

A suprapubic cystostomy is advisable to facilitate the evacuation of mucus, and nephrostomy drainage is recommended. Penrose drains are positioned at the proximal and distal ileal anastomoses and adjacent to the cystostomy.

POSTOPERATIVE CARE AND COMPLICATIONS An antegrade pyelogram is obtained on the seventh to twelfth postoperative day, and the drains are removed over the ensuing 1 to 2 days if there is no extravasation. The nephrostomy is removed if drainage of the ileum is satisfactory. The appearance of an ileal ureter with intravenous pyelography is shown in Figure 7.13.

Obstruction is uncommon if the ileum is not redundant or angulated, but reflux is the rule. A hyperchloremic metabolic acidosis of any degree is treated with a sodium potassium bicarbonate solution. Troublesome obstruction of the bladder outlet by mucus is seen almost exclusively in men and is managed by transurethral resection or incision of the prostate.

RENAL AUTOTRANSPLANTATION

Relocation of a kidney to the pelvis is the preferred method for managing extensive ureteral disease if kidney function is not severely compromised. Atherosclerosis of the pelvic vasculature that precludes satisfactory arterial anastomosis is the primary contraindication. The kidney is removed, perfused, and cooled as described in Chapter 4 for donor transplant nephrectomy. The vascular anastomoses are done as described in the same chapter for the recipient operation. Continuity of the urinary tract is reestablished with a standard ureteroneocystostomy, or the distal ureter may be joined with the renal pelvis. If the entire ureter is diseased, the renal pelvis is anastomosed directly with the bladder.

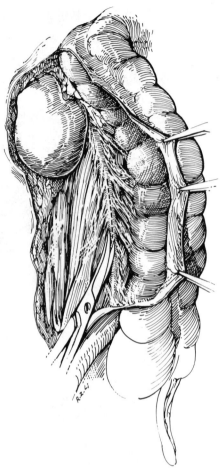

FIGURE 7.14
Ureterolysis

URETEROLYSIS

Ureterolysis refers to mobilization of a functionally obstructed ureter from fibrotic or inflammatory retroperitoneal tissue. Benign retroperitoneal fibrosis, postinflammatory fibrosis, locally invasive malignancies, or radiation therapy may produce sufficient induration of the periureteral tissue to compromise peristalsis. Typically, the lumen of the ureter remains patent and catheters can be passed without difficulty.

Most patients present with vague back pain due to the obstructive uropathy or the fibrotic process, or with laboratory evidence or clinical manifestations of renal insufficiency. Drainage of the affected kidney or kidneys with a double-coiled ureteral stent is advisable to maximize renal function before surgery and to facilitate identification of the ureter intraoperatively.

OPERATIVE TECHNIQUE The optimal operative approach is determined by the laterality and extent of the fibrotic process. Generous transperitoneal exposure is advisable because the constraints of the fibrosis are

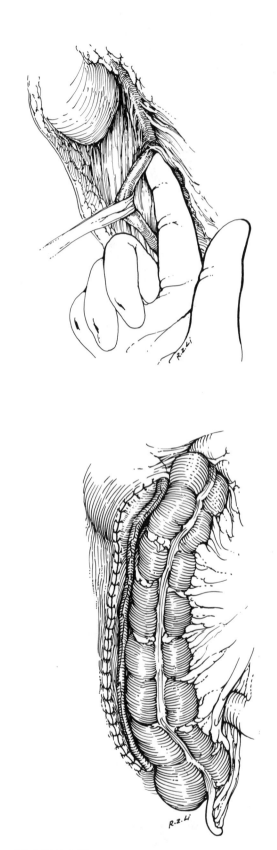

FIGURE 7.15
Intraperitoneal transposition of ureter after ureterolysis

often underestimated before surgery. Ureterolysis is performed in the same manner, regardless of the underlying cause of the encasement.

The most extensive fibrotic processes are caused usually by idiopathic retroperitoneal fibrosis. Bilateral ureteral obstruction is common. The ureters are approached from a lateral direction, as retroperitoneal fibrosis extends from the midline and dissection around the entrapped vena cava or aorta may be hazardous. The ascending or descending colon is reflected medially, and the ureter above and below the entrapped segment is isolated. A plane is established on the adventitia of the normal ureter, and the involved segment is shelled from indurated tissues with blunt or finger dissection (Figure 7.14). At times it is necessary to divide thick fibrotic plaques overlying the ureter. A biopsy of the indurated material is routinely performed to rule out malignancy.

Intraperitoneal transposition of the ureter or ureters helps to prevent recurrent obstruction. This is achieved by manipulating the ureter lateral to the colon and closing the paracolic incision under the ureter (Figure 7.15). Care is taken to avoid angulation of the ureter as it enters and exits the peritoneal space. As the ureteral blood supply and supporting periureteric tissues are disrupted during a ureterolysis, wrapping of the ureter with omentum may facilitate the recovery of normal peristaltic activity. Retrograde pyelograms obtained before and after a successful right ureterolysis with intraperitoneal transposition are shown in Figure 7.16.

Retroperitoneal fibrosis may progress to involve the contralateral ureter after a unilateral ureterolysis. Prophylactic lateral displacement of an unaffected ureter may be advisable.

POSTOPERATIVE CARE AND COMPLICATIONS The double-coiled ureteral stent placed before surgery is not removed for 2 to 4 weeks. The stent helps to maintain the position of the ureter and provides a means for urinary drainage until physiologic peristalsis is restored. If a bilateral ureterolysis has been performed, the stents are removed sequentially over 1 to 2 weeks. An intravenous pyelogram is obtained before removal of the second stent to assess the function of the contralateral ureter.

Acute angulation or incomplete lysis of the ureter

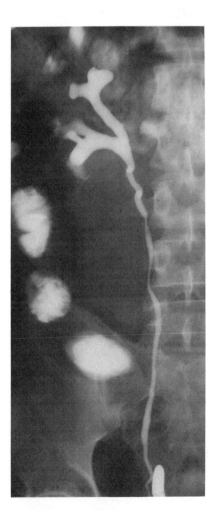
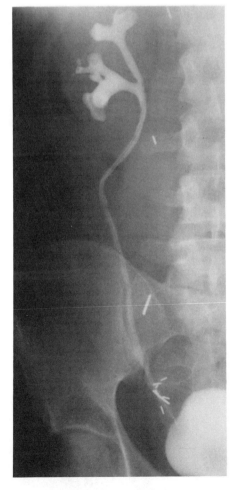

FIGURE 7.16
Retrograde pyelograms demonstrating position of ureter before (left) and after (right) ureterolysis and intraperitoneal transposition for retroperitoneal fibrosis

may lead to persistent obstruction. In some cases meaningful peristaltic activity never returns despite a technically perfect operation. Replacement of a double-coiled ureteral stent provides a temporary solution that, in some cases, may also constitute the most optimal permanent solution. The latter is particularly relevant if the ureteral entrapment is caused by malignant disease or if the patient is elderly.

OPERATIONS FOR URETERAL TRAUMA

The vast majority of ureteral injuries are iatrogenic and occur during endoscopic manipulations or open pelvic operations. Partial ureteral tears or perforations that complicate endoscopic procedures usually heal if a ureteral stent can be negotiated through the injured segment. Complete disruptions necessitate operative intervention but can generally be repaired by primary ureteroureterostomy or ureteroneocystostomy. Injuries recognized at the time of open pelvic surgery are generally amenable to repair using the same techniques.

On occasion, ureteral disruptions that complicate pelvic surgery are recognized initially during the postoperative period. As with vesicovaginal fistulas following gynecologic surgery, reparative interventions are generally feasible if the diagnosis is made within 24 to 48 hours of surgery. With more prolonged diagnostic delays, infection and inflammation generally preclude primary repair. Percutaneous nephrostomy and, if indicated, drainage of the inevitable retroperitoneal urinoma are the treatments of choice. Reconstructive procedures are performed 1 to 2 months later when infection and inflammation have resolved.

Isolated injury to the ureter from violent trauma is unusual. Exploration is almost always required to deal with coexisting intra-abdominal or retroperitoneal injuries. Most traumatic disruptions of the ureter can be managed by debridement of devascularized ureteral tissue, mobilization of the proximal and distal ureter, and ureteroureterostomy or ureteroneocystostomy. As anastomotic leakage may magnify the severity of associated injuries, a double-coiled ureteral stent should always be introduced before the ureter is closed, and the anastomotic site is generously drained.

Nephrectomy is rarely indicated even when an extensive ureteral injury is encountered in an unstable patient. Nephrostomy and ligation of the ureter just proximal to the disruption is an acceptable temporizing measure and permits restoration of ureteral continuity at a later date.

CHAPTER 8

Surgery of the Ureterovesical Junction

The distal ureter that joins with the bladder consists of a 1.5-cm intramural segment that courses through a hiatus of the detrusor muscle and a 1.0-cm submucosal segment that lies between the bladder mucosa and the detrusor muscle. The irregular pattern of the ureteral musculature becomes longitudinal before entry into the detrusor, and the distal 3 cm of the extravesical ureter is surrounded by the fibromuscular Waldeyer's sheath.

The ureteral musculature fans out to form the superficial trigone, which terminates at the verumontanum in the male and the external meatus in the female (Figure 8.1). The deep trigonal muscle is derived from fibers of Waldeyer's sheath and terminates at the bladder outlet. The detrusor muscle lies below the trigone. The trigone is the most stable portion of the bladder and links the ureters with the bladder outlet.

The drainage of urine through the ureterovesical junction is facilitated by contraction of the distal longitudinal ureteral musculature. This activity expands the lumen of the intramural and submucosal ureter. With bladder distention, the trigone and the intramural and submucosal ureter are passively stretched. This narrows the ureteral lumen and prevents the reflux of urine into the ureter. During micturition, contraction of the detrusor muscle and elevated intravesical pressures compress the submucosal ureter to create additional resistance to reflux.

The most common disorders of the ureterovesical junction requiring surgical intervention are vesicoureteral reflux and obstruction. Primary reflux results usually from an inadequate length of the submucosal ureter and is not associated with neurogenic bladder dysfunction or bladder outlet obstruction. The orifice is characteristically located superolateral to the trigone (Figure 8.2). Diverticula next to the ureteral orifice may also produce primary reflux due to inadequate support of the submucosal ureter.

Secondary reflux results from chronic bladder outlet obstruction, neurogenic bladder dysfunction, or iatrogenic injury to the submucosal ureter. Bacteriuria can produce transient reflux due to inflammation and reduced compliance of the submucosal ureter.

Some patients with reflux experience vague flank discomfort. In most cases, however, the condition is asymptomatic. The diagnosis of primary reflux is often established in childhood when urologic investigation is prompted by a urinary tract infection. Depending on the severity and longevity of reflux, dilatation of the ureter and renal collecting system may be observed on the intravenous pyelogram. Renal scarring is seen almost exclusively in individuals who have had acute bacterial nephritis during early childhood.

The diagnosis is made by the radiographic visualization of contrast medium in the lower ureter or entire collecting system during voiding cystourethrography (Figure 8.3). Nuclear cystograms use radionuclides rather than contrast to demonstrate reflux. This study

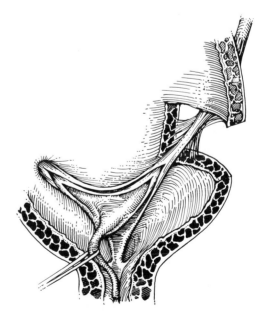

FIGURE 8.1
Superficial and deep trigone arising from ureter and Waldeyer's sheath

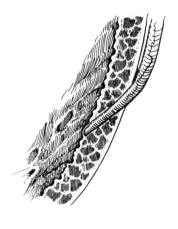

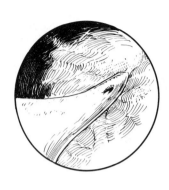

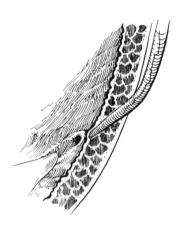

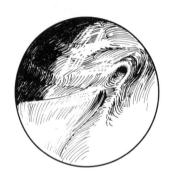

FIGURE 8.2
Side view and endoscopic appearance of normally situated ureteral orifice with adequate submucosal segment (top) and of laterally situated orifice with short submucosal segment (bottom)

is particularly useful for surveillance because the radiation exposure is minimal.

Opinions vary about the advisability and timing of interventions to correct primary reflux that is associated with recurrent renal infections. The controversy is caused by the availability of antimicrobial regimens that are exceedingly effective in preventing bacteriuria and evidence that correction of reflux does not alter susceptibility to urinary tract infection. Uncertainty about the impact of sterile reflux on renal function and the potential for spontaneous resolution of reflux with maturation further muddy the water.

Regardless of a susceptibility to urinary tract infection, most urologists recommend ureteroneocystostomy if reflux is associated with dilatation of the renal collecting system. Reflux that does not produce dilatation of the collecting system but is complicated by infection is managed with prophylactic antibiotics or by ureteroneocystostomy. A submucosal ureter that is short or nonexistent usually indicates that the reflux will not resolve spontaneously and strengthens the rationale for operative intervention. In the absence of

recurring urinary tract infection, reflux of this magnitude requires no treatment.

Congenital obstructions at the ureterovesical junction are caused usually by strictures or adynamic segments adjacent to the detrusor hiatus. Detrusor hypertrophy and fibrosis of the submucosal ureter following iatrogenic injury are the most common acquired causes of obstruction at this site.

URETERONEOCYSTOSTOMY

Ureteroneocystostomy, or reimplantation of the ureter into the bladder, is the operative procedure for correcting vesicoureteral reflux. The object is to lengthen the submucosal ureter by distal relocation of the ureteral orifice, proximal relocation of the detrusor hiatus, or both (Figure 8.4). The creation of a submucosal tunnel to prevent reflux is also applicable to a ureteroneocystostomy that is done for other reasons.

A successful surgical outcome is most likely when the anastomosis is tension-free, the tunneled ureter is

Regardless of the technique of ureteroneocystostomy, the bladder is approached in an extraperitoneal manner through a lower abdominal incision. Stenting of the anastomosis is recommended only if the procedure is technically difficult or bilateral. The bladder is drained with a urethral catheter in the female, but a suprapubic cystostomy is advisable in the male. Penrose drains are usually positioned adjacent to the site of the ureteroneocystostomy and the cystotomy.

Ureteral Advancement

Ureteral advancement, the most technically simple method of ureteroneocystostomy, is performed in a transvesical manner. It is not well suited for the management of dilated ureters and requires sufficient space below the orifice for creation of a submucosal tunnel.

OPERATIVE TECHNIQUE   A cystotomy is performed in the anterior aspect of the bladder, and the mucosa surrounding the affected orifice is circumscribed. A ureteral catheter is introduced and fixed to the edge of the mucosa to facilitate subsequent dissection. The ureter is mobilized from the detrusor hiatus and perivesical attachments for 3 to 4 cm proximal to the bladder (Figure 8.5). Approximately 2 to 3 cm of ureter is drawn into the bladder, and an appropriate site for the new orifice inferomedial to the original orifice is selected. The vesical mucosa is incised, and a submucosal tunnel is developed with a scissors between the mucosal incision and the original orifice. The ureteral catheter is removed, and the ureter is drawn through the tunnel with a stay suture. The posterior edge of the spatulated ureter is fixed to the trigone with a fine absorbable suture placed through the ureter and into the deep musculature. The anastomosis is completed by approximating the vesical mucosa with a full thickness of the free ureteral margins. The mucosal defect at the original orifice is sealed with interrupted

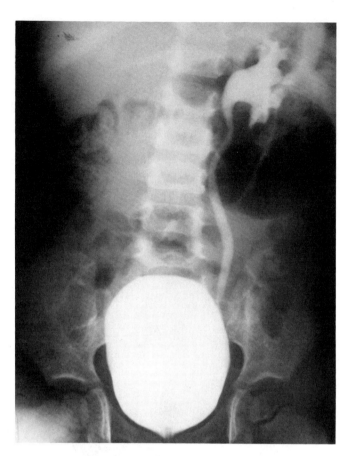

FIGURE 8.3
Cystogram demonstrating left vesicoureteral reflux

supported by firm underlying detrusor muscle, and the submucosal tunnel is four to five times longer than the diameter of the ureter. Tapering or imbrication of a dilated distal ureter may be required to achieve a proper ratio of tunnel length to ureteral diameter. Preservation of the ureteral blood supply and atraumatic handling of the ureter are critical to prevent ischemia and fibrosis.

FIGURE 8.4
Side view of ureter with short submucosal segment (left) and (left to right) establishment of adequate submucosal segment with Politano-Leadbetter, ureteral advancement, and Lich techniques of ureteroneocystostomy

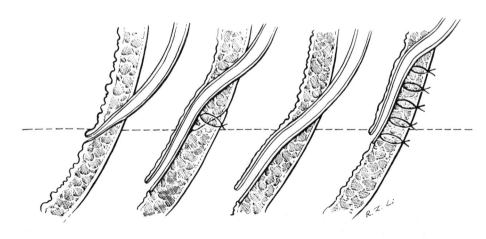

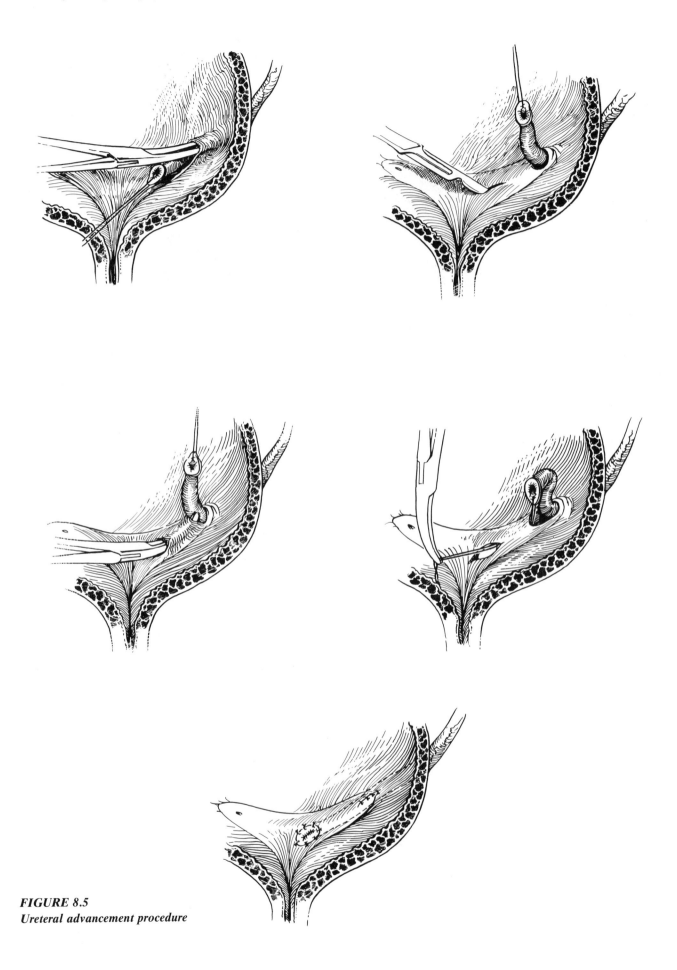

FIGURE 8.5
Ureteral advancement procedure

absorbable sutures, and the bladder is closed in a conventional manner.

Additional length of the submucosal tunnel can be achieved by incising the detrusor for 2 to 3 cm in a superolateral direction from the hiatus. The original hiatus is then closed under the ureter.

Cross Trigonal Advancement

The cross trigonal ureteroneocystostomy is a popular modification of the ureteral advancement technique. It should always be considered when the distance between the orifice and the bladder outlet is insufficient to create a submucosal tunnel of appropriate length.

OPERATIVE TECHNIQUE The basic maneuvers for cross trigonal advancement parallel those of the ureteral advancement procedure, but the submucosal tunnel is developed in an inferior or superior direction across the midline. With bilateral ureteroneocystostomy, one ureter is directed superomedially and the other inferomedially to lie parallel to one another (Figure 8.6). In this situation the bladder mucosa between the orifices may be incised and dissected from the detrusor muscle superiorly and from the trigone inferiorly. The mucosal defects for the new orifices are created as shown in the Figure 8.6, and the transverse mucosal incision is closed with a continuous absorbable suture.

Politano-Leadbetter Procedure

The Politano-Leadbetter technique of ureteroneocystostomy was described originally as a transvesical operation but is commonly done by a combined transvesical-extravesical approach. It involves the creation of a new detrusor hiatus and submucosal tunnel and is the most versatile method of reimplantation.

OPERATIVE TECHNIQUE The circumscribing incision around the ureteral orifice and mobilization of the ureter from the detrusor hiatus and perivesical attachments are performed as described for the advancement procedure. A 2 to 3-cm submucosal tunnel is then developed in a superolateral direction from the original orifice (Figure 8.7). The mucosa is incised at the superior aspect of the tunnel, and a defect in the detrusor muscle is created for the new hiatus. A right-angle clamp is passed through the new hiatus to develop a space behind the bladder which parallels the direction of the submucosal tunnel. The ureteral catheter is removed, a suture attached to the ureter is grasped with the clamp, and the ureter is pulled through the new hiatus. Alternatively, the suture may be grasped at the original hiatus and worked behind the bladder to maneuver the ureter into the new hiatus.

If a combined transvesical and extravesical approach is used, the ureter is brought through the new hiatus under direct vision. This approach may reduce

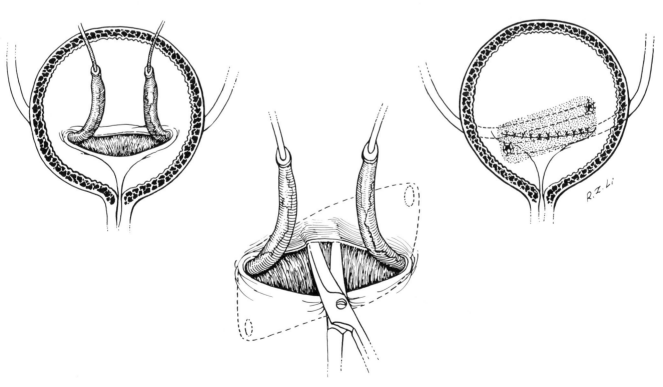

FIGURE 8.6
Cross trigonal advancement procedure

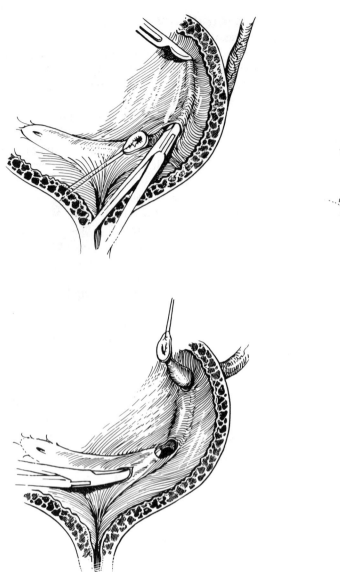
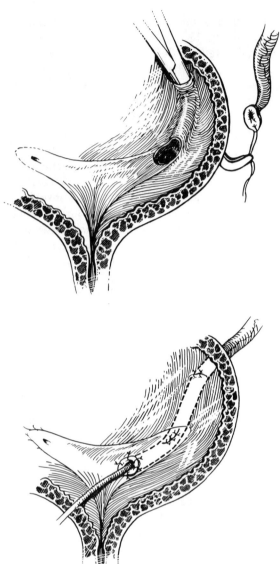

FIGURE 8.7
Politano-Leadbetter procedure

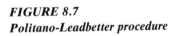

the risk of kinking and is required if tailoring or tapering of the distal ureter is performed.

The original hiatus is closed with interrupted absorbable sutures, and the ureter is drawn through the submucosal tunnel. The tunnel can be lengthened as needed in an inferomedial direction from the original orifice. The ureter is spatulated and fixed to the detrusor muscle and vesical mucosa as described for the advancement operation, and the mucosal incisions are closed.

Lich Procedure

The Lich technique of ureteroneocystostomy does not require disruption of the existing mucosal junction of the ureter and bladder and is performed extravesically.

Most transplant surgeons use this method of reimplantation in recipient operations. However, it is not well suited for the management of dilated ureters because tapering or imbrication is not possible, and the tunnel cannot exceed 2 to 3 cm without the risk of ureteral angulation at the new hiatus.

OPERATIVE TECHNIQUE The distal extravesical ureter is exposed through an extraperitoneal approach and freed from the detrusor hiatus to the level of the mucosa (Figure 8.8). The detrusor muscle underlying the normal course of the ureter is incised for 3 cm and dissected from the bladder mucosa to form a trough. The ureter is positioned in the trough, and the detrusor is closed over the ureter with interrupted absorbable sutures.

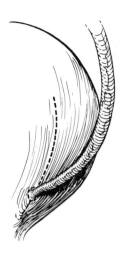
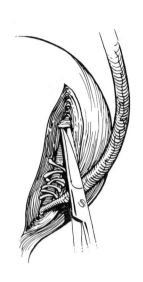
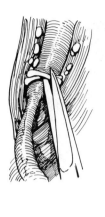
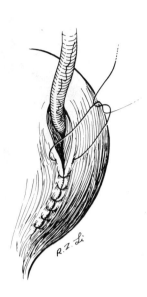

FIGURE 8.8
Lich procedure

Ureteroneocystostomy with Ureteral Duplication

With complete duplication of the renal collecting system, reflux may occur in one or both ureters. The ureter that drains the lower pole is usually involved when there is reflux to a single ureter only. The orifice is almost always lateral to the orifice of the upper-pole ureter, and the submucosal segment is shorter.

The distal portions of duplicated ureters generally share a common sheath and blood supply and should be managed as a single unit during ureteroneocystostomy (Figure 8.9). The principles and techniques

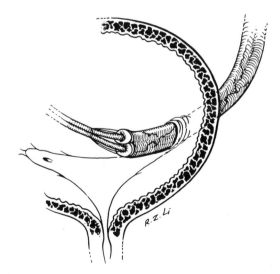

FIGURE 8.9
Ureteroneocystostomy with ureteral duplication

described for reimplantation of a single ureter are applicable to surgery of duplicated ureters.

POSTOPERATIVE CARE AND COMPLICATIONS

The Penrose drains are usually removed after 1 to 2 days. A ureteral stent, if used, is removed after 3 to 4 days, and the urethral catheter or suprapubic tube is removed after 6 to 7 days. When the ureter has been tapered or imbricated, the stent is left indwelling for about 7 days. Perioperative antimicrobial therapy is advisable, and oral antibiotics are administered at full dosage for 2 weeks following hospital discharge. Low-dose prophylactic therapy is warranted for 1 to 2 months if there is a susceptibility to bacteriuria.

A voiding cystourethrogram and an intravenous pyelogram are obtained 2 to 3 months after surgery. Persistent reflux does not necessarily represent an unsuccessful procedure, as residual noncompliance of the submucosal ureter may limit the antireflux capabilities of the reimplantation.

Anastomotic obstruction in the early postoperative period usually is due to angulation of the ureter as it enters the detrusor hiatus or to compression of the ureter by a new hiatus of inadequate size. Distal ureteral fibrosis caused by ischemia is a potential reason for late obstruction but can be corrected usually with a minimal ureteral meatotomy.

Reflux that persists for more than 6 months is generally permanent. This complication results from an inadequate tunnel, fibrosis of the distal ureter, or unrecognized neurogenic bladder dysfunction.

On occasion, reflux develops in a previously

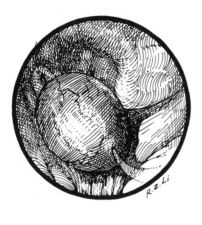

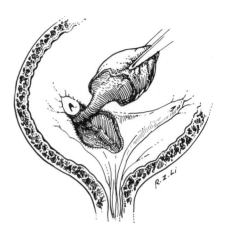

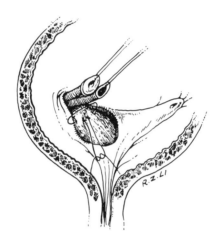

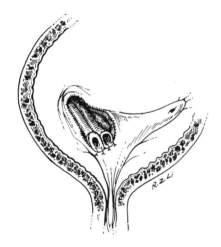

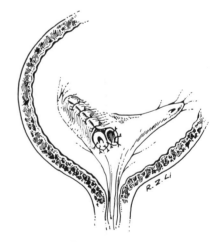

FIGURE 8.10
Ureteroneocystostomy with ureterocele and ureteral duplication

nonrefluxing contralateral ureter. This may result from postoperative inflammation and resolve spontaneously. Persistence of the reflux usually indicates that the submucosal tunnel is of borderline length. For this reason, bilateral ureteroneocystostomy should be considered when the submucosal tunnel of a nonrefluxing contralateral ureter appears abnormally short during preoperative cystoscopy.

OPERATIONS FOR URETEROCELES

A ureterocele is a cystic dilatation of the submucosal ureter. The orifice of a ureterocele may be in the normal location, or it may be situated ectopically at or distal to the bladder outlet. Ureteroceles with ectopic orifices are generally associated with complete ureteral duplications and almost always involve the ureter draining the upper pole.

The diagnosis is usually made with an intravenous pyelogram. Small ureteroceles appear as "cobra head" deformities of the intravesical ureter because the contrast density in the ureter is greater than that in the bladder. The opacification of large ureteroceles, however, is usually delayed, and a negative filling defect at the base of the bladder is observed. The presence or absence of reflux in the affected or contralateral ureter is assessed by voiding cystourethrography.

Small ureteroceles are usually asymptomatic, nonobstructive, and require no treatment. Obstruction is seen with large ureteroceles when the orifice is stenotic or an ectopic orifice is compressed by the bladder outlet. Large ureteroceles may also prolapse into the urethra or obstruct the contralateral ureter, an ipsilateral duplicated ureter, or both.

Obstructive ureteroceles can be decompressed by endoscopic incision of the orifice with scissors. Reflux, however, is a possible sequela. Excision and ureteroneocystostomy is recommended for the treatment of most large ureteroceles.

OPERATIVE TECHNIQUE The bladder is approached through an extraperitoneal lower abdominal incision. A cystotomy is performed, and the ureterocele is grasped with a Babcock clamp. Mucosa adjacent to the ureterocele is incised, and the ureterocele is dissected from the underlying trigonal musculature (Figure 8.10). The ureter is then mobilized from the detrusor hiatus and retroperitoneal attachments.

The integrity of the detrusor hiatus and the bed of the ureterocele are assessed by palpation. If the hiatus is dilated, several sutures are placed to reduce the defect. An attenuated detrusor muscle should be reinforced by imbrication. The ureterocele is amputated and the distal ureter is fixed to the trigone. Because mucosa overlying the ureterocele is excised, mucosa adjacent to the trough is dissected from the detrusor and sutured over the ureter. A formal ureteroneocystostomy should be undertaken if a satisfactory tunnel cannot be created with these maneuvers. In cases of duplication, both ureters are mobilized from the detrusor hiatus and retroperitoneal attachments in their common sheath and advanced as a single unit.

Alternatives to excision and ureteroneocystostomy include pyelopyelostomy and ureteropyelostomy. Nephrectomy or partial nephrectomy is advisable when meaningful renal function cannot be salvaged.

CHAPTER 9

Surgery of the Bladder

The bladder is an expansile muscular reservoir that stores urine at low pressure and empties by coordinated contraction of the detrusor and relaxation of the outlet. The posterosuperior surface is covered by peritoneum. The urachus extends from the apex of the bladder to the umbilicus in the preperitoneal space. The anterolateral aspects lie behind the symphysis and the pubic arch and are stabilized inferiorly by the endopelvic fascia. The retropubic space (or space of Retzius) above the endopelvic fascia is easily developed for extraperitoneal exposure of the bladder. The posterior bladder base in males is separated from the rectum by the seminal vesicles, the vasa deferentia and the ureters (Figure 9.1). In females it lies immediately anterior to the vagina.

The bladder is lined with a transitional epithelium. The muscular wall, or detrusor muscle, is composed of intertwined muscular bundles with no defined layers or orientation. The blood supply is derived from the superior, middle, and inferior vesical arteries, which arise from the hypogastric artery. Branches of the uterine and vaginal arteries in females and of the middle hemorrhoidal artery in males also supply the bladder base. The overlap of arterial profusion is extensive, and transection of the vascular pedicle on one side or the other does not lead to ischemia or dysfunction. Venous blood drains through an extensive adventitial plexus into the hypogastric veins and veins lying anterior to the bladder outlet. Arteries and veins that communicate with the hypogastric vessels are situated in an anterolateral pedicle. Development and transection of these pedicles are necessary during cystectomy or for satisfactory exposure of the inferolateral bladder.

The lymphatics of the bladder drain to the external and internal iliac nodal chains. Sympathetic and parasympathetic innervation is extensive but of minimal surgical importance.

The bladder is approached in an anterior extraperitoneal manner whenever feasible. Additional exposure is attained by sweeping the peritoneum from the superior surface. Cystotomies are preferentially closed in two or three separate layers (Figure 9.2). The mucosa and superficial detrusor muscle are approximated with a continuous 3-0 absorbable suture, and the deep detrusor and perivesical fascia are closed with heavier interrupted absorbable sutures. Additional reinforcing sutures applied to the deep muscle and fascia are advisable at times. Penrose drains or the equivalent are positioned adjacent to the bladder closure and brought out through a stab wound. A suprapubic cystostomy is generally preferred for postoperative bladder drainage in the male and is recommended after extensive reconstructive surgery in either sex. When the integrity of the closure is at all suspect, or when urinary leakage from the suture line can lead to serious complications, the suprapubic tube or urethral catheter is not removed until the absence of extravasation is documented by cystography.

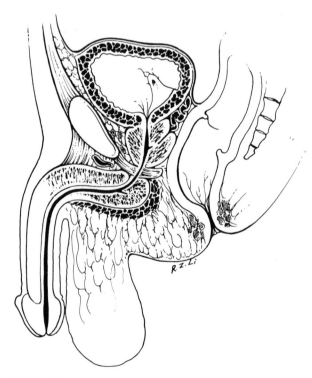

FIGURE 9.1
Relationship of bladder to adjacent pelvic structures in the male

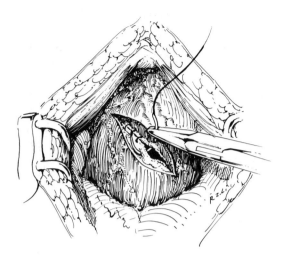

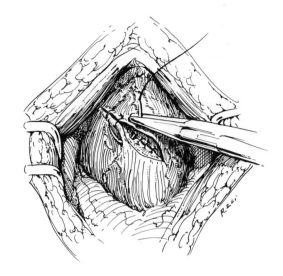

FIGURE 9.2
Two-layered closure of the bladder

SUPRAPUBIC CYSTOSTOMY

Suprapubic cystostomy is the placement of a catheter through the lower abdominal wall for drainage of the bladder. The procedure is indicated when transurethral catheterization is not feasible or is ill-advised.

Percutaneous Cystostomy

Percutaneous cystostomy is an attractive alternative to urethral catheterization in men with acute urinary retention and is the preferred means of bladder drainage after some operative procedures. Percutaneous cystostomy is hazardous if the bladder is not palpable or if the normal pelvic anatomy has been distorted by previous operations. Both situations make entry of the bladder difficult and increase the risks of penetrating the peritoneal cavity.

A variety of tubes designed specifically for percutaneous cystostomy are commercially available. Their caliber range from 8 to 14 F.

OPERATIVE TECHNIQUE The suprapubic area is shaved and prepared with an antiseptic solution. The skin is anesthetized with lidocaine 2 cm above the symphysis pubis in the midline, and a small stab wound is made. A tract to the bladder is then injected with about 25 ml of lidocaine. A spinal needle is advanced at a slightly downward angle toward the bladder to assess the feasibility of bladder puncture and to determine the proper angle of catheter insertion. A cystostomy is never attempted if the bladder cannot be penetrated with the needle.

The cystostomy tube, which has a hollow metal obturator, is held as shown in Figure 9.3 and slowly advanced through the abdominal wall and retropubic space. When urine appears at the hub, the catheter is advanced for an additional 2 cm and the obturator is withdrawn while the catheter is advanced further. The tube is sutured or taped to the skin and connected to a sterile urinary drainage appliance.

Injury to the intra-abdominal pelvic viscera is the principal complication of percutaneous cystostomy

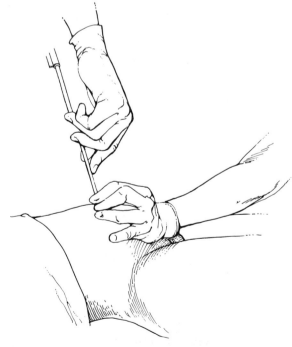

FIGURE 9.3
Insertion of percutaneous cystostomy tube

and is manifested usually by peritoneal or intestinal symptoms. Laceration or penetration of the bowel, or disruption of mesenteric vessels, may occur during unsuccessful attempts at catheter placement or during seemingly perfect positioning of the catheter in the bladder lumen.

Open Cystostomy

Placement of a suprapubic catheter by open surgery is recommended when a percutaneous cystostomy is not possible, a large caliber tube is required for the evacuation of blood, or prolonged or indefinite drainage is anticipated. The procedure can be performed with local anesthesia, but a general or regional anesthetic is preferable. The techniques described for placement of a catheter within the bladder lumen are also applicable to cystostomy drainage used in conjunction with other bladder operations.

OPERATIVE TECHNIQUE   The anterior rectus sheath is exposed with a vertical or transverse suprapubic incision (Figure 9.4). The fascia is divided in the midline, the rectus muscles are separated, and the transversalis fascia is opened to permit entry into the retropubic space. The bladder is distended with saline infused through a urethral catheter, and the peritoneum is swept superiorly from the dome.

A small cystotomy is made between traction sutures or Allis clamps at the most anterosuperior aspect of the bladder. A Malecot catheter or an equivalent is introduced, and the defect is closed around the tube with a heavy absorbable pursestring suture. The ends of the suture are tied around the catheter for added stability. The catheter is brought through the incision or a separate stab wound and fixed to the skin with a nonabsorbable suture.

It should be emphasized that the site of the cystostomy is in the dome rather than the lower anterior wall of the bladder. This eliminates postoperative bladder spasm caused by contact between the catheter and the trigone.

CUTANEOUS VESICOSTOMY

The cutaneous vesicostomy is a means of tubeless bladder drainage. It is well suited for infants or small children in diapers who have dilated bladders due to chronic outlet obstruction or neurogenic dysfunction. The procedure is not appropriate when there is coexisting ureteral obstruction that does not resolve with vesical decompression and is technically difficult if the bladder is thick-walled or small. A vesicostomy is generally closed when the child matures. Intermittent catheterization or alternative forms of urinary diversion may be required, depending on the status of the renal function and on the nature of the underlying vesical disorder.

OPERATIVE TECHNIQUE   The bladder is approached through a small transverse incision midway between the symphysis and the umbilicus (Figure 9.5). The anterior rectus sheath and rectus muscles are incised in the direction of the incision, and a wedge of rectus fascia is removed. The peritoneum is swept from the dome of the bladder, which is then pulled into the wound and opened transversely. The detrusor muscle is attached to the margins of the anterior rectus sheath using interrupted absorbable sutures, and the edge of the cystotomy is fixed to the skin with interrupted absorbable sutures.

To close a vesicostomy, the exteriorized bladder segment is excised and the defect is closed in two or three layers. The opening in the abdominal wall is debrided and the rectus fascia is reapproximated with interrupted heavy absorbable sutures.

POSTOPERATIVE CARE AND COMPLICATIONS   A vesicostomy does not require intubation or the application of a urinary collection appliance. Peristomal dermatitis may develop if the diaper is not changed frequently, and the stoma usually contracts as the child grows. Prolapse of the bladder is seen only when the vesicostomy is made in the anterior aspect of the bladder rather than in the dome.

PARTIAL CYSTECTOMY

Partial, or segmental, cystectomy is an attractive surgical treatment for solitary invasive bladder tumors situated in the fundus of the bladder. Patients who are elderly or in a poor general medical condition are ideal candidates. Coexisting carcinoma-in-situ and a small bladder capacity are relative contraindications. A short course of preoperative pelvic radiation therapy (2000 rad in 5 days) may decrease the risks of seeding the wound with viable tumor cells when the bladder is opened. When radical cystectomy remains a therapeutic option if the tumor is more extensive than anticipated and not amenable to segmental resection, the patient is prepared as described in the section about this procedure.

OPERATIVE TECHNIQUE   Cystoscopy is performed immediately before surgery, and the tumor is outlined with electrocautery 2 cm beyond the visible margin. Otherwise, precise delineation of the tumor margin after opening the bladder may be difficult. A Foley cath-

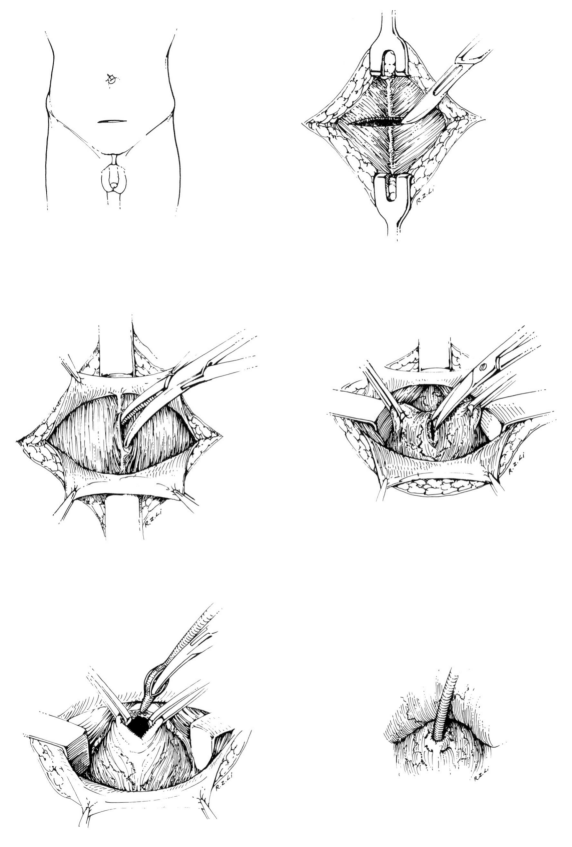

FIGURE 9.4
Open cystostomy

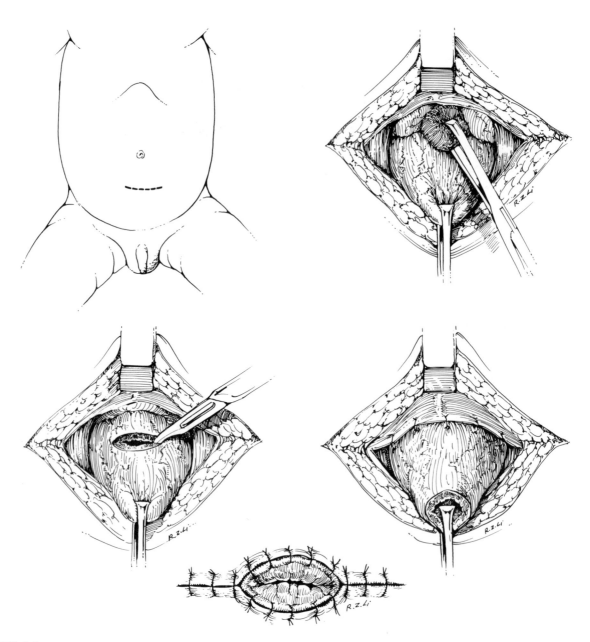

FIGURE 9.5
Cutaneous vesicostomy

eter is inserted transurethrally and remains accessible during the operation.

A lower midline incision is recommended. The abdominal cavity is entered lateral to the urachus, and the peritoneum is incised into the deep pelvis on each side of the umbilical ligaments. The urachus is divided, and the bladder is then freed from the posterior symphysis as described for radical cystectomy. Transection of the ipsilateral anterolateral vascular pedicle is usually required to remove the lateral bladder wall.

Moist sponges are packed next to the bladder to limit contamination by tumor cells. A cystotomy is made between Allis clamps at a point well away from the tumor and extended toward the lesion (Figure 9.6). Narrow blade retractors are introduced to facilitate exposure. The entire bladder wall with adjacent fat and peritoneum is incised with scissors along the identifying line made previously with electrocautery. The surgical specimen, which includes the distal urachus and adjacent peritoneum, is then removed.

Frozen section examination of the bladder margin is always indicated if the tumor appears more extensive than suspected during preoperative bimanual examination and cystoscopy. Bleeding from the transected de-

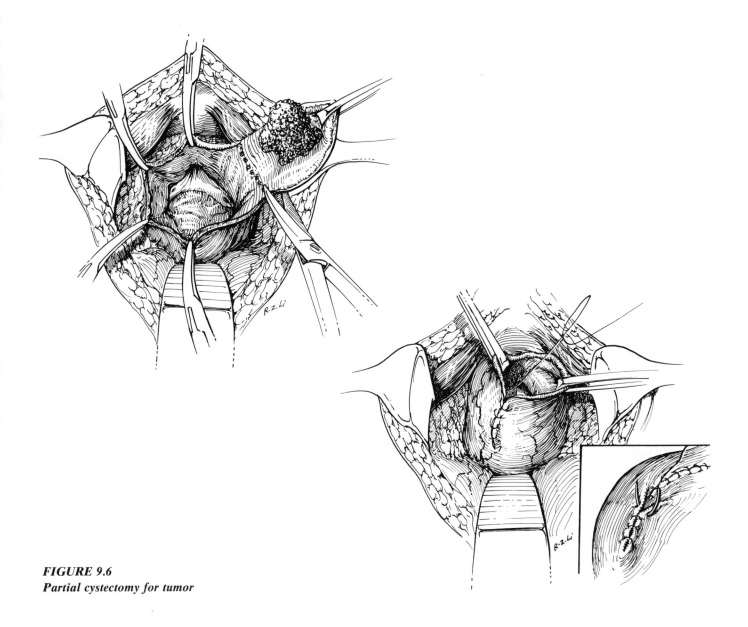

FIGURE 9.6
Partial cystectomy for tumor

trusor muscle is controlled with suture ligatures or electrocautery, and the bladder is closed in two or three layers. Cystostomy drainage is avoided because tumor cells may implant along the drainage tract.

POSTOPERATIVE CARE AND COMPLICATIONS The urethral catheter is removed on the fourth or fifth postoperative day after the integrity of the bladder closure is documented with a cystogram. The Penrose drains are removed on the following day.

Urinary leakage from the cystotomy is the primary postoperative complication and can be managed usually by prolonged catheter drainage. Voiding disturbances are inevitable if a large portion of the bladder has been removed or the bladder capacity before surgery was small. This complication may respond to pharmacologic treatment but is best avoided by proper patient selection. Recurrent urothelial tumors and ex-

travesical recurrences are additional sources of late morbidity. The former are a manifestation of the underlying disease. The latter result from tumor spillage at the time of surgery and are associated with an ominous prognosis.

RADICAL CYSTECTOMY

Radical cystectomy in the male involves removal of the bladder, prostate, and seminal vesicles. In the female the bladder and urethra and usually the anterior vaginal wall, uterus, fallopian tubes, and ovaries are excised. Radical cystectomy is the recommended operative treatment for most invasive transitional cell carcinomas of the bladder, extensive carcinoma-in-situ that is refractory to conservative management, and some urethral carcinomas. Simple cystectomy, or removal of the bladder only, is occasionally performed for benign vesical disorders.

Cystectomy is a major surgical undertaking that necessarily involves urinary diversion or bladder substitution. Potential candidates must be carefully selected. Preoperative radiation therapy (2000 rad over 5 days or 4000 rad over 4 weeks) has been advocated as a component of treatment for transitional cell carcinomas. It is thought that radiation therapy reduces the incidence of local tumor recurrence.

Before surgery the bowel is decompressed and cleansed with a mechanical and antibiotic bowel preparation, and the proper site for an abdominal stoma is chosen with the assistance of an enterostomal therapist.

OPERATIVE TECHNIQUE General anesthesia is required because of the obligate intestinal surgery for the urinary diversion. The patient is placed in a low lithotomy position to permit access to the perineum and rectum. This position also creates an excellent space between the patient's legs for the second assistant. A urethral catheter is introduced and placed in the sterile field.

A midline incision extending from the symphysis pubis to a point several centimeters above the umbilicus is most satisfactory. After dividing the transversalis fascia but before entry of the peritoneal cavity, the bladder is freed from the posterior symphysis to the level of the puboprostatic or pubocervical ligaments. The pelvic peritoneum and bladder are then reflected medially to expose the external iliac vessels and obturator fossa, as described for an extraperitoneal pelvic lymphadenectomy (Chapter 17). In men an 8- to 10-cm segment of vas deferens is excised on each side, and the gonadal vessels are mobilized superiorly. In women the round ligament is divided at the internal inguinal ring.

The abdominal cavity is entered lateral to the urachus just below the umbilicus, and the intraperitoneal contents are palpated. If there are no contraindications to cystectomy, such as unsuspected hepatic or extensive retroperitoneal metastases, the urachus is cross-clamped and transected. The proximal end is secured with a nonabsorbable ligature. A large clamp is applied to the distal end for retraction of the bladder throughout the operation. The peritoneum is then incised into the deep pelvis on each side of the umbilical ligaments (Figure 9.7). The net result of these preliminary maneuvers is complete mobilization of the superior and anterolateral aspects of the bladder.

A self-retaining retractor is positioned and, if desired, a pelvic lymphadenectomy is performed as described in Chapter 17. Exposure of the pelvic sidewalls is enhanced by retraction of the clamped urachus to the contralateral side.

The right paracolic gutter and the posterior peritoneum are incised, and the cecum, ascending colon, and small intestine are reflected superiorly and packed in the upper abdomen. The peritoneum lateral to the sigmoid colon is also opened to expose the left ureter. In women the peritoneum covering the anterior and posterior surfaces of the broad ligament is incised, and the avascular plane below the fallopian tube and ovarian vessels is developed. The ovarian vessels and infundibulopelvic ligament are isolated, doubly clamped, transected, and ligated. Retraction of the ovary and tube medially facilitates ureteral mobilization.

The ureters are isolated at the bifurcation of the common iliac arteries and mobilized with blunt dissection to a point midway between the renal pelvis and the common iliac artery on the left and to a point somewhat lower on the right. Care should be taken to preserve the surrounding fat and areolar tissues. Each ureter is divided several centimeters proximal to the ureterovesical junction. A segment of the proximal ureter is sent for frozen section examination to rule out carcinoma. The ureters are then packed superiorly in the retroperitoneal space.

The bladder is retracted to the contralateral side, and the endopelvic fascia is opened in its deepest recess along the direction of its fibers. The anterolateral vascular pedicle of the bladder, which emanates from the hypogastric vessels, is then developed. Isolation of individual vessels within the vascular pedicle is time-consuming and unnecessary. Rather, a defect is made with blunt dissection in the areolar tissue medial to the bifurcation of the common iliac vessels. The index finger is inserted, and a plane is established behind the pedicle to the level of the endopelvic fascia. The fingertip can be brought through the defect in the endopelvic fascia when the pedicle has been isolated in its entirety.

The integrity of the vascular pedicle is dependent on the superior vesical artery, and transection of this vessel before establishing the posterior plane is not recommended. The lateral aspect of the pedicle is substantially less thick and more easily divided than that adjacent to the bladder. Therefore, it is advisable to develop the pedicle laterally by working tissue between the thumb and index finger. The contralateral anterolateral pedicle is then isolated in an identical manner.

The bladder is retracted to the contralateral side, and the pedicle is perforated with a right-angle clamp several centimeters below the superior margin and as laterally as possible. The intervening tissue is doubly

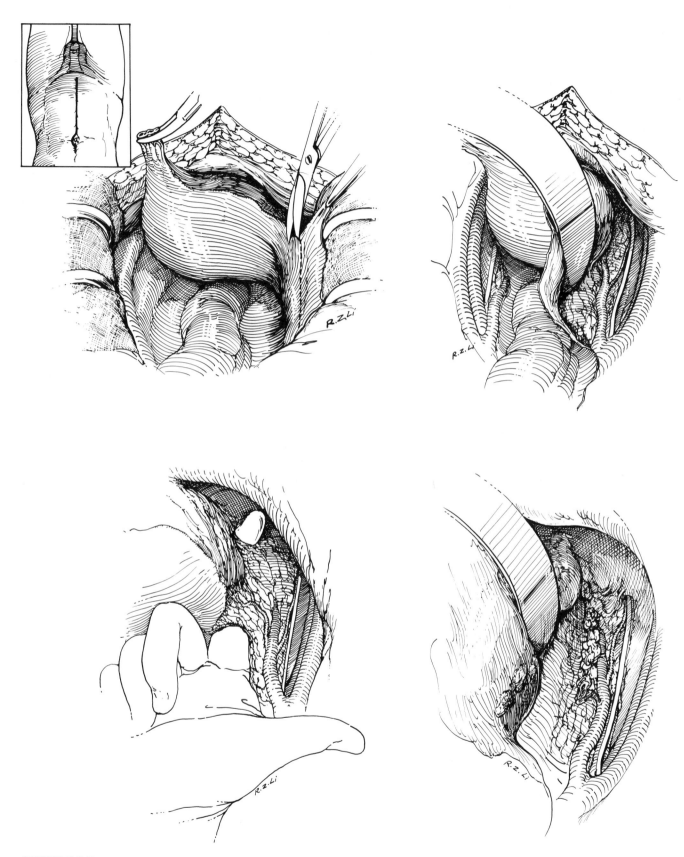

FIGURE 9.7
Mobilization of bladder and transection of anterolateral vascular pedicle in radical cystectomy

clamped, transected, and ligated with nonabsorbable sutures. This process is repeated until the pedicle is divided to the level of the endopelvic fascia. The contralateral pedicle is then transected in the same manner.

At this point the methods of dissection in men and women diverge. In men the peritoneum is incised in the deepest recess of the cul-de-sac. The incision is extended superolaterally on each side to join the lateral peritoneal incision (Figure 9.8). The rectosigmoid is then retracted superiorly with the hand, the bladder is pulled anteriorly with a large blade retractor, and the rectum is swept off Denonvilliers' fascia and the underlying seminal vesicles and prostate gland by extension of the fingers. At times this plane cannot be established without undue force. In these circumstances the dissection is deferred until the membranous urethra has been transected. The prostate can then be separated from the rectum in a retrograde manner under direct vision.

The posterolateral vascular pedicles arising from the hemorrhoidal arteries and coursing immediately laterally to the rectum are developed during the preceding maneuvers. Although these pedicles are less prominent than their anterolateral counterparts, serial clamping, transection, and ligation are required.

The remainder of the operation involves mobilization of the prostate and transection of the membranous urethra. If the preservation of erectile function is of concern, the puboprostatic ligaments, dorsal venous complex, urethra, and posterolateral vascular pedicle of the prostate are managed as described in Chapter 11 for the nerve-sparing radical prostatectomy. When potency is not an issue, the incorporation of some components of the nerve-sparing procedure is still desirable.

The index finger is inserted through the endopelvic fascia to free the anterolateral prostate from the levator ani muscles. The plane between Denonvilliers' fascia and the rectum is then extended to the membranous urethra, and tissue situated lateral to the urethra is perforated with the tips of the index and middle fingers. A urethrectomy, if indicated, is performed as detailed in Chapter 14 before further dissection. Otherwise, with scissors the puboprostatic ligaments are divided adjacent to the periosteum of the symphysis pubis, the apex of the prostate is exposed, and a large right-angle clamp is passed under the dorsal venous complex. The complex is secured with a heavy nonabsorbable suture and transected proximal to the tie. The membranous urethra is then retracted from the urogenital diaphragm and transected under direct vision. It is advisable to apply a large clamp to the urethra just proximal to the point of transection to prevent tumor spillage. In addition, to reduce the viability of poten-

tially contaminating tumor cells, the bladder can be filled with a 10% formalin solution. After 10 minutes the fluid is drained and the urethra is transected. The posterolateral vascular pedicles of the prostate are then transected and secured with nonabsorbable sutures, and the specimen is removed.

The pelvis is liberally irrigated with sterile water to help identify bleeding sites. Water lyses red blood cells, and the pulsatile flow of arterial bleeding and the cloudy appearance of venous bleeding are easily recognized. Bleeding from the urogenital diaphragm is usually controllable with heavy absorbable suture ligatures. If hemorrhage from this site is excessive, a 24 F Foley catheter with a 30-ml balloon is introduced transurethrally and placed on traction. The pelvis is packed with multiple, opened small sponges to encourage hemostasis, and attention is turned to the urinary diversion.

In women a combined pelvic and perineal approach is advantageous during the remaining portions of the operation. The posterolateral vascular pedicle, which includes the uterine vessels and cardinal ligament, is developed beyond the cervix and transected as described for men. The urethra is then freed from the posterior symphysis to the level of the meatus. From a perineal approach the vaginal introitus above the meatus is incised sharply to expose the lower edge of the symphysis pubis, and the plane between the urethra and the symphysis is entered. The uterus is retracted anteriorly with a tenaculum and the rectosigmoid is pulled superiorly with the hand. A sponge-on-ring forceps is inserted into the posterior fornix of the vagina, and the vagina wall is incised with a scalpel from the pelvic approach (Figure 9.9). This incision is then extended down the anterolateral aspects of the vagina to meet the introital incision, and the specimen is removed. If the anterior wall of the vagina is to be preserved, the urethra may be dissected from the vaginal wall with a combined pelvic and perineal approach.

Reconstruction of the vagina is initiated by separating the posterior vaginal wall from the rectum. The superior margin of the vagina is folded anteriorly, and the free edge is fixed to the anterior introitus with interrupted absorbable sutures. The opposing lateral margins of the folded vagina are approximated with interrupted heavy absorbable sutures. A small defect may be retained for placement of large Penrose drains. The pelvis is then liberally irrigated, residual bleeding vessels are secured, and the pelvis is packed with sponges.

POSTOPERATIVE CARE AND COMPLICATIONS   If used, the pelvic Foley catheter drain in men or the Penrose drain in women is removed on the first postoperative day. Postoperative complications resulting from the cystectomy rather than the obligatory urinary diversion par-

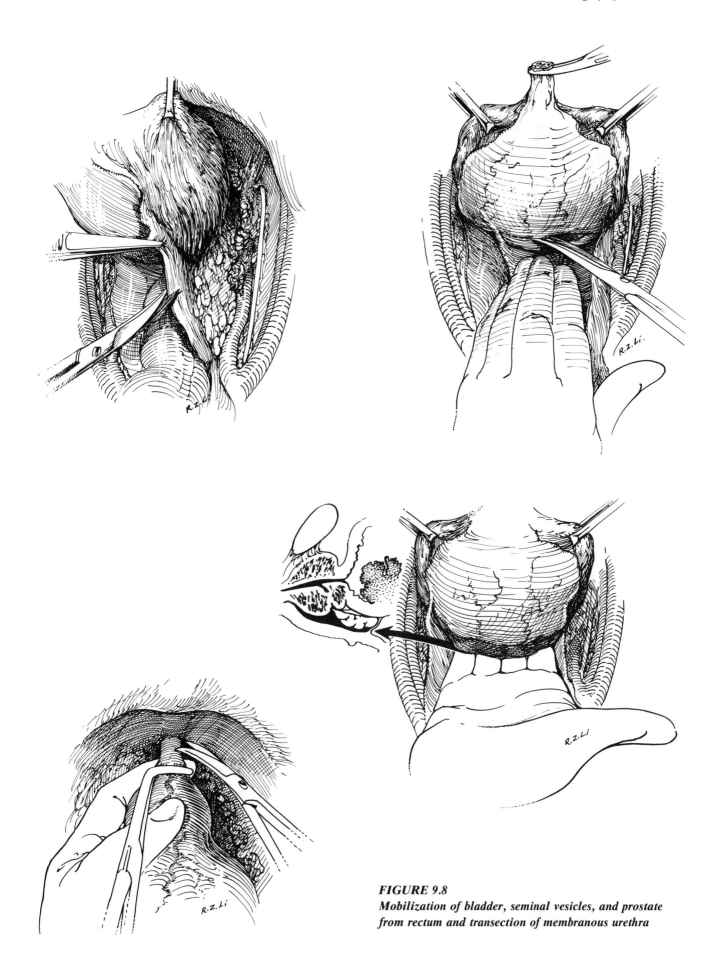

FIGURE 9.8
Mobilization of bladder, seminal vesicles, and prostate from rectum and transection of membranous urethra

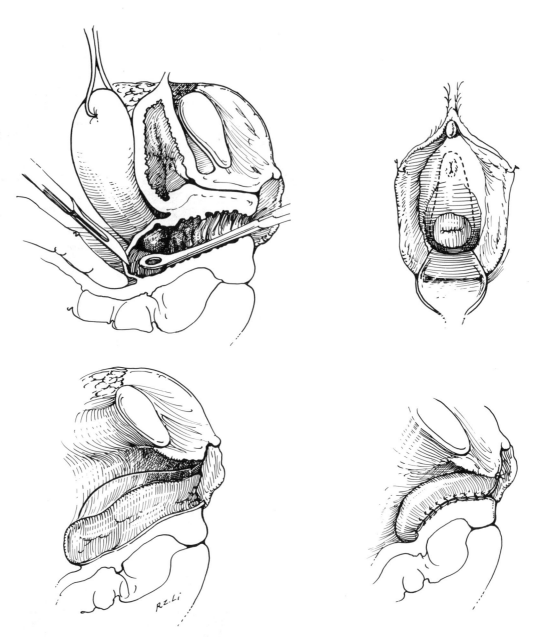

FIGURE 9.9
Excision of anterior vagina and vaginal reconstruction

allel those of all major pelvic operations and include hematoma, abscess, and venous thrombosis with pulmonary embolism.

AUGMENTATION CYSTOPLASTY

Augmentation cystoplasty is performed by incorporating an isolated segment of small or large intestine into the bladder wall. Severe interstitial cystitis, tuberculous cystitis, and neurogenic bladder dysfunction are the primary conditions that produce bladder contrac-

ture of a magnitude that necessitates operative intervention. Augmentation cystoplasty does not generally involve segmental resection of the bladder. However, the anastomosis must be capacious to facilitate complete emptying of the intestinal segment. In addition, when pain is a major manifestation of the vesical disorder, it is advisable to remove the entire supratrigonal bladder. This more extensive procedure, however, should not be confused with bladder substitution, where the trigone as well as the fundus of the bladder are replaced with intestine.

The functional results of bladder augmentation using

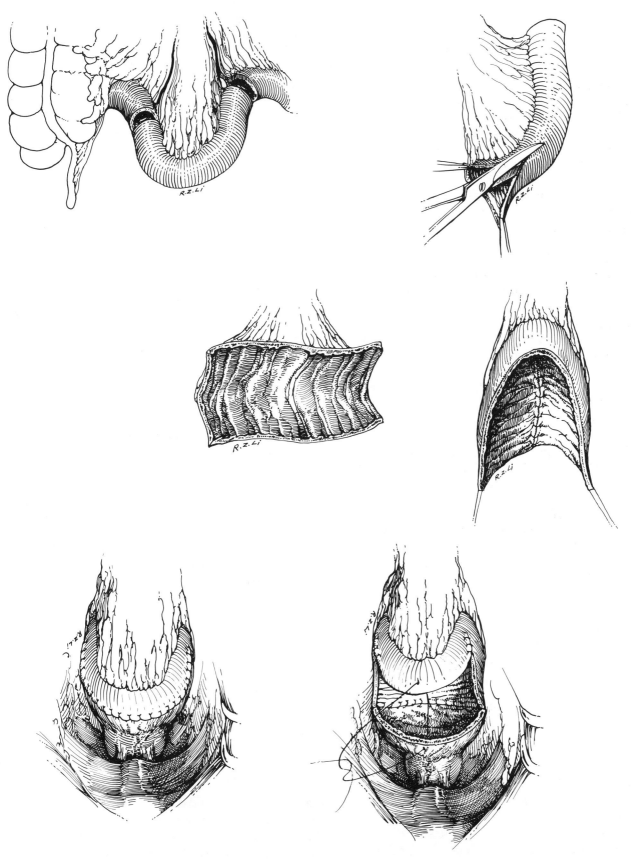

FIGURE 9.10
Augmentation cystoplasty using reconfigured ileum

different bowel segments are similar. Disorders that may result from the transposition of bowel to the urinary tract are discussed in Chapter 10.

Ileal Cystoplasty

Augmentation of the bladder with ileum has been performed by end-to-side anastomosis of an intact tubular segment. However, it is desirable to reconfigure the ileal segment to recreate the normal bladder contour.

OPERATIVE TECHNIQUE   A 20-cm segment of distal ileum is isolated, and intestinal continuity is restored anterior to the segment. The proximal and distal mesenteric incisions must be sufficiently long to permit displacement of the segment into the pelvis without tension. The entire segment is then opened along the antimesenteric border, the luminal margins are folded downward, and the opposed posterior edges of the ileal sheet are approximated with a continuous absorbable suture (Figure 9.10). The base of the partially constructed "cup" is anastomosed with the adjacent posterior bladder margin, and the apex of the anterior edge is reflected to the anterior bladder margin. This brings the free superolateral edges of the ileal sheet together on each side. These edges are joined with a continuous absorbable suture, and the remaining free anterior margin of the ileum is approximated with the anterior bladder wall.

The bladder is drained with a urethral catheter and a suprapubic cystostomy brought through the detrusor muscle.

Sigmoid Cystoplasty

By virtue of the proximity of the sigmoid colon to the bladder, extensive mobilization and long mesenteric incisions are not required when this segment is used for cystoplasty.

OPERATIVE TECHNIQUE   A 15-cm segment of sigmoid colon lying adjacent to the dome of the bladder is isolated and intestinal continuity restored behind the segment. The entire segment is incised longitudinally along a tinea on the antimesenteric border. Because of the larger lumen of the colon (as compared with the ileum), reconfiguration as described for an ileal cystoplasty is not necessary. The sheet of colon is rotated 90°, and the posterior margins of the intestinal sheet and the bladder are approximated with a continuous absorbable suture (Figure 9.11). The sheet is then folded anteriorly and anastomosed with the anterior edge of the bladder. The reconstruction is completed by approximating the lateral opposing edges of the bowel on each side.

Alternatively, the ends of the colonic segment may be closed after longitudinal incision of the tinea (Figure 9.12). The segment is then rotated 90°, and the

preformed "cup" is anastomosed with the bladder in a circumferential manner.

Cecal Cystoplasty

The technique of bladder substitution using the ileocolonic segment is described in Chapter 10. With augmentation cystoplasty the procedure is modified by excision of the distal ileum and closure of the ileocecal valve. The segment is then rotated 180°, the lumen is enlarged as needed with a spatulation, and the intestinal margins are anastomosed with the edges of the bladder.

POSTOPERATIVE CARE AND COMPLICATIONS

The suprapubic tube is removed after 7 to 10 days if extravasation is not seen on cystography. The Penrose drains are removed the following day.

Persistent urinary leakage at the suture lines is the most common postoperative complication. Incomplete bladder emptying and difficulties with evacuation of mucus are notable late complications. The latter are more common in men than in women and can usually be managed by transurethral incision of the bladder outlet.

OPERATIONS FOR STRESS INCONTINENCE IN WOMEN

Stress urinary incontinence is the most common cause of involuntary loss of urine in adult women. It results from the transmission of increased intra-abdominal pressure to the bladder and a rise in the intravesical pressure sufficient to overcome urethral continence mechanisms. Most patients lose varying amounts of urine during coughing and sneezing, but the condition may progress to incontinence during walking or abrupt standing and, in some cases, to total incontinence. It is critical to differentiate stress incontinence from urgency incontinence. Urgency incontinence is the involuntary loss of urine after the patient experiences the desire to urinate; it is not correctable with surgery. Some degree of urgency incontinence, however, often coexists with stress incontinence.

Elevation of the bladder base and restoration of the posterior urethrovesical angle almost always corrects stress incontinence. The suprapubic vesicourethral suspension (the Marshall-Marchetti-Krantz procedure), endoscopic suspension of the vesical neck (the Stamey procedure), or variations of the two will predictably achieve this objective. Mild urinary stress incontinence may resolve also after anterior colporrhaphy. However, this operation does not restore the posterior urethrovesical angle, and elevation

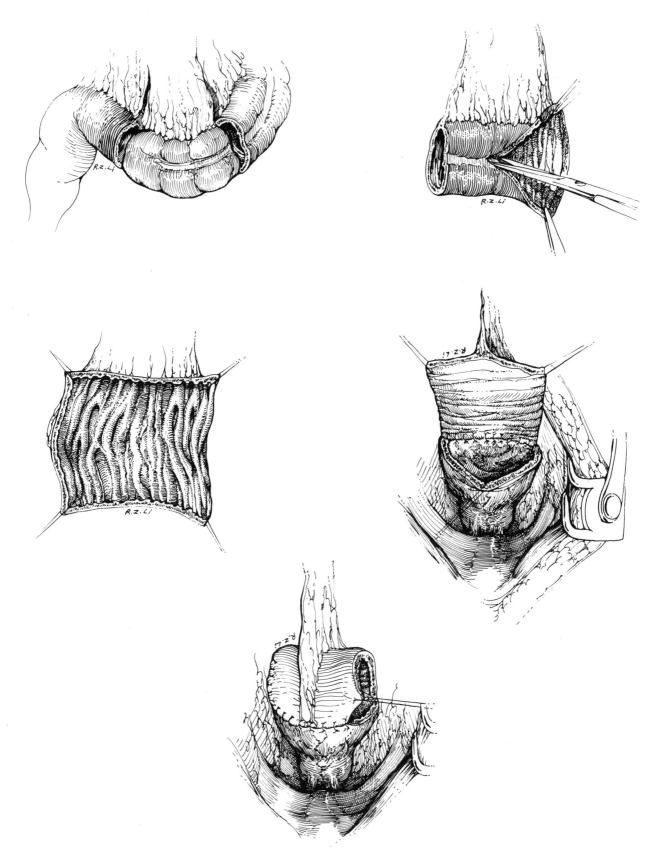

FIGURE 9.11
Augmentation cystoplasty using reconfigured sigmoid colon

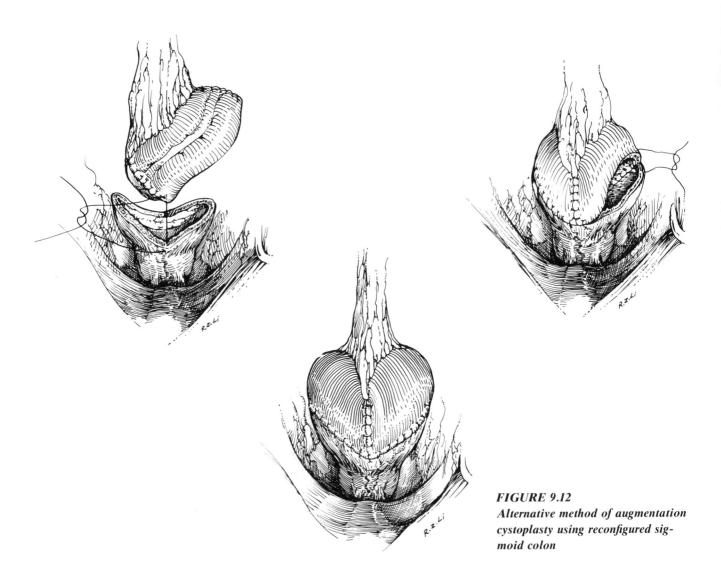

FIGURE 9.12
Alternative method of augmentation cystoplasty using reconfigured sigmoid colon

of the bladder base results solely from the excision of redundant and attenuated vaginal tissues.

Suprapubic Vesicourethral Suspension

The suprapubic vesicourethral suspension is an open pelvic operation involving suture fixation of the periurethral tissues and bladder outlet to the symphysis pubis. It is the standard of comparison for all other treatments of stress urinary incontinence.

OPERATIVE TECHNIQUE The patient is placed in the supine or low lithotomy position and draped to allow access to the vagina. The bladder is catheterized, and the retropubic space is approached through a midline or transverse lower abdominal incision. The bladder and urethra are separated from the posterior symphysis pubis to a point approximately 1 cm from the meatus. Sharp dissection is usually necessary if there have been previous operations for stress incontinence. The endopelvic fascia is incised to permit superior displacement of the bladder without tension, and fat is cleared from the anterior urethra and bladder base.

Three or four heavy absorbable sutures are placed in the anterior vaginal wall on each side of the urethra (Figure 9.13). An additional suture may be applied to each side of the bladder outlet, which is identified by palpation of the Foley catheter balloon. To determine the appropriate site for suture placement in the posterior symphysis, the bladder base is elevated by insertion of two fingers in the vagina. After all the sutures are properly positioned, they are sequentially tied in a distal to proximal manner. Upward displacement of the anterior vagina reduces tension while tying the sutures. A Penrose drain is positioned in the retropubic space before wound closure. It is advantageous to drain the bladder with a percutaneous or open cystostomy rather than a urethral catheter.

Suture fixation of the periurethral vagina and bladder outlet to Cooper's ligament is an alternative

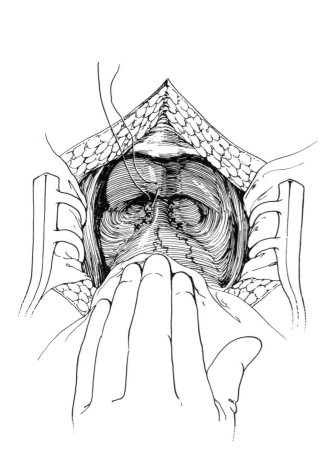

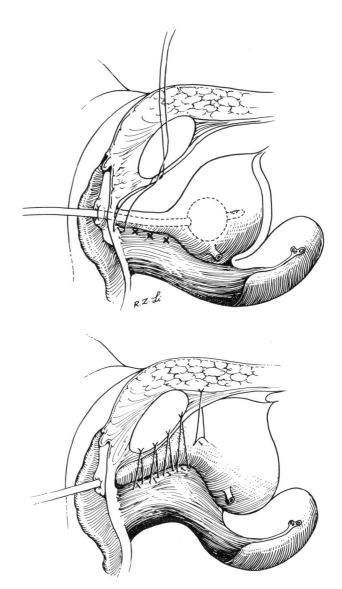

R.Z.Li

FIGURE 9.13
Suprapubic vesicourethral suspension

method of suprapubic suspension that is favored by some surgeons (Figure 9.14). However, substantial mobility of the anterior vaginal wall and urethra is required for satisfactory approximation with the ligament.

Postoperative care parallels that detailed in the next section about endoscopic suspension of the vesical neck. With the exception of the general complications inherent to open pelvic surgery, early and late complications are also similar to those of endoscopic suspension.

Endoscopic Suspension of the Vesical Neck

With the endoscopic suspension of the vesical neck and variations thereof, elevation of the bladder outlet is accomplished with suspending sutures between the rectus fascia and fascial tissues adjacent to the bladder outlet. Documented sterility of the bladder urine before surgery is mandatory, and prophylactic parenteral antibiotics are administered in the perioperative period.

OPERATIVE TECHNIQUE   The patient is placed in a low lithotomy position and the lower abdomen, perineum, vagina, and upper thighs are thoroughly prepped. Drapes are applied to permit access to the lower abdomen and vagina. The anus is covered with an adherent plastic drape or towel.

Two transverse suprapubic incisions about 3 cm in length are made two fingerbreadths above the symphysis and two fingerbreadths lateral to the midline. They are carried to the anterior rectus fascia and packed with moist gauze. A curvilinear vaginal incision is then made below the meatus, and the anterior vaginal wall is dissected from the urethra and bladder base (Figure 9.15). The tubing and balloon of an indwelling Foley catheter are used as landmarks during this and subsequent maneuvers.

A commercially available Stamey needle is thrust

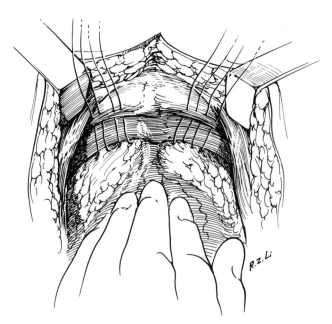

FIGURE 9.14
Suprapubic vesicourethral suspension with suture fixation to Cooper's ligament

through the rectus fascia at the medial aspect of one of the suprapubic incisions and worked immediately behind the symphysis pubis. The tip of the needle is palpated with an index finger in the vaginal wound, guided to a position just lateral to the urethrovesical junction, and pushed into the vaginal wound (Figure 9.16). The Foley catheter is removed, and the urethra and bladder are examined with a cystoscope. Indentation of the bladder outlet during back-and-forth movement of the correctly placed needle is easily observed. Similarly, penetration of the urethra or bladder or po-

sitioning of the needle at the midurethra rather than the bladder outlet is readily apparent.

The Foley catheter is reinserted and a No. 2 monofilament nylon suture is threaded through the eye of the needle. The needle and suture are then pulled into the suprapubic incision. The needle is passed again 2 cm lateral to the initial tract, and proper placement is documented by cystoscopy. The free end of the suspending suture in the vaginal incision is threaded through a 1-cm length of 5-mm Dacron vascular graft, threaded through the eye of the needle, and pulled into the suprapubic incision. The Dacron bolster is grasped with an Allis clamp during the latter maneuver. This helps to situate the bolster in the appropriate position lateral to the bladder neck and prevents twisting of the suspending suture.

After an identical procedure is performed on the contralateral side, the vaginal wound is vigorously irrigated with an antibiotic solution and closed with a continuous absorbable suture. This closure is always done before the suspending sutures are tied because elevation of the anterior vaginal wall makes exposure problematic. The two ends of each suspending suture are tied together without undue tension, and the suprapubic incisions are closed in a routine manner. The end result of the endoscopic suspension is shown in Figure 9.17.

The bladder is filled with irrigant, and a percutaneous cystostomy tube is introduced for postoperative drainage. The vagina is packed with gauze covered with an antibiotic ointment.

POSTOPERATIVE CARE AND COMPLICATIONS   On the first postoperative day the vaginal packing is removed. Pelvic discomfort is relatively minor, although a pulling sensation in the lower abdomen is not unusual when the patient is standing.

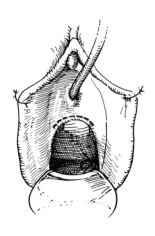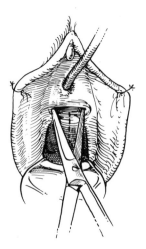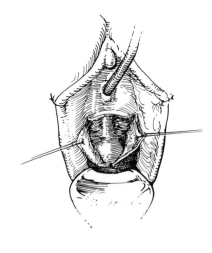

FIGURE 9.15
Vaginal incision for endoscopic suspension of the vesical neck

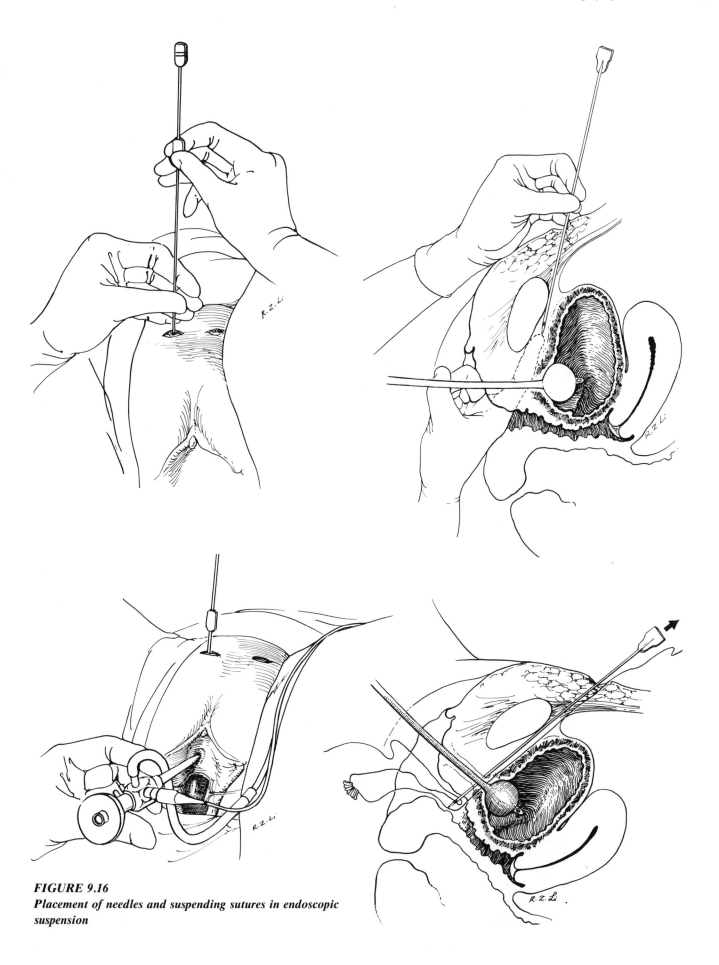

FIGURE 9.16
Placement of needles and suspending sutures in endoscopic suspension

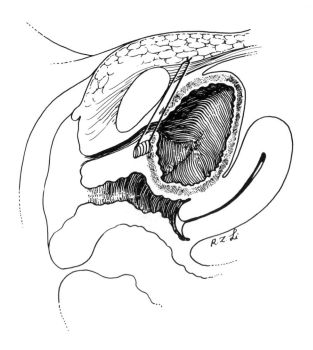

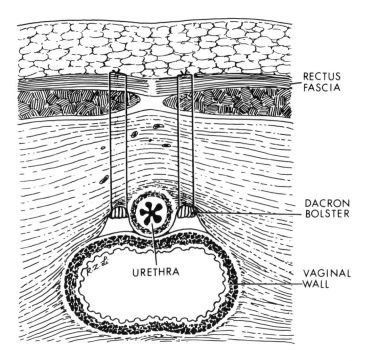

FIGURE 9.17
End result of endoscopic suspension

Voiding trials are initiated on the first or second day after surgery. The patient is taught how to clamp and unclamp the suprapubic tube and is forewarned that urinary retention is common. She should be reassured that the problem is not associated with an adverse functional outcome. The tube is occluded, and spontaneous micturition is attempted when a sensation of bladder fullness is appreciated. A calibrated plastic container is placed in the commode to collect voided urine.

After a successful or unsuccessful attempt at micturition, the suprapubic tube is unclamped and the residual volume is measured. It is important for the patient to understand and participate actively in this process. Hospital discharge on the fourth or fifth postoperative day is the rule, and the procedure must be continued at home if bladder emptying is not satisfactory.

Regardless of voiding status, oral antibiotics are administered for the first 2 weeks after hospital discharge. Sitz baths are instituted 1 week after surgery to encourage healing of the vaginal incision. The suprapubic tube is removed when the residual urine volume is less than one-half the voided urine volume.

Early treatment failures are uncommon and result usually from either improper patient selection or improper surgical technique. Urinary retention for 2 to 3 months after surgery occurs infrequently but is particularly distressing to the patient who is treated for less than severe incontinence. Transection of one suspend-

ing suture by opening a suprapubic wound under local anesthesia often leads to prompt restoration of bladder emptying and rarely impacts on the ultimate success of the operation. However, if transection of the remaining suture is necessitated by continued urinary retention, recurrent stress incontinence is inevitable.

Wound infection or infection and erosion of the Dacron grafts are surprisingly infrequent. Recurrence of stress urinary incontinence after an initially favorable result is reported to occur in approximately 10% of patients.

ARTIFICIAL URINARY SPHINCTERS

Artificial urinary sphincters are used primarily to correct severe stress incontinence in men. Injury to the membranous urethra during prostatic surgery is the usual cause of the condition. In women artificial sphincters are indicated for the management of severe incontinence due to sphincteric incompetence that is not curable by more conservative surgical interventions. Incontinence associated with neurogenic bladder dysfunction is managed pharmacologically and is not amenable to treatment by sphincter implantation.

Several devices that function in the same general manner are available. A cuff is positioned around the bulbous urethra or bladder outlet and is connected by tubing to a fluid reservoir and pump assembly (Figure

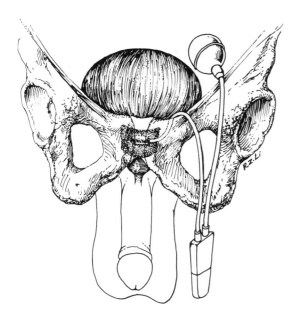

FIGURE 9.18
Artificial urinary sphincter

9.18). The cuff is deflated during micturition and then inflated to compress the urethra and increase outlet resistance. Instructional courses sponsored by the manufacturers of artificial sphincters are available to interested urologists and are highly recommended for the inexperienced.

OPERATIVE TECHNIQUE   Documented sterility of the urine and perioperative parenteral antimicrobial therapy are mandatory. When the cuff is to be positioned around the bladder outlet, a low midline incision is made. The bladder outlet and base of the prostate in men, and the bladder outlet only in women, are mobilized to allow circumferential placement of the cuff. The pump is positioned in the scrotum or in the labium majorum on the side of manual dominance, and the reservoir is inserted into a pocket developed behind the rectus muscle. The cuff, reservoir, and pump are filled with diluted contrast medium and the tubing is connected. The apparatus is tested to be certain that the tubing is not kinked and that there is enough fluid in the system for adequate distention of the cuff.

Placement of the cuff around the bulbous urethra necessitates perineal as well as suprapubic exposure. The urethra is more easily mobilized than the bladder outlet, but the risks of perforation are greater.

POSTOPERATIVE CARE AND COMPLICATIONS   The cuff is not activated for 4 to 6 weeks after surgery to encourage healing. Erosion of the cuff, infection, and device malfunction are the primary complications; each occurring in about 5 to 10 percent of cases. Because of the relative paucity of supporting tissues around the bladder outlet of women, the risks of erosion are greater than that in men. Cuff erosion or infection of any component usually necessitates removal of the entire apparatus. Malfunction of the system requires operative intervention to replace the defective part.

Y-V PLASTY OF THE VESICAL OUTLET

Expansion of the bladder outlet by Y-V plasty is done usually to correct bladder neck contractures in men. The circumferential scarring results almost exclusively from transurethral resection or open enucleation of the prostate. The procedure is not recommended unless conservative management with transurethral incision proves unsuccessful. Historically, Y-V plasties were commonly performed in otherwise healthy girls with frequent urinary tract infections or vesicoureteral reflux. The concept that abnormal bladder outlet resistance contributes to these disorders, however, has now been abandoned.

OPERATIVE TECHNIQUE   The anterior bladder and prostate are exposed through a lower abdominal incision. A Y-shaped incision extending through the fibrotic bladder outlet to a point just proximal to the puboprostatic ligaments is made as shown in Figure 9.19. The apex of the compliant bladder wall is fixed to the end of the prostatic incision with a heavy absorbable suture. The resulting V-shaped defect is then closed in two layers.

A Penrose drain is placed in the retropubic space, and the bladder is drained with a suprapubic or urethral catheter. The catheter is removed after 7 to 10 days when a cystogram demonstrates the absence of extravasation.

OPERATIONS FOR VESICOVAGINAL FISTULAS

Fistulas between the bladder and the vagina result usually from unrecognized injury to the posterior bladder during hysterectomy. Necrosis of locally extensive pelvic malignancies may also lead to fistula formation, but in these cases surgical correction is rarely possible.

Postoperative fistulas are manifested by varying degrees of vaginal discharge beginning immediately or as long as 1 to 2 weeks after surgery. The diagnosis is established by demonstrating extravasation of contrast medium into the vagina with cystography. Small fistulas that escape radiologic detection are identified by the placement of cotton balls or of a tampon into the vagina and the instillation of a methylene blue solution into the bladder. After several hours the vaginal packing is removed, and the material from the apex of the vagina is almost always stained blue. The location and

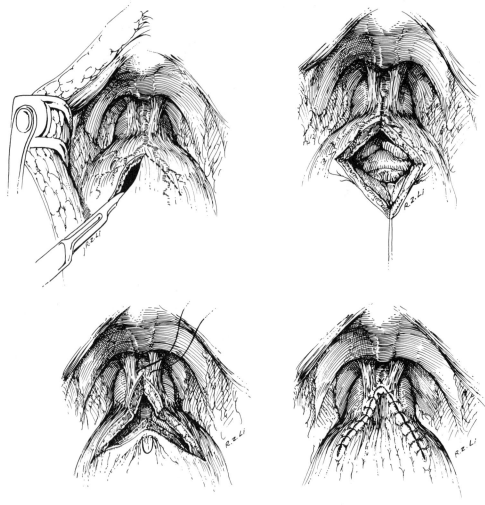

FIGURE 9.19
Y-V plasty of bladder outlet in the male

size of the fistula are assessed with cystoscopy. An intravenous pyelogram is mandatory to eliminate the possibility of coexisting ureteral injury.

The success of a vesicovaginal fistula repair depends largely on the timing of the surgery. Fistulas detected within 1 to 2 days of surgery are generally amenable to immediate intervention. Local inflammation and infection that develop during more prolonged diagnostic delay, however, usually preclude successful closure. Resolution of this process requires 1 to 2 months. Catheterization during the interval may reduce the magnitude of urinary leakage, but most patients require pads or diapers. The urologist must resist the temptation of premature intervention to placate an understandably unhappy patient.

Vaginal Repair

Small fistulas situated away from the ureteral orifices are generally amenable to vaginal repair.

OPERATIVE TECHNIQUE   The patient is placed in the lithotomy position, and the vaginal vault is exposed by suture fixation of the labia minora laterally, retraction of the vaginal side walls with blade retractors, and inferior displacement of the posterior vault with a weighted retractor. Healthy vaginal mucosa adjacent to the fistula is incised circumferentially, and a plane is developed with a scissors between the vaginal wall and the bladder (Figure 9.20). The fistulous tract of the bladder is then circumscribed and the fistula is removed en bloc.

The bladder defect is closed with interrupted absorbable sutures. The vaginal mucosa is approximated with interrupted absorbable sutures so that the suture line is at right angles to the bladder closure. Interposition of labial tissue between the bladder and vagina augments the integrity of the repair. A percutaneous cystostomy is recommended for urinary drainage.

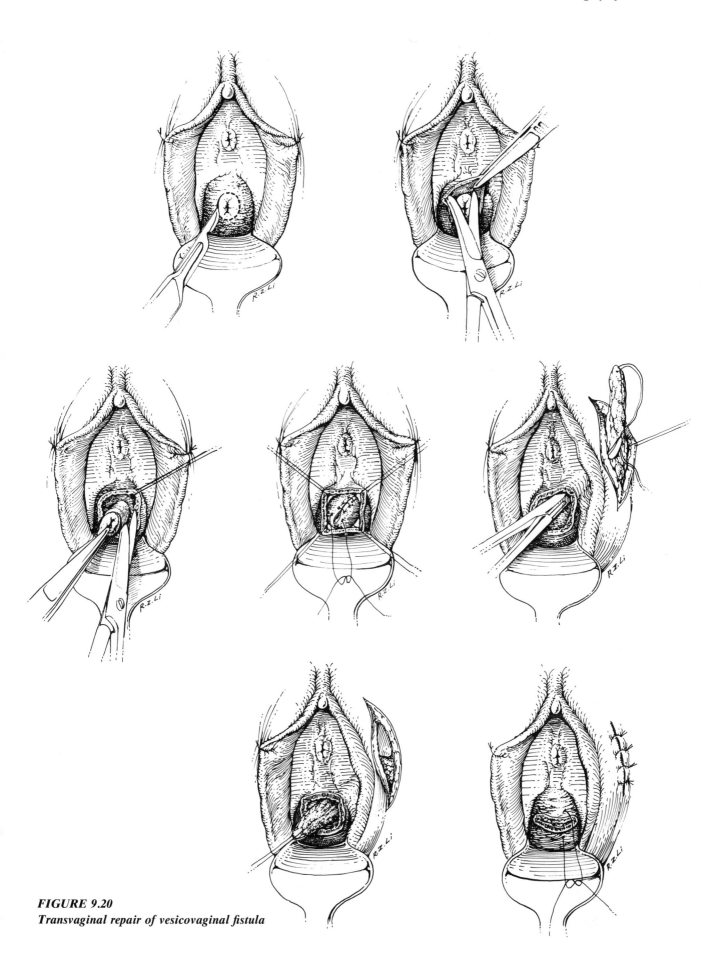

FIGURE 9.20
Transvaginal repair of vesicovaginal fistula

Transvesical Repair

Fistulas that are large, inaccessible by a vaginal approach, or located next to a ureteral orifice are repaired in a transvesical fashion.

OPERATIVE TECHNIQUE   Ureteral catheterization before surgery is recommended if the fistula encroaches on an orifice. The low lithotomy position permits transvaginal manipulation of the anterior vaginal wall, which may help to delineate the plane between the vagina and bladder. A transverse or midline lower ab-

dominal incision provides satisfactory transperitoneal exposure. However, the midline incision is mandatory if omental interposition is contemplated.

A cystotomy is made in the posterior dome of the bladder. The full thickness of bladder and the overlying peritoneum is then incised to a point adjacent to the fistula (Figure 9.21). In some cases the entire fistula can be circumscribed and removed without further dissection. Otherwise, the bladder is mobilized from the vagina, and the fistulous tracts in the bladder

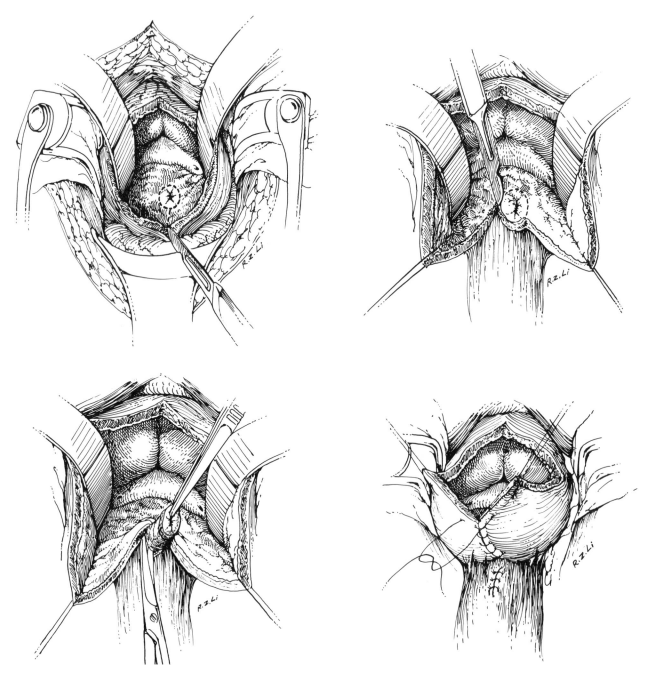

FIGURE 9.21
Transvesical repair of vesicovaginal fistula

and vagina are circumscribed and excised individually. The bladder is closed in two or three layers, and the peritoneum is sealed with a continuous absorbable suture. The vagina is closed in one layer with interrupted absorbable sutures. Urinary drainage with a suprapubic cystostomy is recommended.

Interposition of omentum between the bladder and vagina may be desirable if the repair is compromised by indurated or friable tissues. On occasion the omentum is sufficiently long to reach the deep pelvis without mobilization. Usually, however, the omentum must be separated from the transverse colon and the stomach (Figure 9.22). The gastroepiploic arcade between the stomach and the omentum is preferably divided on the left because the right vascular pedicle is larger and more dependent. The straight gastric

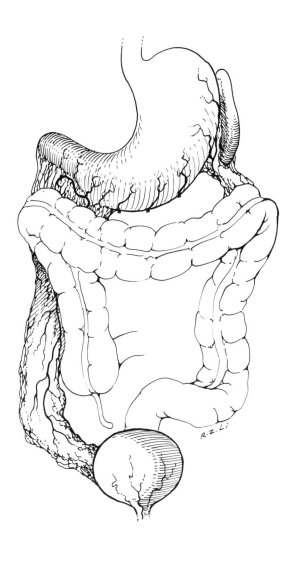

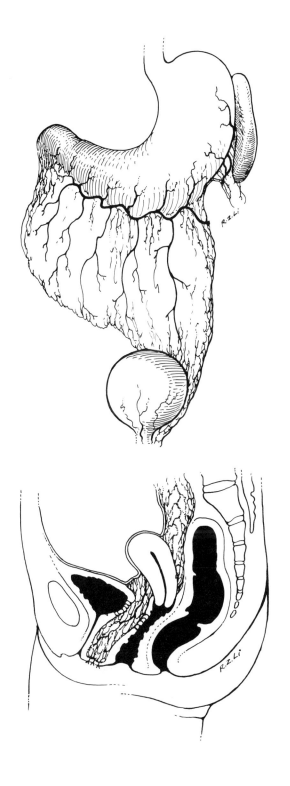

FIGURE 9.22
Interposition of omentum in vesicovaginal fistula repair

vessels between the stomach and the arcade are individually transected and ligated.

The omentum is positioned in the retroperitoneum behind the ascending colon and the cecum; between the bladder and vagina the omentum is sutured into a space sufficiently large to accommodate two or three fingers. Dissection of the anterior vagina from the urethra and bladder outlet using a perineal approach and attachment of the omentum to the vaginal mucosa help to prevent upward migration.

POSTOPERATIVE CARE AND COMPLICATIONS

A cystogram is performed on the seventh to tenth postoperative day, and the suprapubic catheter is removed if extravasation is not observed. Persistent urinary leakage usually resolves after 2 to 4 weeks of catheter drainage. Intercourse should be avoided for 1 to 2 months after surgery.

OPERATIONS FOR VESICOENTERIC FISTULAS

Communication between the bladder and bowel results usually from inflammatory or neoplastic disorders of the intestine. The urine is invariably infected with one or more bacterial types, and irritative voiding symptoms are the most common presenting complaint. Pneumaturia and the finding of bowel contents in the urine are almost pathognomonic. The site of the bladder fistula is determined by cystoscopy and appears usually as a focal area of bullous edema. At times thick material with the consistency of toothpaste can be expressed with suprapubic pressure. A pelvic mass may be palpable on bimanual examination.

Depending on the size of the fistula, contrast material may opacify the bowel during cystography. Contrast studies of the small and large intestine usually demonstrate the fistulous site in the bowel and the nature of the underlying intestinal disease. An intravenous pyelogram is required to rule out ureteral involvement.

Few vesicoenteric fistulas close spontaneously. Operative management focuses on treatment of the intestinal component of the fistula and of the associated intestinal disease. Repair of the vesical component is generally straightforward.

OPERATIVE TECHNIQUE
The bowel is cleansed with a mechanical and antibiotic preparation unless contraindicated by a high-grade obstruction. Parenteral antimicrobial therapy in the perioperative period is mandatory. Preoperative catheterization of the ureter facilitates identification during surgery and is recommended if the fistula or associated inflammation encroaches on the ureter.

A lower midline incision that can be extended superiorly as needed for exposure of the entire large and small intestine is desirable. Induration and inflammation surrounding the fistula are the rule, and abscesses are not infrequent. Adherent bowel is separated from the bladder and the fistulous tract is transected. A cystotomy is made adjacent to the vesical component of the fistula, and the tract is excised with a circumscribing full-thickness incision of the bladder wall. A suprapubic cystostomy is performed and the bladder is closed in two or three layers. The diseased segment of bowel is then removed and intestinal continuity is restored. If the quality of the intestinal anastomosis is questionable, a proximal diverting colostomy is performed.

When there is minimal inflammation and the fistula is easily identified, the vesical and enteric components may be excised en bloc with a segment of adjacent bladder and the segment of involved intestine (Figure 9.23). At the other extreme, primary repair may be hazardous if there are extensive abscesses or if the patient is debilitated or unstable. A staged procedure with initial proximal colostomy and secondary repair of the fistula is advisable in these circumstances.

BLADDER DIVERTICULECTOMY

Bladder diverticula result usually from chronic bladder outlet obstruction. These acquired outpocketings consist of bladder mucosa that has herniated through the detrusor muscle, and they are surrounded by varying degrees of fibrous tissue. Congenital diverticula are not common and consist of detrusor muscle as well as mucosa.

Most diverticula are asymptomatic, and treatment is limited to correction of the bladder outlet obstruction that accompanies the acquired variety. Large diverticula, however, may empty incompletely and require excision because of voiding disturbances or stone formation. In addition, diverticula containing carcinomas that are not amenable to transurethral resection or fulguration and diverticula that cannot be examined completely by cystoscopy in bladders with transitional cell carcinoma should be removed. A diverticulectomy can be performed in a transvesical or extravesical fashion.

OPERATIVE TECHNIQUE
For the transvesical approach the bladder is exposed through an extraperitoneal lower abdominal incision. The peritoneum is swept superiorly from the dome, and a cystotomy is made on the anterior surface. Mucosa surrounding the outlet of the diverticulum is circumscribed and dissected sharply from the detrusor muscle (Figure 9.24). The deepest recess of the diverticulum is then grasped

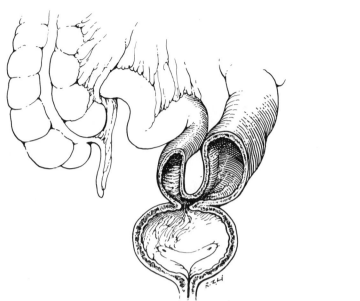
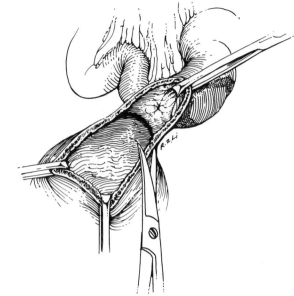

FIGURE 9.23
Repair of vesicoenteric fistula

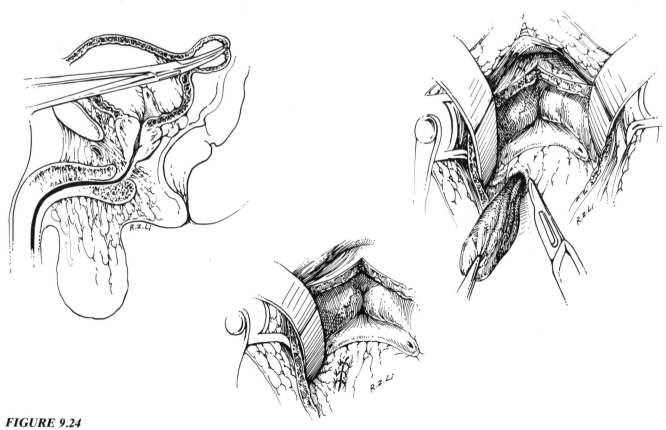

FIGURE 9.24
Transvesical diverticulectomy

with a clamp and the diverticulum is drawn into the bladder. It is amputated flush with the detrusor muscle, and the resultant vesical defect is closed in two or three layers with absorbable sutures.

A transperitoneal approach is usually necessary for the extravesical diverticulectomy. Partial transection of the anterolateral vascular pedicle of the bladder is often required for satisfactory exposure of diverticula emanating from the inferolateral bladder. The outlet of the diverticulum adjacent to the detrusor muscle is isolated and incised to allow introduction of the finger. This facilitates dissection of the diverticulum from surrounding pelvic structures. When completely mobilized, the diverticulum is amputated flush with the detrusor muscle, and the vesical defect is closed in two or three layers (Figure 9.25). A suprapubic cystostomy is used for bladder drainage and is generally removed after 5 to 7 days.

OPERATIONS FOR BLADDER TRAUMA

Rupture or perforation is the only manifestation of bladder trauma that requires surgical intervention. Most iatrogenic injuries occur during endoscopic procedures and result in extraperitoneal extravasation of irrigant. With blunt trauma the extravasation is usually extraperitoneal if there is an associated pelvic fracture and intraperitoneal if there is no bony disruption (Figure 9.26). The nature of bladder perforation with penetrating trauma is variable and is not infrequently accompanied by injury to other pelvic viscera.

Traumatic perforation of the bladder causes suprapubic discomfort and an inability to void. Suspected bladder injuries are investigated initially with a retrograde urethrogram to rule out coexisting urethral damage. The bladder is catheterized if the urethra is intact, and a cystogram is performed in the anteroposterior and lateral projections. An x-ray obtained after drainage is advisable to detect minor degrees of extravasation. An intravenous pyelogram should also be obtained to eliminate the possibility of associated renal or ureteral injury.

Extraperitoneal extravasation results in a diffuse, sunburst pattern confined to the pelvis (Figure 9.27). With intraperitoneal extravasation, contrast medium is seen between loops of bowel within the abdominal cavity.

Intraperitoneal ruptures of any cause, extraperitoneal ruptures following trauma, and perforations from penetrating injuries are best managed by pelvic exploration and open repair. Extraperitoneal ruptures caused by iatrogenic injury can be treated usually by transurethral bladder drainage alone.

OPERATIVE TECHNIQUE Parenteral antimicrobial therapy is instituted immediately after diagnosis. The pelvis is preferably explored through a transabdominal lower midline incision that can be extended superiorly as needed. After abdominal exploration the peritoneum is reflected from the bladder, and the perforation is debrided and closed in two to three layers. A cystotomy may be required to repair ruptures near the base of the bladder. In this situation the closure is generally performed in a transvesical fashion. A suprapubic cys-

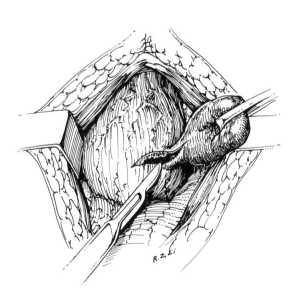
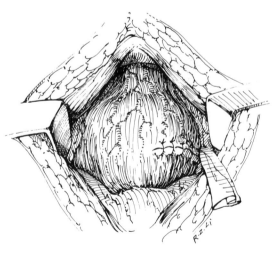

FIGURE 9.25
Extravesical diverticulectomy

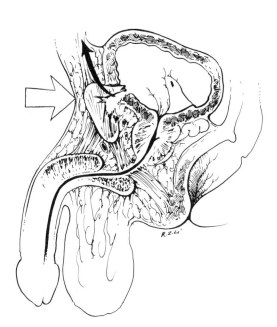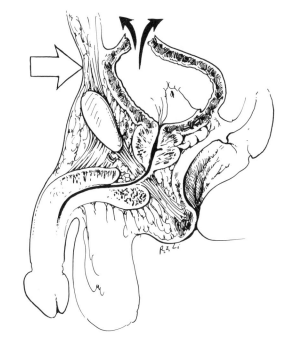

FIGURE 9.26
Extraperitoneal and intraperitoneal rupture of the bladder

tostomy is recommended for bladder drainage, and Penrose drains are positioned next to the site or sites of bladder closure.

POSTOPERATIVE CARE AND COMPLICATIONS A cystogram is performed 5 to 7 days after surgery. In the absence of extravasation, the suprapubic tube is clamped and removed 1 to 2 days later if voiding function is satisfactory. Persistent extravasation is uncommon if all perforations are identified and closed at surgery.

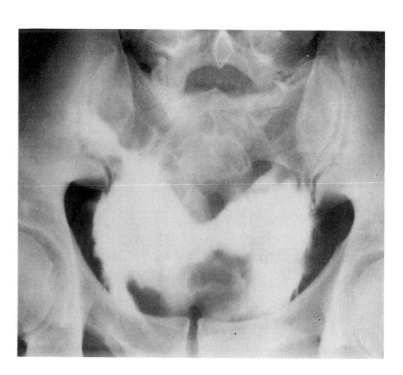

FIGURE 9.27
Cystogram demonstrating extraperitoneal rupture of the bladder

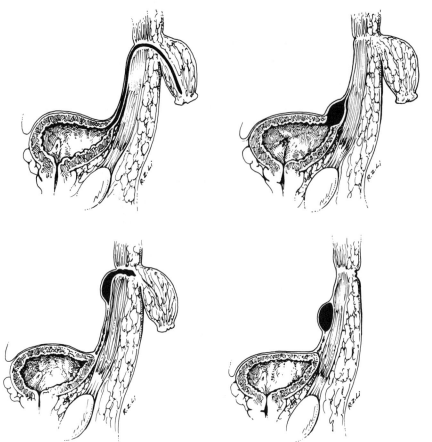

FIGURE 9.28
Urachal disorders

OPERATIONS FOR URACHAL DISORDERS

The urachus is a remnant of the fetal tubular connection between the bladder and allantois. It extends from the apex of the bladder to the umbilicus and lies between the transversalis fascia and the peritoneum. The lateral umbilical ligaments, which are remnants of the umbilical arteries, are situated on each side.

Disorders of the urachus are unusual. Delayed closure results in a vesicoumbilical fistula and urinary leakage at the umbilicus (Figure 9.28). Incomplete obliteration of the urachus adjacent to the bladder produces a diverticulum, whereas incomplete obliteration adjacent to the umbilicus leads to inflammation and drainage. Isolated cysts along the course of the urachus present as mass lesions, which may be symptomatic or infected.

Malignant tumors of the urachus are usually adenocarcinomas and arise next to the bladder. They are generally asymptomatic until the bladder is infiltrated,

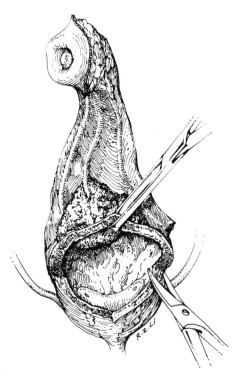

FIGURE 9.29
Excision of urachus and adjacent bladder for carcinoma

and local extension at diagnosis is common. With cystoscopy, urachal carcinomas appear as irregular sessile lesions at the dome of the bladder.

OPERATIVE TECHNIQUE Excision of the entire urachus is recommended for the treatment of benign disorders. Incision and drainage of infected sinuses or cysts, however, should usually precede the extirpative procedure. The urachus is approached through an extraperitoneal lower midline or transverse incision. It is transected at the umbilicus, dissected from the peritoneum, and excised with a small portion of the bladder dome.

With malignant tumors of the urachus, the umbilicus, urachus, umbilical ligaments, adjacent peritoneum, and dome of the bladder are removed en bloc (Figure 9.29). Partial or complete excision of the adjacent rectus muscle may be required for satisfactory management of invasive tumors.

Urinary Diversion and Bladder Substitution

Supravesical diversion of the urinary stream or replacement of the bladder with intestinal segments is an integral component of extirpative bladder surgery. Urinary diversion is employed also when the bladder is not removed, but disease or dysfunction is so severe that reparative procedures are not feasible.

Cutaneous ureterostomy and implantation of the ureters into the intact sigmoid colon (ureterosigmoidostomy) were the primary methods of supravesical diversion before the ileal conduit was introduced in 1950. Stomal stenosis, however, was a common complication of cutaneous ureterostomy and limited its application to individuals with a short life expectancy. Ureterosigmoidostomy was associated with prohibitive mortality in the preantibiotic era. The general infectious complications inherent to intestinal surgery were more easily avoided and controlled with the availability of effective antibiotics, but the incidence of pyelonephritis caused by an admixture of urine and fecal material remained substantial.

The ileal conduit was the by-product of unsuccessful efforts by Bricker and associates to construct a continent intra-abdominal urinary reservoir after removal of the bladder and rectosigmoid. Although technically more complex than ureterosigmoidostomy, the ileal conduit separated the urinary and fecal streams, and the incidence of acute renal infection was greatly reduced. In addition, the hyperchloremic acidosis observed in most patients with ureterosigmoidostomy was unusual. Acceptance of a cutaneous stoma by physicians and patients was facilitated by the development of external urinary appliances capable of watertight fixation to the peristomal skin. By the early 1960s the ileal conduit was established as the preferred form of urinary diversion regardless of the status of the sigmoid colon and rectum.

Stomal stenosis and deterioration of renal function following uneventful diversion with the ileal segment were unusual in early experiences. However, these complications were subsequently seen in a disturbingly high proportion of patients who survived more than 10 years after surgery. Free reflux of infected urine between the conduit and the ureters was implicated as the primary cause of renal damage. To overcome these problems, the colon conduit was introduced in the late 1960s. Diversion with this intestinal segment permits the construction of nonrefluxing ureterointestinal anastomoses, and the large-caliber stomas are less susceptible to contracture. The procedure seemed highly desirable for patients with a long life expectancy, but the true advantages of the colon conduit compared with the ileal conduit remain controversial.

The urologic community is now witnessing a new era in the field of urinary diversion that ultimately may lead to safe and effective methods for complete functional restoration of the lower urinary tract after extirpative surgery.

CUTANEOUS URETEROSTOMY

Cutaneous ureterostomy is now used almost exclusively as a temporizing measure in infants with massive dilatation of the upper urinary tract. It is particularly well suited for unstable infants with sepsis or uremia. After the underlying cause of the ureteral dilatation has been identified and corrected, continuity of the urinary system can often be restored. In some cases, however, irreparable conditions necessitate permanent supravesical urinary diversion. In adults, percutaneous nephrostomy and internal ureteral stents have by and large replaced cutaneous ureterostomy as a means for decompression of the upper urinary system.

The optimal technique for cutaneous ureterostomy is based on the necessity for unilateral or bilateral diversion and on the anticipated nature of subsequent management.

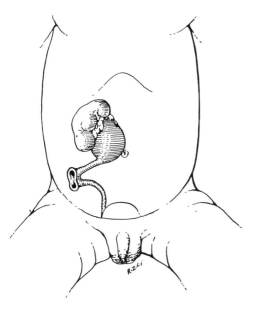
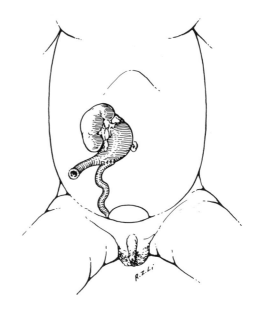

FIGURE 10.1
Loop cutaneous and Y-ureterostomies

Loop Cutaneous Ureterostomy and Y-Ureterostomy

Ureteral integrity is preserved with the loop cutaneous and Y-ureterostomy (Figure 10.1). This simplifies subsequent reconstruction of the urinary system.

OPERATIVE TECHNIQUE The dilated ureter is exposed through a subcostal extraperitoneal flank incision. Mobilization of the proximal ureter to the renal pelvis is necessary to straighten potentially obstructive kinks. For a loop ureterostomy the ureter is brought through the incision and attached to the external oblique muscle with interrupted fine absorbable sutures. The exteriorized ureter is incised for 1 cm, and the margins are sutured to the skin (Figure 10.2). The abdominal incision on each side of the stoma is closed in separate layers, taking care to avoid angulation or compression of the ureter.

With the Y-ureterostomy the upper ureter is transected and the distal end is anastomosed with the renal pelvis. The proximal end is brought through a defect in the abdominal wall, and an end stoma is created using techniques described later in this section.

The loop ureterostomy is closed by excision of the exteriorized segment and ureteroureterostomy. The Y-ureterostomy is closed by removal of the proximal ureteral segment.

End Cutaneous Ureterostomy

End cutaneous ureterostomies are generally used for temporary drainage when restoration of ureteral continuity is not contemplated. Specific indications include the decompression of an obstructed, duplicated system when partial nephrectomy or pyelopyelostomy is planned, or bilateral urinary diversion before anticipated renal transplantation. When bilateral diversion is necessary, two end stomas—one stoma made by joining both ureters at the level of the skin—or a transureteroureterostomy with one end stoma may be constructed (Figure 10.3).

OPERATIVE TECHNIQUE With unilateral procedures, the ureter is approached through an extraperitoneal flank incision. A transabdominal midline approach is preferred for bilateral cutaneous ureterostomy. The ureter is freed to the renal pelvis and then mobilized distally and transected at a level that permits tension-free manipulation through an appropriate site in the abdominal wall. The ureteral vasculature is the only blood supply to the stoma and must be preserved. The distal ureter is ligated.

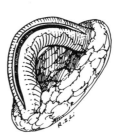
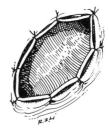

FIGURE 10.2
Stoma of loop cutaneous ureterostomy

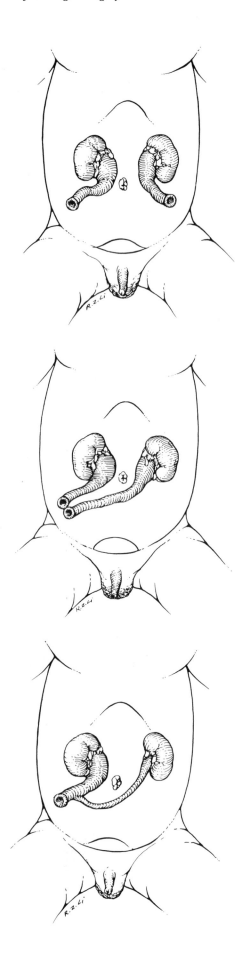

A V-shaped skin incision is made at the site of the stoma, and the ureter is brought through a defect created in the underlying abdominal musculature. The ureter is spatulated on the side adjacent to the skin flap, everted, and fixed to the skin with absorbable sutures (Figure 10.4). The skin flap is then elevated into the spatulation and approximated with the edges of the ureter. When both ureters are diverted by transureteroureterostomy, the single end cutaneous stoma is constructed in the same manner.

If both ureters are joined at the skin to form a single midline or lateral stoma, the medial ends are spatulated and joined at the apex with a single absorbable suture (Figure 10.5). The ureters are then everted and fixed to the skin, and the free ureteral margins are approximated with interrupted absorbable sutures.

POSTOPERATIVE CARE AND COMPLICATIONS

Intubation of the ureter for at least 7 days is advisable to ensure adequate drainage. Urinary collection appliances are not necessary if the patient wears diapers.

Acute necrosis of the stoma and late stomal stenosis are more frequent with cutaneous ureterostomy than with urinary diversions constructed with intestinal segments. The dilated ureter contracts after relief of an obstruction, and retraction of the stoma is also common. Finally, revision of a ureteral stoma is problematic because it is difficult to mobilize the ureter to obtain additional length.

CUTANEOUS PYELOSTOMY

Exteriorization of a markedly dilated renal pelvis is an alternative technique for temporary supravesical diversion in young children. The renal pelvis is approached through an extraperitoneal flank or lumbar incision and brought to the skin through a separate defect in the posterolateral abdominal wall. The wall of the pelvis is secured to the muscle, and the free edges of a pyelotomy are sutured to the skin.

URETEROSIGMOIDOSTOMY

The most technically simple method of urinary diversion involving an intestinal component is the ureterosigmoidostomy, but it is associated with the most

---

FIGURE 10.3
Bilateral end cutaneous ureterostomy, bilateral end cutaneous ureterostomy with single stoma, and transureteroureterostomy with end cutaneous ureterostomy

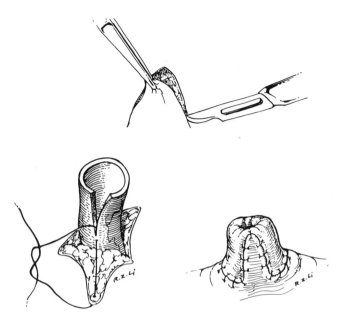

FIGURE 10.4
Stoma of end cutaneous ureterostomy

distressing long-term complications. An incompetent anal sphincter is an absolute contraindication; relative contraindications are anticipated noncompliance with lifelong observation, prior pelvic radiation therapy, renal insufficiency, and dilatation of the ureters.

OPERATIVE TECHNIQUE As with all elective intestinal surgery, a thorough mechanical and antibiotic bowel preparation and perioperative antimicrobial therapy are mandatory. An antimicrobial retention enema administered the night before surgery and intravenous hydration to replace fluid loss during bowel preparation are advisable.

A lower midline incision provides satisfactory exposure. If cystectomy is a component of the operation, it is performed first. If the bladder is not removed, the right ureter is approached through an incision in the pelvic peritoneum at the level of the common iliac artery. The left ureter is exposed by medial reflection

of the sigmoid colon. Each ureter is mobilized proximally and distally, transected as close to the bladder as possible, and positioned adjacent to the sigmoid colon.

The ureterocolonic anastomoses are performed through posterolateral teniae in the distal sigmoid colon that lies in the midline. The tenia is incised transversely and the mucosa is freed from its undersurface for 4 to 5 cm. The tenia is then divided near its lateral border, and a disc of mucosa is removed from the lowermost portion of the trough (Figure 10.6). A ureteral stent is advanced to the renal pelvis, and the spatulated ureter is anastomosed with the colonic mucosa using through-and-through interrupted absorbable sutures. The tenia is closed over the ureter with interrupted nonabsorbable sutures. The resultant tunnel should be sufficiently capacious to allow the introduction of a clamp alongside the ureter. Tight, potentially obstructive tunnels must be revised. Peritoneum lying lateral to the colon may be reflected over each anastomosis and sutured to the serosa.

Nonrefluxing anastomoses can be constructed also with a transcolonic approach. The anterior sigmoid colon is opened with an 8-cm longitudinal incision. Posterolateral submucosal tunnels 3 to 4 cm in length are then developed in a manner reminiscent of that described for the Politano-Leadbetter ureteroneocystostomy. A defect in the colonic musculature is established at the superior aspect of the tunnel, and the ureter is drawn into the lumen. The ureter is spatulated and anastomosed with the colonic mucosa using interrupted absorbable sutures. The contralateral anastomosis is done, ureteral stents are advanced to the renal pelves, and the anterior colon is closed in two layers.

A rectal tube is inserted through the anus and sutured to the perianal skin. The ureteral stents are left in the lumen of the rectum or positioned within the rectal tube. Penrose drains are placed next to the anastomoses, tunneled through the retroperitoneal space, and brought out through an anterolateral stab wound.

POSTOPERATIVE CARE AND COMPLICATIONS The rectal tube and Penrose drains are removed after 8 to 10 days when injection of liquid contrast medium demonstrates the absence of extravasation. The ureteral stents are sequentially removed over the following 2 days. Oral antibiotics at full dosage are administered for 2 to 4 weeks, and suppressive low-dose therapy with trimethoprim should be given indefinitely. The stools are watery, but incapacitating diarrhea is unusual.

Leakage at the ureterocolonic anastomoses is the postoperative complication of greatest concern. Both fecal matter and urine contaminate the pelvis, and abscess formation is inevitable. Operative intervention is required for all but the most minor leaks, and

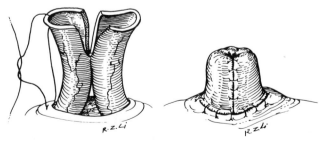

FIGURE 10.5
Stoma of joined bilateral end cutaneous ureterostomy

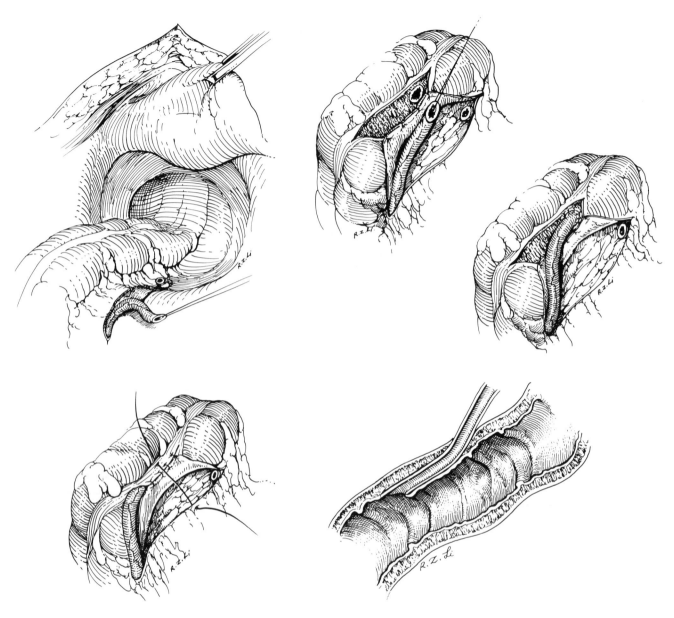

FIGURE 10.6
Tunneled ureterocolonic anastomosis

construction of an alternative form of diversion is generally required.

The late complications of ureterosigmoidostomy include anastomotic obstruction, recurrent renal infection, infected renal calculi, and a hyperchloremic metabolic acidosis from the absorption of urinary chloride and the excretion of bicarbonate. Benign or malignant colonic tumors arising next to the ureteral anastomoses develop in as great as 40 percent of patients, and intermittent proctosigmoidoscopy is mandatory. This unique carcinogenesis is not seen with other forms of urinary diversion with intestinal seg-

ments and is apparently induced by the combination of urine and feces.

ILEAL CONDUIT

The ileal conduit, or ureteroileocutaneous diversion, remains the standard for permanent urinary diversion in the adult. Significant postoperative morbidity and early complications are unusual, the incidence of late complications is well defined, and most urologists are adept at the procedure.

The proper location for a right lower quadrant stoma is marked the day before surgery by an experienced enterostomal therapist. The site should not encroach on scars, skin creases, the umbilicus, or bony prominences and must be visualized by the patient. The bowel is cleansed as described for ureterosigmoidostomy, although an antibiotic enema is unnecessary.

OPERATIVE TECHNIQUE If a cystectomy is performed, the low lithotomy position is recommended (see Chapter 9). Otherwise, the supine position is appropriate. A midline incision extending from the symphysis pubis to a point above the umbilicus provides adequate exposure.

The conduit is made with a 15- to 20-cm section of distal ileum. The length of the segment should always be slightly longer than anticipated and trimmed at the end of the procedure if the conduit is redundant. Conduits that are too short cannot be lengthened. The distal end of the ileal segment is located about 10 cm from the ileocecal valve (Figure 10.7). The distal mesenteric incision, which determines the mobility of the ileal segment, extends for 10 to 15 cm between the ramifica-

tions of the ileocolic and right colic arteries. The proximal mesentery is incised for 2 to 3 cm only. The bowel is transected between noncrushing clamps and the ileal segment is positioned posteriorly. Intestinal continuity is restored with a standard small-bowel anastomosis, and the mesenteric defect is closed with interrupted sutures. When end-to-side ureteroileal anastomoses are to be done, the proximal end of the ileal segment is closed in two layers.

If a cystectomy is not performed, the cecum is reflected superiorly by incision of the paracolic gutter and posterior peritoneum. The right ureter and encompassing fibrofatty tissue are mobilized distally and transected adjacent to the bladder. The distal ureter is secured with a nonabsorbable suture. The left ureter is exposed by medial reflection of the sigmoid colon, mobilized proximally and distally, and divided as close to the bladder as is feasible. A tunnel is then created with blunt dissection behind the mesentery of the sigmoid colon that connects the right and left peritoneal incisions. The size of the tunnel should be sufficient to accommodate four fingers. The left ureter is grasped

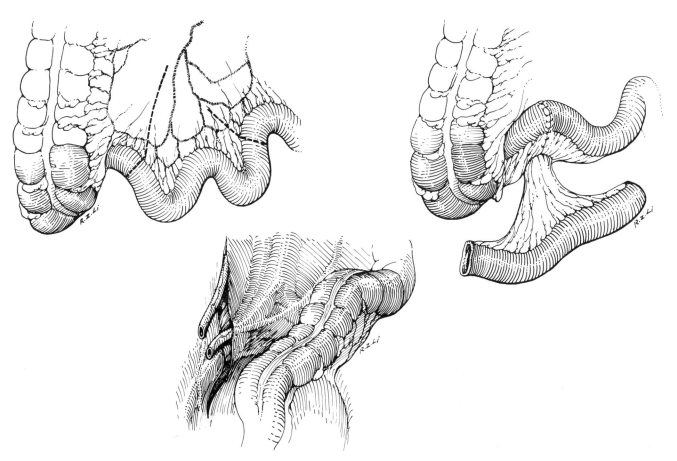

FIGURE 10.7
Isolation of bowel segment and ureters for ileal conduit

with a Babcock clamp and drawn into the right peritoneal incision, taking care to avoid twisting or angulation.

For end-to-side ureteroileal anastomoses, the proximal end of the conduit is positioned under the medial edge of the right peritoneal incision and secured with several interrupted sutures. This stabilizes the conduit during subsequent maneuvers.

We prefer a two-layered ureteroileal anastomosis. The first layer is created with fine interrupted absorbable sutures placed through-and-through the ureter and bowel. The suture through the ileum should include a generous amount of serosa and muscularis, but just the edge of the mucosa. The second layer reinforces and seals the anastomosis and is made with interrupted fine nonabsorbable sutures that encompass periureteral fibrous tissue and the serosa of the ileum.

The left ureteroileal anastomosis is performed first. The conduit is reflected superomedially and a 0.5-cm transverse seromuscular incision is made about 1 cm from the end of the conduit (Figure 10.8). The incision should be longer if the ureter is dilated. The ileal mucosa is gently dissected from the muscularis with a hemostat, and the disc of mucosa that bulges through the incision is excised.

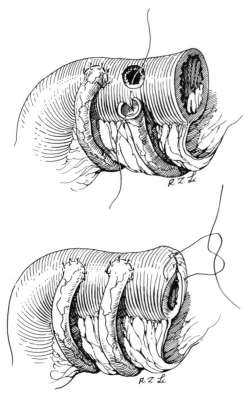

FIGURE 10.8
End-to-side ureteroileal anastomoses

The medial end of the ureter is spatulated for 0.5 cm, and the ureter is attached to the ileum with a reinforcing suture at the 6 o'clock position. The apex of the ureteral spatulation is then approximated to the ileal defect with a through-and-through suture at the 6 o'clock position, two through-and-through sutures are placed at the 4 and 8 o'clock positions, and two reinforcing sutures are applied at the 4 and 8 o'clock positions. A soft pediatric feeding tube or single-coiled ureteral stent is introduced into the distal end of the conduit, identified at the partially completed anastomosis, and advanced to the left renal pelvis. The first layer of the anastomosis is completed with sutures at the 10, 12, and 2 o'clock positions. These sutures are not tied until all are properly positioned. The anastomosis is completed with two or three additional reinforcing sutures.

The right ureteroileal anastomosis is performed in an identical manner 1 cm distal to the left anastomosis. The left posterior peritoneal incision and the right posterior peritoneal defect located below the conduit are then closed with interrupted sutures.

An end-to-end ureteroileal anastomosis is well suited for dilated ureters. The medial end of each ureter is spatulated for 1 cm, and the posterior margins of the spatulations are joined with a continuous fine absorbable suture (Figure 10.9). The anterior edge of the right ureteral spatulation is then approximated with the posterior border of the ileal lumen. The anastomosis is completed by approximating the margins of the ureteral lumens and the anterior edge of the left ureteral spatulation with the ileum. Ureteral stents are used at the discretion of the surgeon.

The abdominal defect for the stoma is made at the predetermined site in the right lower quadrant. A disc of skin 1 to 2 cm in diameter is removed, and the subcutaneous fat is separated bluntly to expose the anterior rectus sheath. A cruciate incision is made in the sheath, the underlying muscle fibers are divided with electrocautery, and a cruciate incision is made in the posterior sheath and peritoneum (Figure 10.10). The defect should be sufficiently capacious to admit two fingers.

The distal conduit is grasped with a Babcock clamp and brought through the abdominal wall. To create a protruding stoma, about 3 cm of ileum should extrude without tension. The conduit is fixed with seromuscular sutures to the peritoneum, and the stoma is everted with four heavy absorbable sutures. Each suture encompasses the skin edge or subcutaneous tissue, the serosa and muscularis of the conduit at the level of the skin, and a full thickness of the free end of the conduit. Additional interrupted absorbable sutures are placed to seal the edges of the skin and the everted ileum. The ureteral stents are then sutured to the peristomal skin.

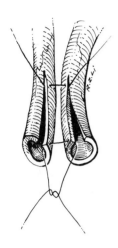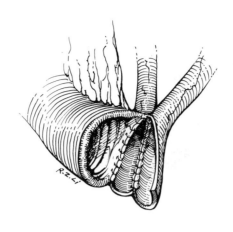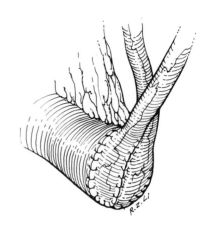

FIGURE 10.9
End-to-end ureteroileal anastomosis

In obese patients, or in patients with a short ileal mesentery, tension-free manipulation of the conduit above the skin may not be possible. A loop stoma is recommended in these circumstances (Figure 10.11). The distal end of the conduit is closed in two layers, and a knuckle of the conduit is pulled through the abdominal defect. With the conduit positioned 3 cm above the level of the skin, the wall is fixed to the anterior rectus sheath with interrupted seromuscular sutures. The antimesenteric border of the distal arc is incised transversely for 270° at the level of the skin and the proximal component of the arc is everted. This component is sutured to the skin in the manner described for an end stoma. The edge of the recessed distal component is fixed to the skin with simple interrupted absorbable sutures.

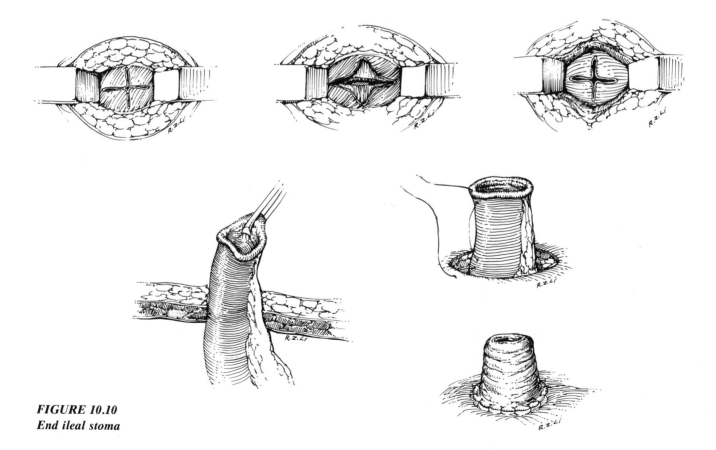

FIGURE 10.10
End ileal stoma

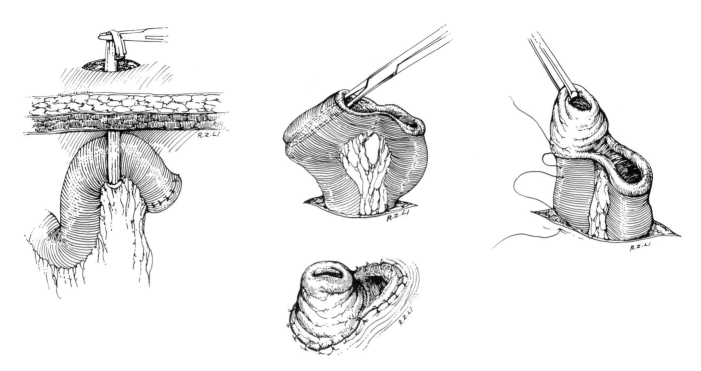

FIGURE 10.11
Loop ileal stoma

An ileal conduit generally lies just anterior to the cecum (Figure 10.12). Internal herniation of small intestine behind the conduit is unlikely, and fixation of the conduit to the peritoneum proximal to the abdominal defect is not necessary. When ureteral stents are not used, a 24 F multi-eyed catheter is introduced through the stoma and secured to the skin. This facilitates the evacuation of urine until normal peristaltic activity resumes. We do not drain the retroperitoneal space.

POSTOPERATIVE CARE AND COMPLICATIONS A "loopogram" is performed on the fifth to seventh postopera-

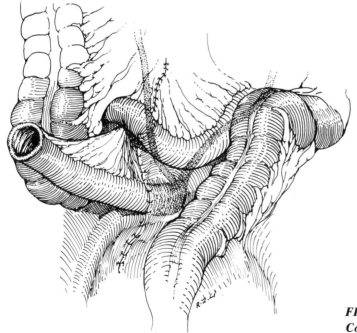

FIGURE 10.12
Completed ileal conduit

tive day. If the conduit is watertight, the ureteral stents are removed sequentially over 2 days. The patient, and if appropriate, close family members are instructed in the application and care of the urinary appliance during the early postoperative period.

Leakage or obstruction at the ureterointestinal anastomoses and, infrequently, disruption or obstruction of the bowel anastomosis are the cause of most major complications. Anastomotic leaks are managed by bilateral percutaneous nephrostomy or the placement of ureteral stents. Resolution of the complication is unusual if it persists longer than 2 to 3 weeks and operative revision is warranted. Ischemia or infarction of the conduit is unusual but should be suspected if the stoma develops a persistent bluish discoloration.

An intravenous pyelogram is performed 2 to 3 months after surgery if convalescence is uneventful. Some degree of ureteral dilatation is often seen at this time, but the excretion of contrast material should be prompt.

Stomal stenosis and obstruction of the ureteroileal anastomoses are the most common late complications. The latter should always be suspected if there is acute pyelonephritis, elevation of the serum creatinine level, or flank pain. Renal calculi develop in about 15 to 30 percent of patients and bacteriuria is inevitable. Suppressive antimicrobial therapy, however, is of little or no benefit. A hyperchloremic metabolic acidosis is unusual if the serum creatinine is 2.0 mg/dl or less. Mild renal insufficiency from an interstitial nephritis is seen 10 to 20 years after surgery in a large proportion of patients.

COLON CONDUIT

A colon conduit is more difficult to construct than an ileal conduit and is rarely indicated in the patient with a short life expectancy. The sigmoid rather than the transverse colon is used for the conduit unless the condition of the distal ureters mandates high ureteral anastomoses. Inflammatory disorders of the large intestine are contraindications to a colon conduit.

The bowel is cleansed before surgery as described for ureterosigmoidostomy, and the stomal site is marked by an enterostomal therapist.

OPERATIVE TECHNIQUE   As with other diversions performed in conjunction with cystectomy, the bladder is removed first. The sigmoid colon is then reflected medially, a 15- to 20-cm segment is isolated, and intestinal continuity is restored. The bowel anastomosis is situated anterior to the isolated segment if a left lower quadrant stoma is planned and posterior to the segment if a midline or right lower quadrant stoma is planned (Figure 10.13). Satisfactory mobility of the conduit requires incision of the distal mesentery to a point overlying the sacrum and, usually, division of the superior hemorrhoidal artery. The proximal mesentery is incised for 2 to 3 cm only.

The proximal lumen of the conduit is closed in two layers. For a right-sided stoma the proximal end is secured to the sacral promontory. The left ureter is brought medially under the mesentery of the sigmoid colon, and the right ureter is brought medially under the posterior peritoneum. For a left-sided stoma the proximal conduit is fixed to the ipsilateral psoas muscle, and the right ureter is drawn through a tunnel under the sigmoid mesentery. The left ureter lies naturally at the base of the conduit. Nonrefluxing ureterocolonic anastomoses at staggered sites in one or two teniae are created as described for ureterosigmoidostomy and are supported with ureteral stents.

The abdominal wall defect for the stoma is made as described for an ileal conduit but should be slightly larger and admit three fingers. The techniques described for creation of a protruding end ileal stoma are also used for the colonic stoma. Drainage of ureterocolonic anastomoses is not necessary.

Postoperative care and complications parallel those described for an ileal conduit. The late complications of stomal stenosis, renal insufficiency, and renal stones, however, are probably less common than with the ileal conduit.

CONTINENT URINARY RESERVOIRS

Continent urinary reservoirs are constructed from intact or reconfigured bowel, have capacities of 400 to 1200 ml, and are emptied by periodic catheterization of an abdominal stoma. Continence is provided usually by intussusception of the ileum proximal to the stoma. Reflux is prevented by tunneled ureterocolonic anastomoses or intussusception of ileum distal to refluxing ureteroileal anastomoses. The intraluminal pressures of reservoirs made with reconfigured bowel are substantially less than those constructed from intact intestinal segments.

Experiences with the five forms of continent reservoirs described in this section have been the largest and the longest. However, each has been subject to continual technical modifications that promise to improve reservoir function and reduce the incidences of postoperative and late complications.

Cecal Reservoir

The storage component of the cecal reservoir is made from intact cecum and ascending and transverse colon. Intussusception of the ileum through the ileocecal valve creates a continence mechanism, and tunneled

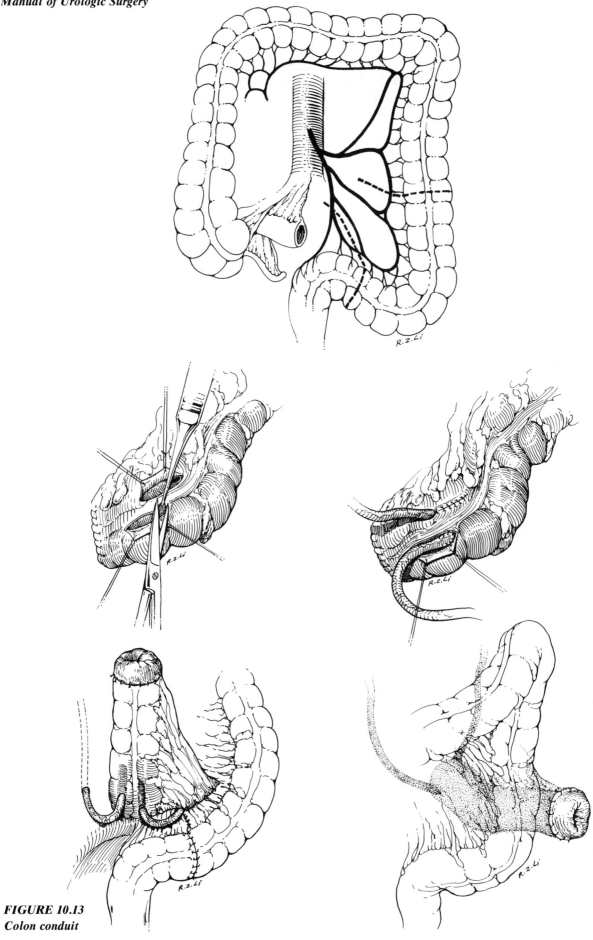

FIGURE 10.13
Colon conduit

ureterocolonic anastomoses serve as the antireflux mechanisms.

OPERATIVE TECHNIQUE The posterior peritoneum is incised from the cecum to the duodenum. The right gutter is incised to the hepatic flexure, and the hepatocolic ligament is transected and secured with ligatures. The mesentery of the transverse colon situated 10 cm distal to the hepatic flexure is divided for 5 cm; the mesentery of the ileum situated about 15 cm from the ileocecal valve is divided for 15 cm between the right colic and ileocolic arteries (Figure 10.14). The bowel segment is isolated and intestinal continuity is established by ileocolostomy. Spatulation of the antimesenteric border of the ileum is required so that the circumference approximates that of the colon. The mesenteric defect between the transverse colon and ileum is closed to prevent internal herniation.

The superior aspect of the reservoir is closed in two layers, and the left ureter is brought under the sigmoid mesentery and positioned behind the cecum. An appendectomy is performed as necessary, and the mesentery is excluded from the most distal 8 cm of the ileum. This facilitates the intussusception. The anterior wall of the cecum is opened, and a Babcock clamp is introduced through the ileocecal valve. The ileum is grasped at the midpoint of the mesenteric exclusion, and with gentle traction an intussusception protruding about 5 cm into the cecum is achieved with remarkable ease. Dilatation or incision of the ileocecal valve is not necessary. A bluish discoloration of the intussusception is not unusual but may be unsettling to the surgeon.

The intussusception is made permanent with three rows of staples spaced at 90° intervals. Staples are not applied to the intussusception adjacent to the posteroinferior lumen of the cecum. A small defect is then made in the wall of the cecum over the end of the intussusception for introduction of the stapling device. The opposed mucosa of the cecum and intussusception are each incised longitudinally and the valve is anchored to the cecal wall with a fourth row of staples. The small cecostomy is closed in two layers. The emerging reservoir outlet is then secured to the ileocecal valve and surrounding cecal wall with multiple interrupted seromuscular sutures.

The ileocolonic segment is reflected upward, and a tunneled left ureterocolonic anastomosis is performed in a medially situated tenia using the techniques described for a ureterosigmoidostomy. The right ureter and a laterally situated tenia are exposed by reflecting the segment to the patient's left, and the right nonrefluxing anastomosis is performed. Double-coiled stents are advanced to the renal pelves and the cecostomy is closed in two layers. The reservoir is inflated with a methylene blue solution to help identify small leaks and to document competence of the intussuscepted valve.

Using the techniques described for the ileal conduit, a defect in the right lower abdominal wall is prepared for the reservoir outlet. The outlet is pulled through the defect, and the reservoir is anchored to the retroperitoneum. A clockwise rotation of the reservoir is generally required to prevent angulation of the left ureter as it enters the tunneled anastomosis. The cecum adjacent to the reservoir outlet is secured to the posterior peritoneum and rectus sheath with multiple seromuscular sutures. During these maneuvers and during abdominal closure, the stoma is intermittently catheterized to ensure that the outlet does not become angulated. A slightly protruding or flat stoma is then made using conventional techniques.

In patients with preexisting ileal conduits the reservoir is made in the same manner, but the conduit is intussuscepted through a posteromedial tenia. This obviates construction of new enteroureteral anastomoses and creates an antireflux mechanism distal to the preexisting anastomoses.

Patched Cecal Reservoir and Indiana Reservoir

A patched cecal reservoir differs from the cecal reservoir in that transverse colon is not included, a patch of ileum is incorporated into the ascending colon, and ileal plication rather than ileal intussusception is used as a continence mechanism. The ileal patch reduces the magnitude of intraluminal pressure spikes created by physiologic contraction of the reservoir.

During the past several years the originators of the patched reservoir have favored a modification whereby a reconfiguration of the colonic segment rather than an ileal patch is employed to reduce intraluminal pressures. This "Indiana" reservoir is more easily constructed.

OPERATIVE TECHNIQUE The ascending colon is divided about 20 cm from the cecum. Inclusion of the proximal transverse colon is not necessary because reservoir capacity is increased by the addition of the ileal patch. The ileum is then transected 15 and 30 cm proximal to the ileocecal valve, and intestinal continuity is reestablished (Figure 10.15). The proximal ileal segment, which is used for the patch, is incised on the antimesenteric border. The anterosuperior colonic segment is also incised to accommodate the patch. Tunneled ureterocolonic anastomoses are performed over ureteral stents, and the reservoir is closed by approximation of the corresponding edges of the open colon and ileal patch. Preexisting ileal conduits are opened along the antimesenteric border and used for the patch.

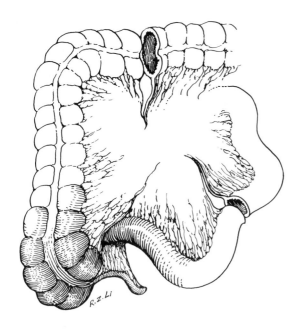

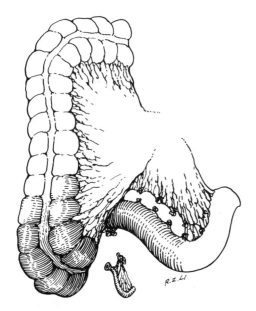

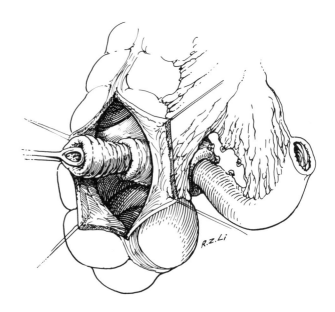

FIGURE 10.14
Cecal reservoir

The terminal ileum is plicated over a 12 F catheter, the reservoir is anchored to the posterior peritoneum, a defect in the abdominal wall is created for the ileal outlet, and a flat stoma is made. Intussusception of ileum through the ileocecal valve can be used in addition to the ileal plication to achieve continence.

With the Indiana reservoir an intestinal segment identical to that used for the cecal reservoir is isolated. The anterior wall of the transverse and ascending colon is incised to a point 3 to 5 cm from the most dependent portion of the cecum (Figure 10.16). The reservoir is closed by folding the opened sheet of colon anteriorly and approximating the edges of adjacent

bowel. The ureterocolonic anastomoses and reservoir outlet are constructed as described for the patched cecal reservoir.

Kock Reservoir

The Kock reservoir is made entirely from reconfigured ileum and is an ingenious but technically complex modification of the continent ileostomy procedure. Continence is provided by ileal intussusception, and reflux is prevented by another ileal intussusception distal to refluxing end-to-side ureteroileal anastomoses.

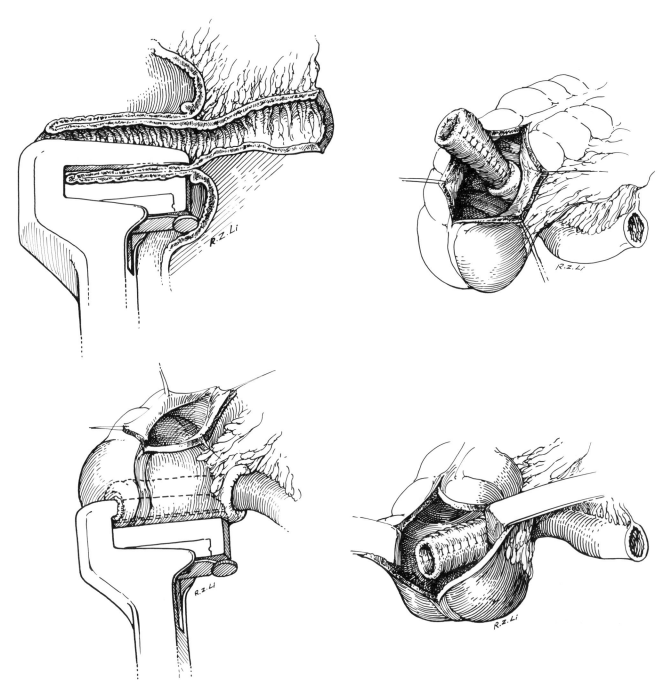

FIGURE 10.14
Cecal reservoir (continued)

OPERATIVE TECHNIQUE An 80-cm segment of ileum is required to construct the reservoir. The proximal ileal mesentery is divided for 5 cm, but the distal mesenteric incision should extend 10 to 15 cm to allow mobility of the reservoir. The bowel segment is isolated, intestinal continuity is reestablished, and the proximal end of the ileal segment is closed.

The proximal and distal 20-cm sections of the ileal segment are used for the afferent and efferent inlets and intussusceptions, respectively; the 40-cm central section is used for the storage reservoir. The central segment is folded at its midpoint, and the two opposed limbs are joined with a continuous seromuscular suture and opened along the antimesenteric border (Figure 10.17). The incisions adjacent to the afferent and efferent limbs should be staggered so that the two intussusceptions do not abut one another after completion of the reservoir. The mesentery is excluded from 8 cm of the afferent and efferent limbs immediately adjacent to the central segment. Additional defects are

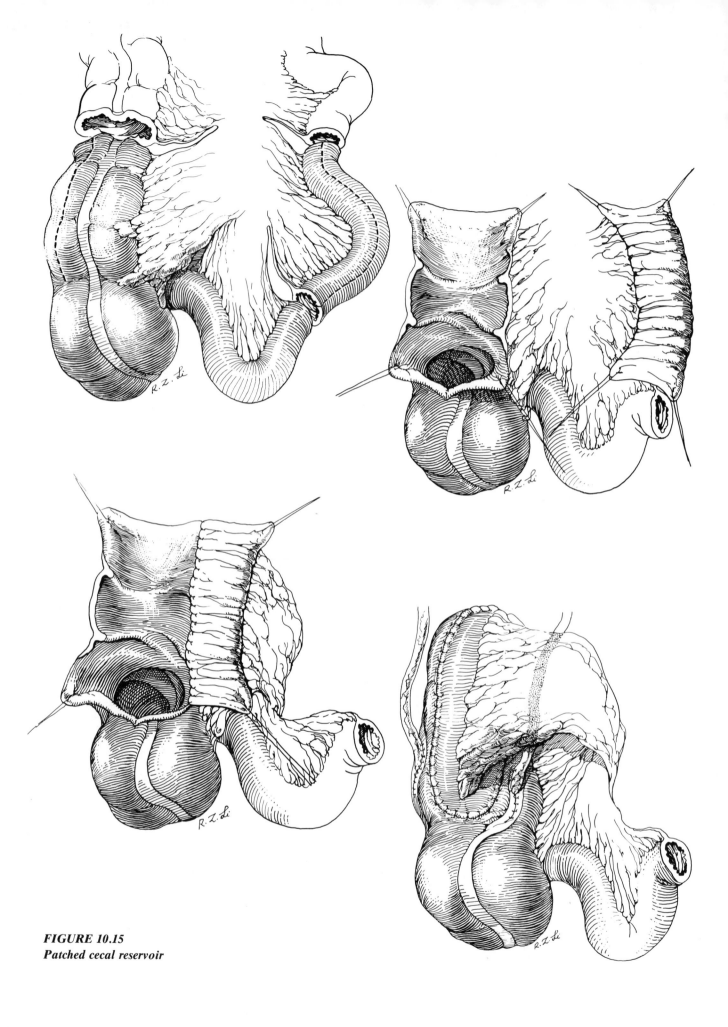

FIGURE 10.15
Patched cecal reservoir

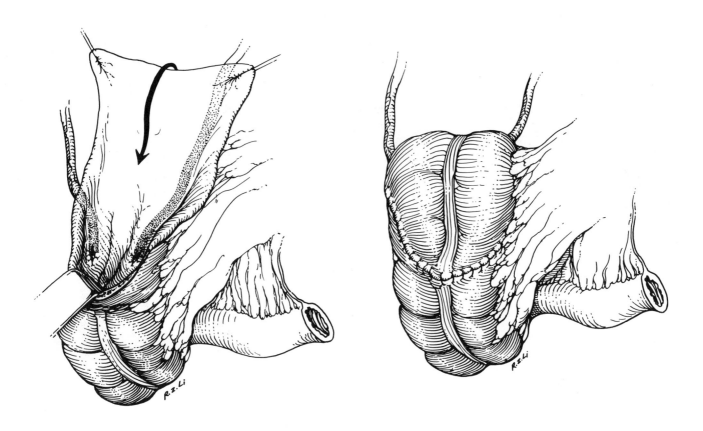

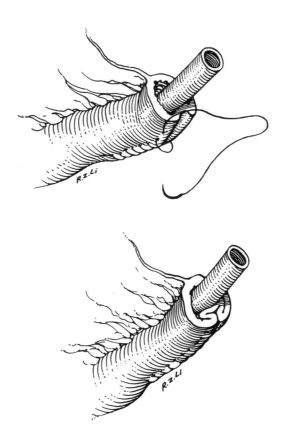

FIGURE 10.16
Indiana reservoir

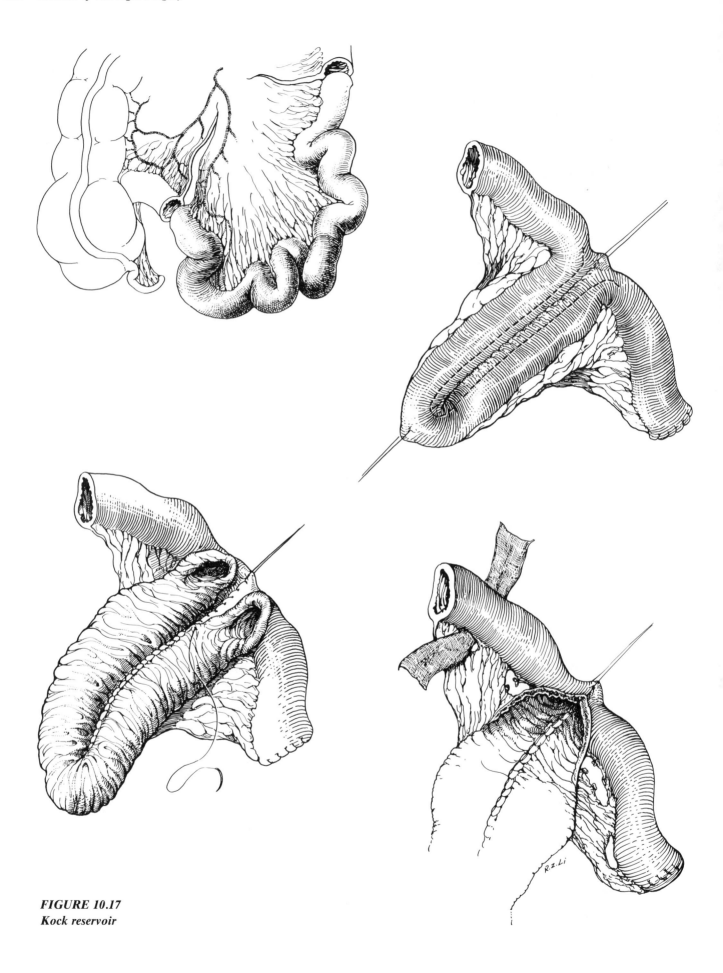

FIGURE 10.17
Kock reservoir

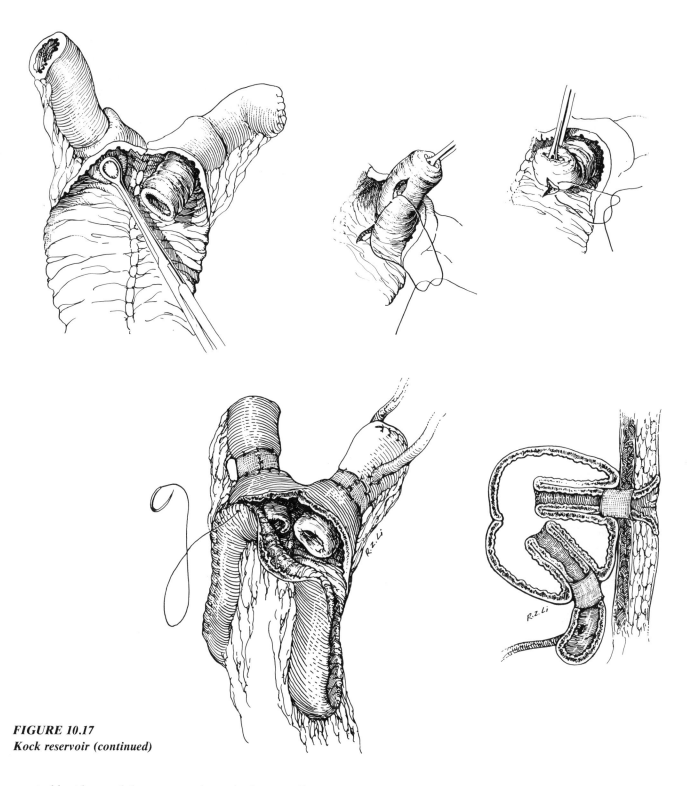

FIGURE 10.17
Kock reservoir (continued)

created just beyond the mesenteric exclusions to allow placement of supporting synthetic mesh collars. The limbs are then intussuscepted, the supporting collars are positioned and secured with sutures, and the valves are attached to the reservoir wall with staples or sutures. The reservoir is closed by folding the intestinal plate superiorly and approximating the adjacent free margins.

The afferent inlet is anchored to the sacral promontory, and end-to-side ureteroileal anastomoses are performed over ureteral stents that extend through the intussusception. A defect in the abdominal wall is prepared, the collar around the efferent outlet is sutured to the anterior rectus sheath, and a flat stoma is constructed.

In patients with preexisting ileal conduits, the

conduit is shortened and anastomosed in an end-to-end fashion with the afferent inlet.

Mainz Reservoir

A Mainz reservoir is made from reconfigured sheets of distal ileum, cecum, and ascending colon. Continence is provided usually by an ileoileal intussusception proximal to the stoma. Reflux is prevented by tunneled ureterocolonic anastomoses.

OPERATIVE TECHNIQUE   A 50-cm length of distal ileum and a 15-cm length of cecum and ascending colon are isolated and intestinal continuity is restored. The proximal 20 cm of the ileal segment is left intact, but the distal 30 cm and the entire colonic segment are opened on the antimesenteric border (Figure 10.18). The sheets of colon and ileum are then positioned as shown in Figure 10.18, and the opposing margins are joined with continuous sutures.

Tunneled ureterocolonic anastomoses are made over ureteral stents at either the edge of the colon, as shown in Figure 10.18, or in the more inferior colonic tenia. The mesentery of the proximal intact ileal segment is excluded for a distance of 8 cm and an ileoileal intussusception is performed. It is stabilized with sutures or staples as well as a supporting collar. The reservoir is closed by folding the medial margin of the attached sheets of colon and ileum laterally and approximating the adjacent free edges. The reservoir is then anchored to the retroperitoneum; a defect in the abdominal wall is prepared; the base of the intussusception and collar are secured to the abdominal wall; and a stoma is created.

POSTOPERATIVE CARE AND COMPLICATIONS
The essentials of postoperative care are similar for all types of continent reservoirs. A drainage tube that

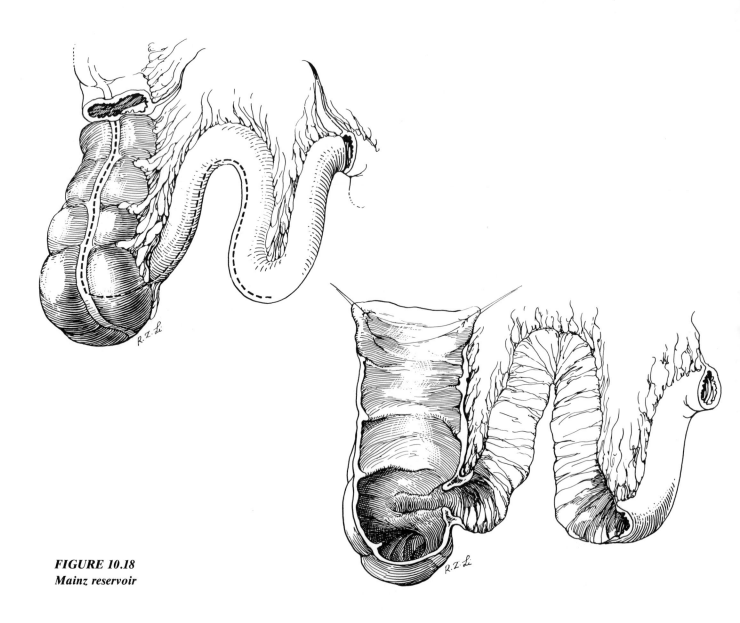

FIGURE 10.18
Mainz reservoir

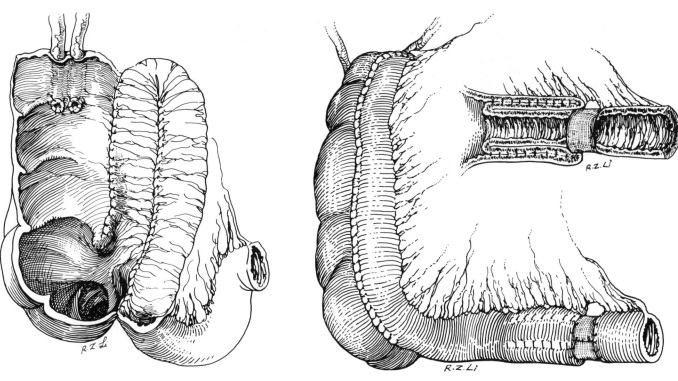

FIGURE 10.18
Mainz reservoir (continued)

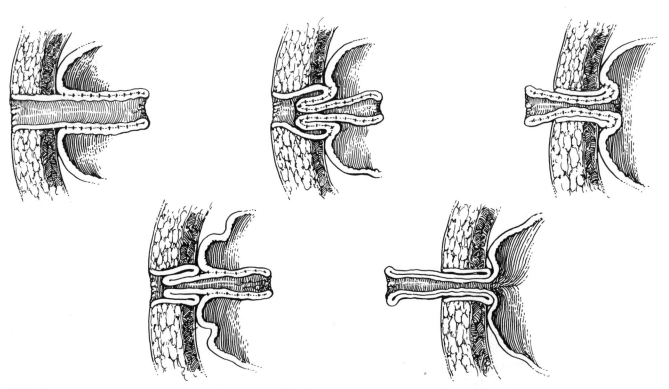

FIGURE 10.19
Prolapse (top) and slippage (bottom) of intussuscepted ileal continence mechanism

exits through the stoma or through a stab wound in the reservoir is irrigated every 4 hours with 50 ml of saline to evacuate mucus. The patient should be instructed in this procedure before leaving the hospital. The ureteral stents, which should preferably drain into the reservoir, and the reservoir drainage tube are left intact at discharge. The patient returns 3 to 4 weeks after surgery for radiographic investigations of the reservoir and upper urinary tracts. Oral antimicrobial therapy is advisable during this interval. If no leaks are detected with a "cystogram" and the intravenous pyelogram is unremarkable, the reservoir catheter is removed and the ureteral stents are extracted with routine cystoscopic methods. When logistically feasible, we remove the stents in a sequential manner over a 2- to 3-day period.

The patient is instructed in the technique of self-catheterization, which should be performed initially at 2- to 3-hour intervals. During the ensuing weeks the frequency of catheterization is gradually decreased. Oral antimicrobial therapy is advisable during the next 1 to 2 months, and the reservoir is intermittently irrigated to remove mucus. A gauze pad only is applied to the stoma.

Leakage at the reservoir suture lines is the most common postoperative complication. However, most defects close with extended drainage.

Malfunction of the continence mechanism and catheterization difficulties are the principal late complications. Valve prolapse or slippage is the most common problem and usually leads to incontinence (Figure 10.19). Mesenteric exclusion, the use of supporting collars of synthetic mesh, staple fixation of the intussusception, and, most important, attachment of the intussusception to the reservoir wall have all been introduced during recent years and should help to reduce the incidence of prolapse or slippage. Catheterization difficulty almost always precedes prolapse or sliding, but may result also from supra- or infrafascial angulation of the reservoir outlet.

Ureteral obstruction or reflux, renal infection, electrolyte imbalance, stone formation, and intestinal malabsorption are not common. Carcinogenesis of the transposed bowel is not anticipated, but bacteriuria is to be expected.

BLADDER SUBSTITUTION PROCEDURES

Bladder substitutes are urinary reservoirs made from bowel that are positioned in the pelvis and anastomosed with the bladder outlet or proximal urethra. They empty by either spontaneous micturition or intermittent transurethral catheterization. The general methods for construction of the storage component and antireflux mechanism parallel those of continent reservoirs. However, because selection criteria restrict clinical application, experience with bladder substitution is less than with continent reservoirs.

Preexisting urinary incontinence or anticipated injury to the urinary sphincter during extirpative surgery are relative contraindications to bladder substitution procedures. Artificial urinary sphincters or intussusceptions proximal to the reservoir outlet have been used to overcome this problem. Among patients with bladder cancer, biopsy-proven involvement of the urethra precludes bladder substitution. Tumor extension beyond the bladder outlet, which increases the possibilities of residual or recurrent disease at the urethral anastomosis, and atypia of the urethral mucosa or diffuse carcinoma in situ of the bladder, which increase the risks of urethral recurrences, are relative contraindications.

Bladder substitution procedures, like continent reservoir procedures, are most conveniently categorized by the segment and configuration of bowel that is used to develop the reservoir. The methods for construction of bladder substitutes from intact bowel are relatively straightforward, and the techniques for making substitutes from reconfigured bowel parallel those described for continent reservoirs. Descriptions of operative procedures, therefore, are limited to the ileal bladder substitute.

Ileal Bladder Substitute (Camey Procedure)

The ileal bladder substitute was developed and popularized by Dr. Maurice Camey of Paris. Because of the simplicity of the operation and abundant clinical experiences, it is the standard of comparison for other substitution procedures.

OPERATIVE TECHNIQUE A 40-cm segment of ileum that can be brought to the urogenital diaphragm at its midpoint is used for the reservoir (Figure 10.20). The segment is isolated, intestinal continuity is established anterior to the segment, and the mesenteric defect is closed. The outlet of the reservoir should be sufficiently large to accommodate the little finger and is created by excising a disc of muscularis and mucosa from the the antimesenteric border. The anastomosis between the reservoir outlet and the urethra is made with through-and-through absorbable sutures in a manner similar to the vesicourethral anastomosis after radical retropubic prostatectomy.

Each end of the ileal segment is incised 3 to 4 cm along the antimesenteric border to provide exposure for construction of the ureteroileal anastomosis. A 4-cm strip of mucosa is excised from the posterior lumen of the ileum beginning about 2 cm below the edge of the bowel. The ureter is brought through a defect made at the superior aspect of the trough. The

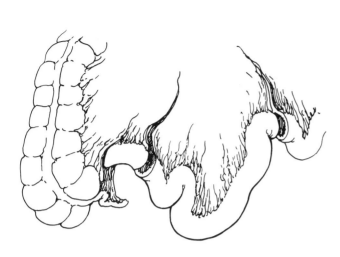

FIGURE 10.20
Ileal bladder substitute (Camey procedure)

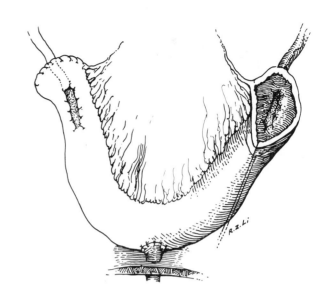

anterior ureter is spatulated, and the posterior margin is sutured to the inferior margin of the trough. The ileal mucosa is then approximated with the lateral borders of the ureter making no attempt to construct a submucosal tunnel.

Ureteral stents are advanced to the renal pelves, and a multi-eyed urethral catheter is placed in the *right* limb of the reservoir. This positioning facilitates the drainage of mucus that is pushed by peristalsis from

the left to the right limb. The ends of the intestinal segment are closed in two layers, and the reservoir is anchored to the pelvic side wall and retroperitoneum in a U-shaped configuration.

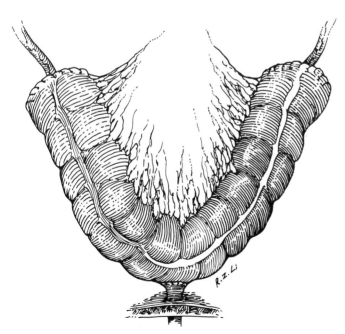

FIGURE 10.21
Sigmoid bladder substitute

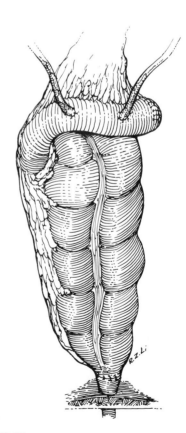

FIGURE 10.22
Ileocolonic bladder substitute

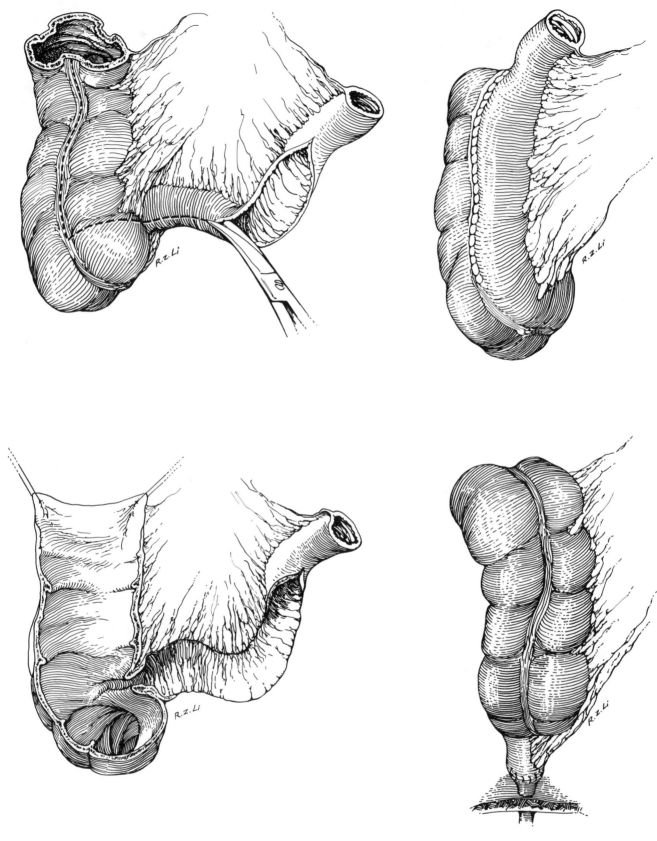

FIGURE 10.23
Bladder substitute from reconfigured ileocecal segment

Sigmoid Bladder Substitute

Bladder substitutes from intact sigmoid colon are usually constructed in a manner identical to that described for an ileal bladder substitute (Figure 10.21). However, the ureterocolonic anastomoses are created with a tunneling technique. Some workers prefer to orient the sigmoid vertically so that the enterourethral anastomosis is made in an end-to-end manner.

Ileocolonic Bladder Substitutes

The capacities of bladder substitutes made from the ileocolonic segment are generally larger than those made from intact ileal or sigmoid segments. In addition, the ileocecal valve can serve as an effective anti-

reflux mechanism. The most common technique of reservoir construction involves a 180° rotation of the intestinal segment and anastomosis of the ascending colon to the urethra. The ureters are anastomosed to the ileum in an end-to-side or end-to-end manner (Figure 10.22). To enhance the antireflux properties of the ileocecal valve, the ileum may be intussuscepted through the valve as described for the continence mechanism of the cecal reservoir.

Bladder Substitutes of Reconfigured Bowel

Like continent urinary reservoirs, bladder substitutes created from reconfigured intestinal segments have lower intraluminal pressures than those constructed

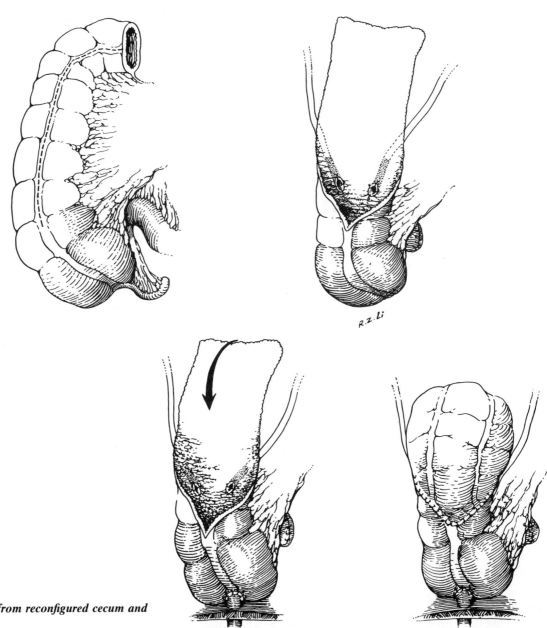

FIGURE 10.24
Bladder substitute from reconfigured cecum and ascending colon

from intact segments. A large number of techniques for reorganizing sheets of intestine have been reported.

A method of bladder substitution using a reconfigured ileocolonic segment is shown in Figure 10.23. The technique is reminiscent of the Mainz method of reservoir construction. However, the number of suture lines is reduced because the partially incised ileal segment is sutured directly to the margins of the colonic segment. The reservoir is rotated 180° to permit direct end-to-end anastomosis of the ileal outlet and urethra. The ureters are anastomosed to the colonic segment with conventional tunneling techniques.

A relatively simple reconfiguration of the cecum and ascending colon that resembles the Indiana reservoir is shown in Figure 10.24. The reservoir is formed from the cecum and ascending and proximal transverse co-

lon. The superior aspect of the colon is incised on the antimesenteric border to a point 5 to 8 cm from the most dependent portion of the cecum. Nonrefluxing ureterocolonic anastomoses are made in the posterior cecum, and the most dependent cecum is anastomosed with the urethra. The reservoir is closed by folding the opened sheet of colon downward and approximating the adjacent bowel margins.

The Kock reservoir may also be adapted for bladder substitution. The reservoir is positioned in the pelvis, and the efferent outlet is anastomosed with the urethra. Because the efferent intussusception is not capable of voluntary relaxation, catheterization is required for drainage. This obviates the need for artificial sphincter implantation in patients with incompetent urinary sphincters.

The Kock reservoir has also been modified for

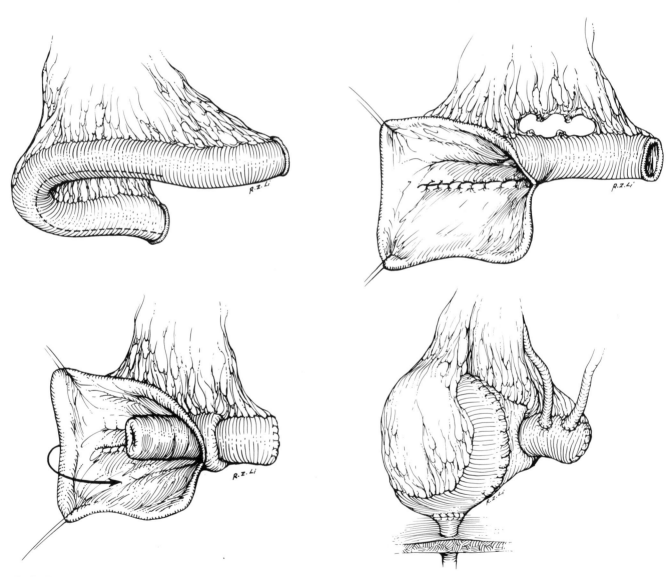

FIGURE 10.25
Bladder substitute from reconfigured ileum (Hemi-Kock substitute)

bladder substitution by elimination of the efferent intussusception and outlet. The afferent inlet and intussusception are developed from the proximal 15 cm of a 45-cm ileal segment (Figure 10.25). End-to-side ureteroileal anastomoses are made in this limb. The storage component is created from the distal 30-cm section. Two 15-cm segments are opposed, opened on the antimesenteric border, and joined by approximation of the adjacent margins. The reservoir is closed by folding the ileal sheet medially and approximating the bowel edges. An opening made in the most dependent aspect of the storage reservoir is anastomosed with the urethra.

The Mainz reservoir is also suitable for bladder substitution by anastomosis of the ileal outlet to the urethra. An ileoileal intussusception in the reservoir outlet could be used if the urinary sphincter is incompetent.

POSTOPERATIVE CARE AND COMPLICATIONS

Urethral catheter drainage is required for several weeks after bladder substitution procedures. The catheter is removed when the cystogram reveals no extravasation. The patient voids by a coordinated relaxation of the perineal musculature and abdominal straining when pelvic fullness or cramping is sensed.

As with continent urinary reservoirs, leakage at the suture lines is the most common postoperative complication. Late complications are related primarily to urinary control. As great as 50 percent of patients with the Camey reservoir and a poorly defined portion of patients with other forms of bladder substitutes experience enuresis. Total incontinence occurs in approximately 10 percent of cases.

Clinically significant ureteral reflux or obstruction, electrolyte imbalance, stone formation, and intestinal malabsorption are not common. Most patients with bladder substitutes do not have bacteriuria. Carcinogenesis in the transposed bowel is not anticipated and has not been observed. However, intermittent urethroscopy and cytologic examination of the urine are required to detect urethral recurrences in patients with bladder substitutes created after cystectomy for transitional cell carcinoma.

CHAPTER 11

Surgery of the Prostate Gland

The prostate is a chestnut-sized glandular organ that lies between the bladder outlet and the urogenital diaphragm and is traversed by the urethra. The symphysis pubis is anterior, the levator ani muscles are lateral, and the rectum is posterior to the prostate (Figure 11.1). It is stabilized by the paired puboprostatic ligaments and by the reflections of the endopelvic fascia. Denonvilliers' fascia covers the posterior prostate as well as the vasa deferentia and seminal vesicles. The lateral pelvic fascia invests the anterior and anterolateral surfaces. Neurovascular bundles posterolateral to the prostate are situated in extensions of this fascial sheet. Erectile function may be preserved if these bundles are not injured during radical prostatectomy. The rectourethralis muscles course between the apex of the prostate and the urogenital diaphragm.

The prostate is encompassed by a thick fibrous capsule. The ejaculatory ducts pierce the posterosuperior margin and enter the urethra at the verumontanum (see Figure 12.1). There are four zones of prostatic parenchyma that differ histologically and functionally (Figure 11.2). The peripheral zone is below and behind the ejaculatory ducts and contains about 70 percent of the glandular tissue. Adenocarcinomas of the prostate usually develop in this zone. The central zone occupies the posterior aspect above the verumontanum and surrounds the ejaculatory ducts. It comprises about 25 percent of the glandular tissue. The transition zone surrounds the urethra above the verumontanum and contains 5 to 10 percent of the glandular tissue. Benign prostatic hyperplasia develops in this zone. Finally, the anterior aspect of the prostate is composed of nonglandular fibromuscular tissue.

The arterial blood supply is derived from the inferior vesical artery, a terminal branch of the hypogastric artery. This artery enters the posterolateral base of the prostate and perfuses the parenchyma and the urethra. A capsular branch, which courses posterolateral to the prostate in the neurovascular bundle, supplies the capsule and peripheral parenchyma. Venous drainage is to

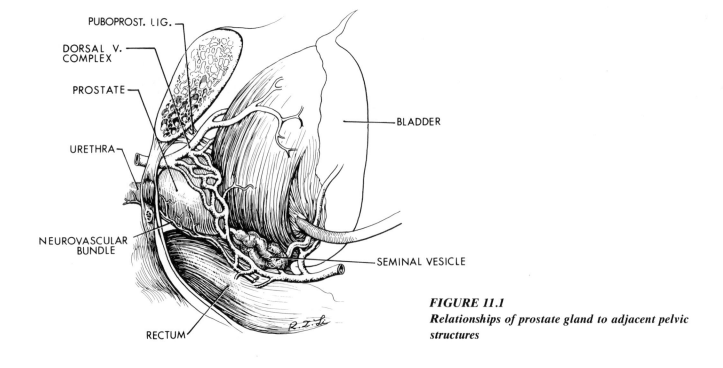

PUBOPROST. LIG.
DORSAL V. COMPLEX
PROSTATE
URETHRA
NEUROVASCULAR BUNDLE
RECTUM
BLADDER
SEMINAL VESICLE

FIGURE 11.1
Relationships of prostate gland to adjacent pelvic structures

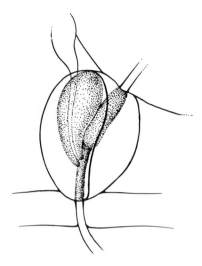

FIGURE 11.2
Zones of the prostate

the dorsal venous plexus and, ultimately, to the hypogastric veins.

Benign prostatic hyperplasia and adenocarcinoma are the primary prostatic disorders of surgical concern.

Operations for Benign Prostatic Hyperplasia

Benign prostatic hyperplasia (BPH) arises from glands in the transition zone and is characterized histologically by varying degrees of stromal, fibrous, muscular, and glandular hyperplasia. Its etiology is unknown, but histologic evidence of BPH is observed in most men older than 50 years of age. There are no reliable medical treatments for the condition.

Expansion of the hyperplastic tissue results in an increased resistance to urinary outflow and palpable enlargement of the prostate gland. The former is manifested by a decrease in the caliber and force of the urinary stream, hesitancy, intermittency, and in some cases acute urinary retention. With chronic outlet obstruction there is hypertrophy of the detrusor muscle. This and incomplete bladder emptying result in urinary frequency, nocturia, and in advanced stages, overflow incontinence and hydronephrosis.

Enlargement of the prostate per se is not an indication for operative intervention. In the absence of a medical reason for prostatectomy, the patient should decide whether intervention is appropriate. This judgment is based on the magnitude of voiding symptoms, the risks of surgery, and the knowledge that the symptoms may or may not increase.

Removal of obstructing hyperplastic tissue, or adenomas, is accomplished by transurethral resection or by enucleation with open surgery. The transurethral approach, which is addressed in Chapter 18, is better tolerated and applicable for most affected patients. When the weight of the hyperplastic tissue is estimated to exceed 50 to 70 g, the open approach may be preferable. However, the criteria for transurethral and open surgery are quite variable and generally reflect the skill and experience of the urologist with the two techniques.

Open prostatectomy is advantageous if there are coexisting vesical calculi that are difficult to remove with transurethral techniques or large symptomatic diverticula that require excision. Conditions that make transurethral resection difficult (e.g., extension of large adenomas into the bladder lumen, small bladder capacity) and skeletal disorders that do not permit the lithotomy position are also indications for open surgery.

Small adenomas can be exceedingly difficult to enucleate and should be managed by transurethral resection whenever possible. Prostatic carcinoma also complicates the operation because the plane between the true prostate (or surgical capsule) and the hyperplastic prostate is often destroyed by infiltrating tumor.

The anatomic and functional status of the upper urinary tract is established before surgery with an intravenous pyelogram. Cystoscopy is also recommended to assess the size and location of hyperplastic tissue and to eliminate the possibility of coexisting but unsuspected urethral or bladder disease. Prostatic adenomas can be enucleated through a suprapubic, retropubic, or perineal approach. The transvesical–capsular approach combines elements of the suprapubic and retropubic operations by means of a vertical incision extending from the bladder into the prostatic capsule. This is a reasonable alternative if direct visualization of both the prostatic fossa and the bladder lumen is desired.

We routinely administer prophylactic antibiotics in the perioperative period and delay the operation if the urine is unexpectedly infected.

SUPRAPUBIC PROSTATECTOMY

The suprapubic prostatectomy provides generous exposure to the bladder lumen and is preferred when there are coexisting surgically correctable vesical disorders. Many urologists also recommend this approach when the adenoma extends into the bladder lumen. Exposure of the prostatic fossa, however, is suboptimal.

OPERATIVE TECHNIQUE The patient is placed in the supine position, and a urethral catheter is introduced and left in the sterile field. Intravenous indigo carmine, 10 ml, is administered shortly after beginning the operation to facilitate the location of the ureteral orifices. The retropubic space is entered through a low abdominal incision, and peritoneum is swept from the dome of the bladder. A transverse cystotomy 2 cm above the base of the prostate is made between stay sutures, and the bladder outlet is exposed by lateral and superior retraction with narrow blade retractors (Figure 11.3). The urethral catheter is removed, and the vesical mucosa surrounding the base of the prostate but well away from the ureteral orifices is incised with a knife or cautery. The retractors are removed, and a finger is forced into the prostatic urethra and thrust anteriorly to "crack" the thin anterior tissue. A plane between the adenoma and the surgical capsule is then developed with finger dissection laterally and posteriorly. The urethral mucosa at the apex of the adenoma is encircled with the fingers and "pinched off." The adenoma is then delivered into the bladder, and residual attachments at the posterior bladder outlet are transected with scissors. If the adenoma is large, two or more "lobes" may be removed separately. Adherence of the adenoma to the capsule may necessitate dissection with scissors.

The prostatic fossa is carefully palpated to ensure that all nodular tissue is removed. Insertion of a finger into the rectum also helps to assess the completeness

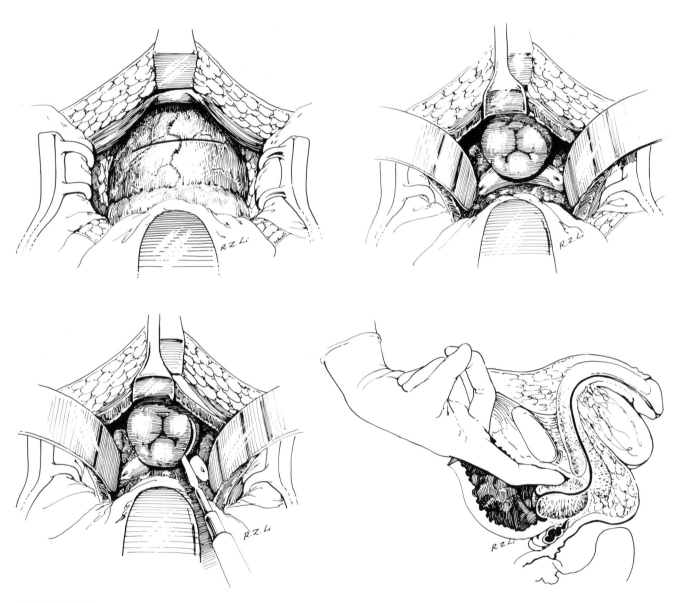

FIGURE 11.3
Suprapubic prostatectomy

of the enucleation. The retractors are replaced into the bladder, and the prostatic fossa is packed with gauze. Deep figure-of-eight heavy absorbable sutures are placed in the bladder outlet at the 4 and 8 o'clock positions to secure the inferior vesical arteries (Figure 11.4). If the bladder outlet is snug, a wedge of tissue in the posterior midline is removed, and the mucosa of the posterior bladder outlet is sutured to the prostatic fossa. The packing is then removed, and the fossa is exposed by lateral retraction of the bladder outlet with narrow blade retractors and continuous suction. It is difficult to manipulate a needle within the prostatic fossa, and hemostasis is achieved with electrocautery.

When hemostasis appears adequate, a 22 F Foley catheter with a 30-ml balloon is introduced transurethrally. The balloon is inflated in the bladder and placed on moderate traction. We prefer to use a suprapubic catheter to supplement bladder drainage when

hemostasis is less than optimal. The cystotomy is closed in two layers and a Penrose drain is placed in the retropubic space.

RETROPUBIC PROSTATECTOMY

The retropubic approach provides excellent exposure of the prostatic fossa that facilitates the control of bleeding vessels.

OPERATIVE TECHNIQUE   The anterior bladder is exposed as described for a suprapubic prostatectomy, but the dissection is extended to the puboprostatic ligaments. Friable veins and fatty tissue overlying the prostatic capsule are swept laterally, and a small sponge is packed between the prostatic capsule and levator ani muscles on each side. Heavy stay sutures are placed just distal to the bladder outlet and just

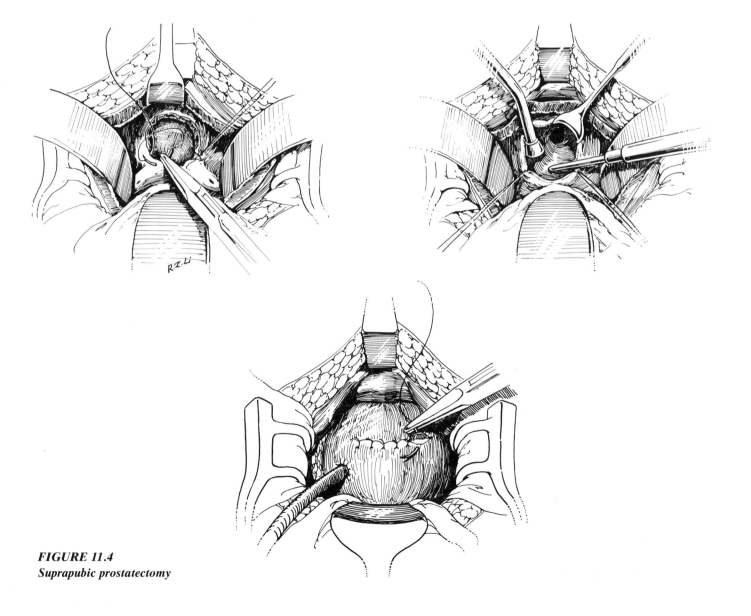

FIGURE 11.4
Suprapubic prostatectomy

proximal to the puboprostatic ligaments to secure veins within the lateral pelvic fascia. The urethral catheter is removed at this juncture, and 10 ml of indigo carmine is administered intravenously to facilitate identification of the ureteral orifices after the adenoma has been removed.

With the use of electrocautery a transverse capsulotomy is made between the stay sutures and is carried into the adenoma (Figure 11.5). A plane between the surgical capsule and adenoma is established around the margins of the capsulotomy with the tips of a scissors. With the index finger the plane of enucleation is developed laterally, posteriorly, and inferiorly. At the

apex of the adenoma the urethra is pinched off or transected with scissors under direct vision. The anterior plane is then developed superiorly, and the mucosa of the anterior bladder outlet is perforated. The adenoma is grasped with a uterine tenaculum or Allis clamp, separated from the posterior bladder outlet with a scissors, and removed (Figure 11.6). The sponges lateral to the prostate are extracted, and the fossa is palpated with a finger to identify residual adenomatous tissue.

A narrow blade retractor is introduced through the capsulotomy and the bladder outlet and pulled superiorly to expose the posterior outlet and prostatic fossa.

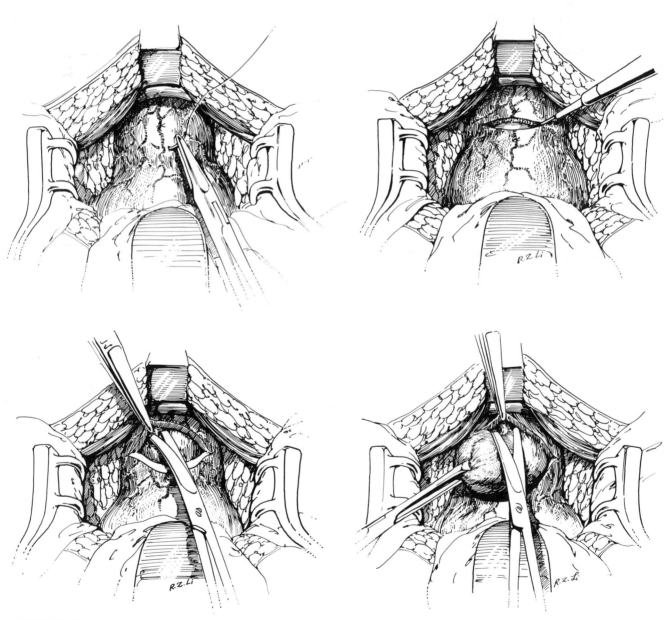

FIGURE 11.5
Retropubic prostatectomy

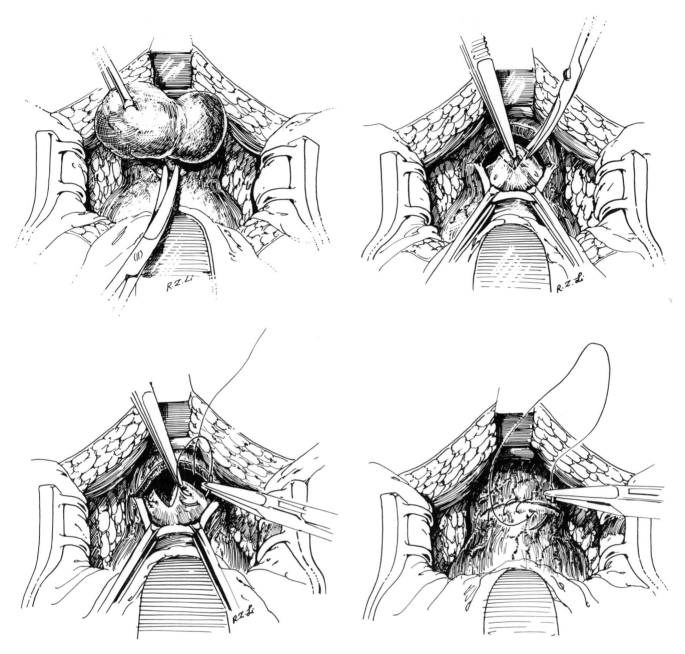

FIGURE 11.6
Retropubic prostatectomy

If bleeding is excessive the fossa is packed with gauze. The trigone and ureteral orifices are identified, and a wedge of tissue is excised from the posteromedial bladder outlet. Heavy absorbable figure-of-eight sutures are placed at the 4 and 8 o'clock positions to secure the inferior vesical arteries, and the margin of the posterior bladder outlet is tacked to the prostatic fossa with interrupted absorbable sutures. All bleeders in the prostatic fossa are fulgurated or secured with ligatures under direct vision.

A 22 F Foley catheter with a 30-ml balloon is intro- duced transurethrally and manipulated into the blad- der. The capsulotomy is closed with two continuous heavy absorbable sutures. The closure is initiated be- yond the lateral aspect of the capsulotomy and pro- gresses to the midline. The second suture is used to close the contralateral side in an identical manner. The bladder is distended with saline to identify leakage at the suture line and a Penrose drain is placed in the retropubic space. A suprapubic cystostomy is gener- ally not necessary but can be performed in the unusual case where hemostasis is suboptimal.

PERINEAL PROSTATECTOMY

The perineal approach to prostatic surgery has lost favor with many urologists largely owing to increased experience with retropubic surgery. Visualization of the prostatic fossa is excellent, but the risks of impotence and rectal injury are probably greater than with the suprapubic or retropubic approaches.

OPERATIVE TECHNIQUE   Adequate exposure for perineal prostatectomy requires an exaggerated lithotomy position. Sandbags are placed under the sacrum so that the perineum has a vertical orientation.

A curved perineal incision is made 2 cm from the perianal skin (Figure 11.7). The lateral extent should lie medial to the ischial tuberosites. The ischiorectal fossae are opened with a scalpel. A finger is inserted into each fossa and worked medially to meet anterior to the rectum in the midline. Subcutaneous tissue and the central tendon are divided, care taken to ligate small arterial bleeders. A curved Lowsley tractor is

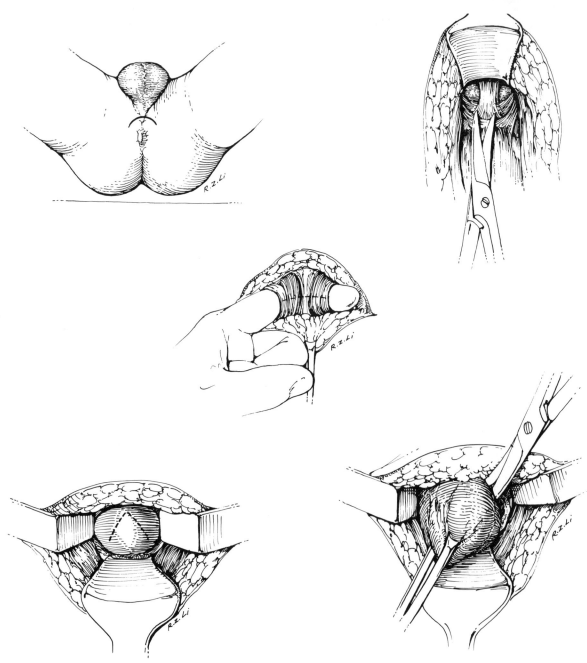

FIGURE 11.7
Perineal prostatectomy

introduced into the bladder to facilitate identification of the membranous urethra and prostate. The rectum is pushed downward and the levator ani muscles are divided at the midline. Fine extensions of the rectourethralis muscle are also transected. The blades of the Lowsley tractor are opened, and the prostate is pulled inferiorly with anterior rotation of the handle. This permits dissection of the rectum from the prostate under direct vision.

The rectum is displaced downward with a small retractor over a protective pad. Lateral and superior retraction of the external anal sphincter also enhances exposure. A transverse or inverted V capsulotomy is made into the substance of the adenoma with electrocautery. The cleavage plane between the adenoma and surgical capsule is established with a scissors under direct vision. The dissection is preferably carried to the apex of the adenoma first, where the urethra is incised with the scalpel. The curved Lowsley tractor is removed, the anterior aspect of the urethra is transected, and a straight Lowsley tractor is inserted through the apex of the adenoma. The adenoma is then enucleated anteriorly and the bladder lumen is entered. The posterolateral cleavage plane is developed to the bladder outlet, mucosal attachments are divided with a scissors, and the specimen is removed.

Figure-of-eight sutures are placed in the bladder outlet at the 4 and 8 o'clock positions to secure the inferior vesical arteries. The prostatic fossa is palpated to identify residual adenoma, and bleeding vessels are cauterized or ligated under direct vision. A wedge of tissue may be excised from the posterior midline of the bladder outlet.

A 22 F Foley catheter with a 30-ml balloon is inserted through the urethra and the bladder outlet, and the capsulotomy is closed with interrupted or continuous heavy absorbable sutures (Figure 11.8). A Penrose drain is placed next to the suture line and brought out through a perineal stab wound. Reapproximation of the levator ani muscles and central tendon is not necessary. The subcutaneous tissue and skin are closed with interrupted heavy absorbable sutures.

POSTOPERATIVE CARE AND COMPLICATIONS

The postoperative care after each of the three techniques of open prostatectomy is similar. The catheter is taped to the thigh with modest traction to compress the bladder outlet and reduce bleeding. Intermittent manual irrigation may be necessary for the evacuation of blood clot. Continuous slow irrigation of the bladder through a three-way catheter helps to clear blood before it coagulates. This management, however, mandates close nursing supervision because obstruction of the drainage lumen leads to overdistention of the bladder and disruption of suture lines. In most cases the urine is clear on the first or second postoperative day. Excessive hemorrhage or recurrent accumulation of clot necessitates endoscopic examination and fulguration of bleeders.

The urethral catheter is removed on the fourth to fifth postoperative day, and if present, the suprapubic catheter is clamped. The Penrose drain is removed 24 hours later if drainage is minimal. Excessive drainage necessitates unclamping of the suprapubic catheter or reinsertion of the urethral catheter.

Oral antibiotics are administered for 1 week after hospital discharge, and the urine is cultured 1 and 4 weeks after discharge. Most patients experience mild but worrisome urgency incontinence for 1 to 2 weeks

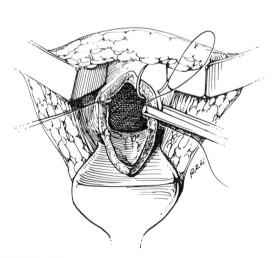

FIGURE 11.8
Perineal prostatectomy

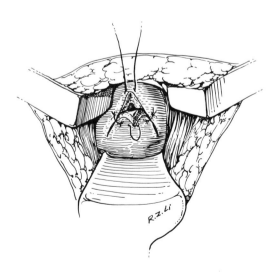

after catheter removal. Transient stress incontinence is not uncommon.

Permanent stress incontinence is the most distressing late complication of open prostatectomy, and results usually from injury to the membranous urethra during enucleation of the apical adenoma. Unrecognized neurogenic bladder dysfunction may also lead to stress or urgency incontinence when the obstructive adenoma is removed. Impotence is remarkably infrequent unless a perineal approach has been used. Bladder neck contractures are uncommon, but inflammation caused by the urethral catheter may lead to the formation of filmy urethral strictures. These can be managed usually by simple urethral dilation. Separation of the skin edges after perineal prostatectomy is not uncommon and is treated with warm sitz baths.

Operations for Prostate Cancer

Prostate cancer is the second most common solid tumor and the third leading cause of cancer deaths among men in the United States. The primary tumor is usually manifested by palpable induration or nodularity of the prostate, and biopsy of the abnormal area is the means of diagnosis. Approximately 10 percent of localized cancers are not palpable and are discovered by histologic examination of tissue that is removed for the management of obstructive symptomatology.

PROSTATE BIOPSY

There are no reliable noninvasive tests for localized prostate cancer. However, tissue is easily procured by needle, aspiration, or transurethral biopsy for histologic investigation. Even with unequivocal evidence of disseminated prostate cancer, treatment is never instituted until the diagnosis is confirmed histologically by biopsy of the primary tumor.

Needle Biopsy

Cylindrical cores of prostatic tissue are obtained by biopsy with a Tru-cut or a Vim-Silverman biopsy needle. The needle is introduced into the prostate with a transperineal or transrectal approach. A spring-loaded biopsy device that discharges a small-caliber needle similar to the Tru-cut needle is now available. This ''Biopty'' apparatus can be used in conjunction with transrectal ultrasonography to permit precise positioning of the needle tract within the prostate. The transrectal approach is also necessary when the Biopty needle is used without ultrasound guidance.

The disadvantages of transrectal prostate biopsy are bacteremia and sepsis caused by contamination of the needle tract with fecal material. Chronic infection and abscess of the prostate, however, are remarkably unusual. The advantage of the transrectal approach is more accurate positioning of the needle over localized prostatic induration.

Hospitalization and anesthesia are not required for a needle biopsy, but a parenteral antibiotic is admin-

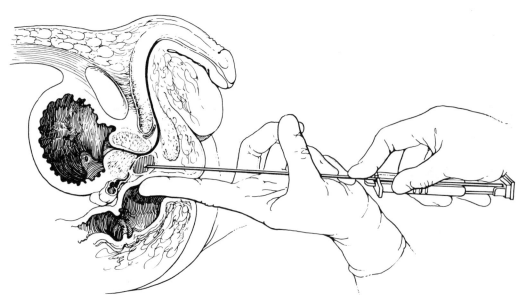

FIGURE 11.9
Transperineal needle biopsy of prostate

stered before the procedure. We also administer an antiseptic enema before transrectal biopsy.

OPERATIVE TECHNIQUE For transperineal biopsy (Figure 11.9) the patient is placed in the lithotomy position and the scrotum is retracted superiorly. The perineum is prepared, and the midline perineal skin and subcutaneous tissues are infiltrated with lidocaine. A small stab wound is made in the midline, and the index finger is inserted in the rectum to guide the needle. The Tru-cut needle in the closed position is advanced through the perineum to a point adjacent to the indurated prostate. The obturator is then thrust into the prostate, the sheath is advanced over the obturator to shear the tissue core, and the needle is twisted and withdrawn in the closed position. The tissue specimen is teased from the needle with a fine forceps or small-gauge needle. The process is repeated to obtain two or three cores approximately 1 cm in length.

Perforation of the posterior urethra or bladder during biopsy is not infrequent but is generally innocuous. Pressure is applied to the perineum for several minutes to tamponade bleeding. Cystoscopy is performed before or after biopsy as indicated.

With transrectal biopsy (Figure 11.10) the needle is passed through the anus on the volar aspect of the index finger, the tip is positioned over the area of induration, and a biopsy of the prostate is done through the rectal wall. The Biopty needle is also introduced through the anus and discharged into the prostate.

POSTOPERATIVE CARE AND COMPLICATIONS A fluoro-quinolone antibiotic at full oral dosage is administered for 3 to 5 days after biopsy. Prostatic and periprostatic inflammation is inevitable, and some urologists believe that radical prostatectomy, if indicated, should be performed within a week of biopsy or delayed for 4 to 8 weeks after biopsy. Implantation of tumor cells in the biopsy tract is extremely unusual.

Aspiration Biopsy

An aspiration biopsy of the prostate is performed in a transrectal manner with a Franzen needle apparatus. A pathologist skilled in the interpretation of cytologic specimens is a prerequisite for the diagnosis of cancer with aspiration techniques.

OPERATIVE TECHNIQUE A needle guide secured to the index finger is introduced into the rectum and positioned over the prostate (Figure 11.11). A malleable fine-gauge needle is then advanced through the guide and into the prostate. A syringe that is fixed in a specially designed holder and attached to the hub of the needle is placed on suction. The aspiration needle is moved back and forth within the prostate, and cellular material is sucked into the needle. The needle is withdrawn, and its contents are smeared on a slide and stained. Examination of the specimen can be done immediately.

Transurethral Biopsy

Transurethral biopsy of the prostate is indicated when radical surgery is not a treatment option, and symptoms of bladder outlet obstruction due to prostatic hyperplasia or carcinoma necessitate surgical

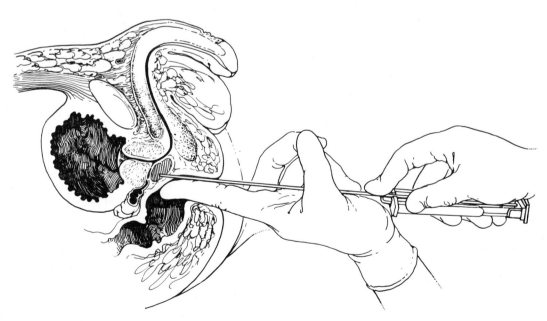

FIGURE 11.10
Transrectal needle biopsy of prostate

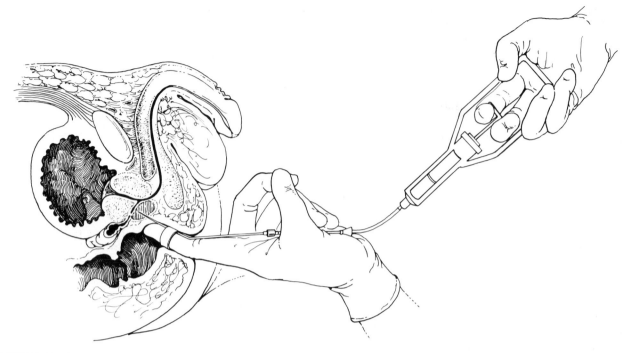

FIGURE 11.11
Aspiration biopsy of prostate

intervention. In the unusual case where multiple attempts at diagnosis by needle biopsy are unrevealing but the suspicion of carcinoma is great, diagnosis may require examination of more extensive portions of the prostate procured by this technique.

RADICAL PROSTATECTOMY

Radical prostatectomy is the most reliable means for eradication or control of localized tumors. The prospects for cure are greatly reduced if there is palpable tumor extention beyond the prostatic capsule or pelvic lymph node metastases. The advisability of surgery in these circumstances is controversial.

Radical prostatectomy is performed through a retropubic or perineal approach and involves removal of the entire prostate, distal vasa deferentia, and seminal vesicles. Radical retropubic prostatectomy allows simultaneous pelvic lymphadenectomy, and techniques for the preservation of potency have been detailed and verified. Impotence almost always follows radical perineal prostatectomy when performed using traditional methods. However, technical modifications that preserve the posterolateral neurovascular bundle reduce the risks of this complication. As with all operations, the preferred approach is dictated by the skills and experience of the surgeon.

Radical Retropubic Prostatectomy

The technique described for radical retropubic prostatectomy includes maneuvers developed by Dr. Patrick Walsh for control of the dorsal venous complex and for preservation of the neurovascular bundles posterolateral to the prostate. The former is invaluable for preventing difficult-to-control hemorrhage, whereas the latter is necessary for the preservation of potency.

Prophylactic antibiotics are administered in the perioperative period, and the operation is delayed if urine culture before surgery demonstrates unexpected infection.

OPERATIVE TECHNIQUE A supine position with the break of the table halfway between the umbilicus and the symphysis pubis is recommended. A Foley catheter is introduced and left in the sterile field. The pelvis is approached through a lower midline incision, and an extraperitoneal pelvic lymphadenectomy is performed as described in Chapter 17. Depending on treatment philosophy, the lymph nodes may be sent for frozen section examination and the operation aborted if metastases are identified. Alternatively, some authorities prefer to omit the lymphadenectomy.

If a radical prostatectomy is undertaken, the table is broken for 30° and rotated into the Trendelenburg position so that the lower abdomen is parallel to the floor. The peritoneal envelope is retracted superiorly with the malleable center blade of a self-retaining retractor. The endopelvic fascia is incised in the deepest recess and opened anteromedially to the puboprostatic ligaments (Figure 11.12). The index finger is insinuated through the defect, and the lateral prostate is freed from the levator ani muscles with blunt dissection. The dorsal venous complex and fatty tissue overlying the prostate are gently separated from the posterior symphysis to expose the puboprostatic ligaments. Down-ward pressure on the base of the prostate with two sponge-on-ring forceps enhances exposure. The puboprostatic ligaments are then transected flush with the periosteum of the symphysis. These ligaments are avascular, and the application of hemostatic clips or sutures is not necessary. After transection of the ligaments, the prostate falls away from the symphysis.

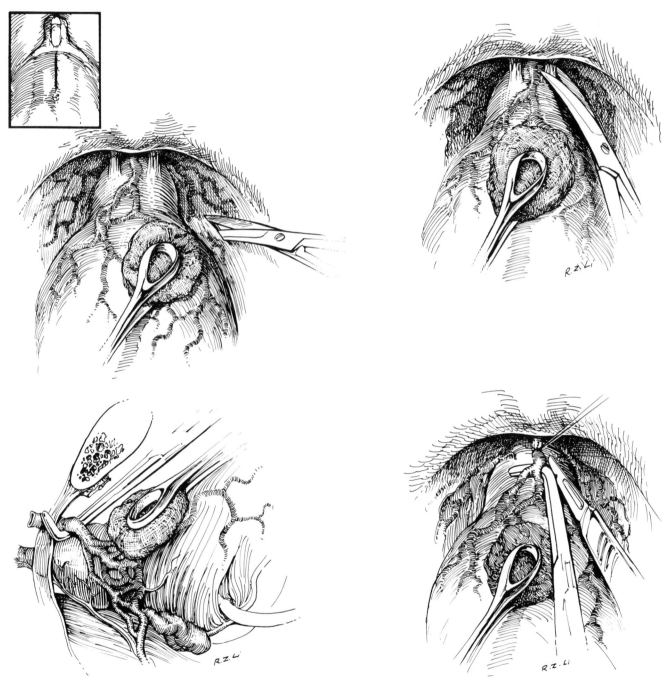

FIGURE 11.12
Incision of endopelvic fascia and transection of puboprostatic ligaments and dorsal venous complex in radical retropubic prostatectomy

However, additional blunt dissection is required to expose the apex of the prostate.

The dorsal venous complex and associated fascial tissue form a palpable plate approximately 2 cm in width and 1 cm in thickness over the apex of the prostate. A large right-angle clamp is introduced under the complex at the 3 o'clock position lateral to the urethra, worked over the anterior aspect of the urethra, and penetrated through the contralateral fascial tissue at the 9 o'clock position. The clamp is gently separated to enlarge the plane, and a 0-silk suture is grasped and drawn through the defect. The suture is tied as distally as possible, the right-angle clamp is repositioned, and the complex is transected proximal to the tie with a long-handled knife. Back bleeding is minimal, but several small arterial bleeders on the anterior surface of the prostate usually require fulguration.

A longitudinal plane is developed with the points of a clamp between the urethra and adjacent fascial tissue that contain the neurovascular bundle. A right-angle clamp is then worked around the apex of the prostate, and an umbilical tape is grasped and drawn through the defect (Figure 11.13). The anterior aspect of the urethra is transected under direct vision to expose the urethral catheter. The catheter is transected just beyond the urethral meatus and pulled into the pelvis, care taken to avoid leakage of fluid from the balloon inflation channel. Retraction of the prostate with the catheter greatly facilitates subsequent maneuvers. The right-angle clamp is repositioned behind the urethra and the posterior aspect is transected under direct vision with a long-handled knife.

The apex of the prostate is retracted superiorly with the catheter, and the midline rectourethralis muscles

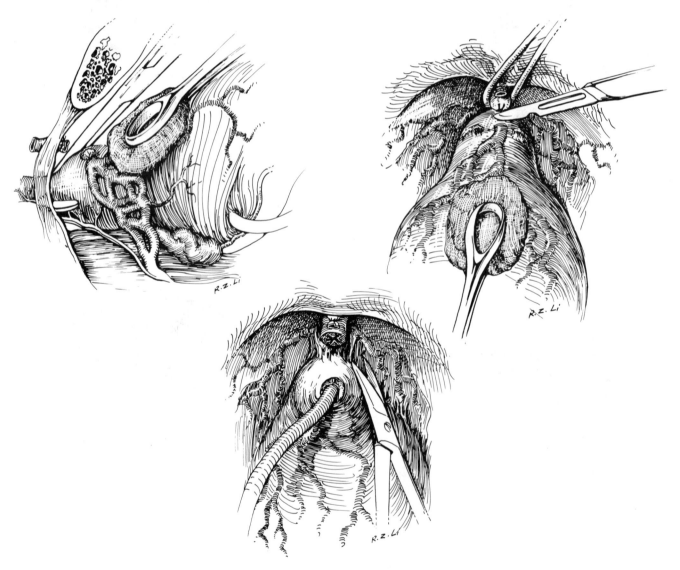

FIGURE 11.13
Transection of urethra and rectourethralis muscles

are transected with a scissors. Small avascular bands of muscle extending between the lateral prostatic capsule and the posterior symphysis are usually encountered and are divided with a scissors.

The index finger is inserted behind the apex, and the posteromedial prostate and investing Denonvilliers' fascia are separated from the rectum (Figure 11.14). One mobilizes the posterolateral prostate by sweeping a finger laterally while hugging the contour of the prostate. This helps to define the posterolateral vascular pedicle that arises from the posterolateral neurovascular bundle. The apex of the prostate is pulled to the contralateral side, and a right-angle clamp is positioned in the notch between the vascular pedicle and the anterolateral prostatic capsule. The pedicle is clamped just above the neurovascular bundle, transected, and secured with a fine nonabsorbable suture. The maneuver is repeated two to three times to divide the pedicle to the base of the prostate. If there is palpable induration of the prostate adjacent to the pedicle,

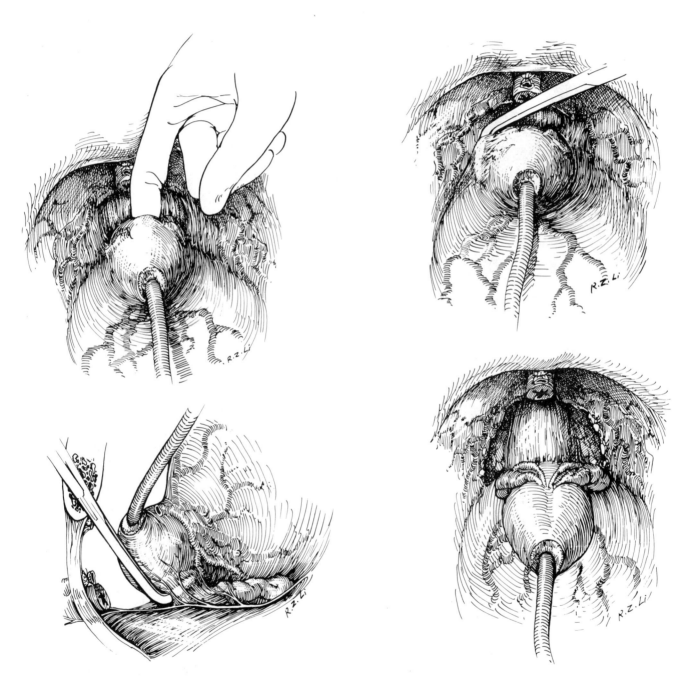

FIGURE 11.14
Dissection of prostate from rectum and division of posterolateral vascular pedicles

the clamp is applied more laterally to include the neurovascular bundle. The prostate is then retracted away from the opposite side, and the contralateral pedicle is transected in an identical manner.

With the apex of the prostate retracted superiorly, the vasa deferentia and the laterally situated seminal vesicles are seen beneath Denonvilliers' fascia. The inferior vesical arteries lying adjacent to the junction of the seminal vesicles and prostate are also accentuated with this maneuver. These vessels, which consti-

tute the superior extent of the vascular pedicle, are clamped, transected, and ligated.

A vertical or transverse incision is made in Denonvilliers' fascia and each vas is isolated and divided between large hemostatic clips. The seminal vesicles are then mobilized from the bladder anteriorly and Denonvilliers' fascia posteriorly, and vessels entering their tips are secured with hemostatic clips. If difficulties are encountered during this component of the operation, it is advisable to delay the dissection until

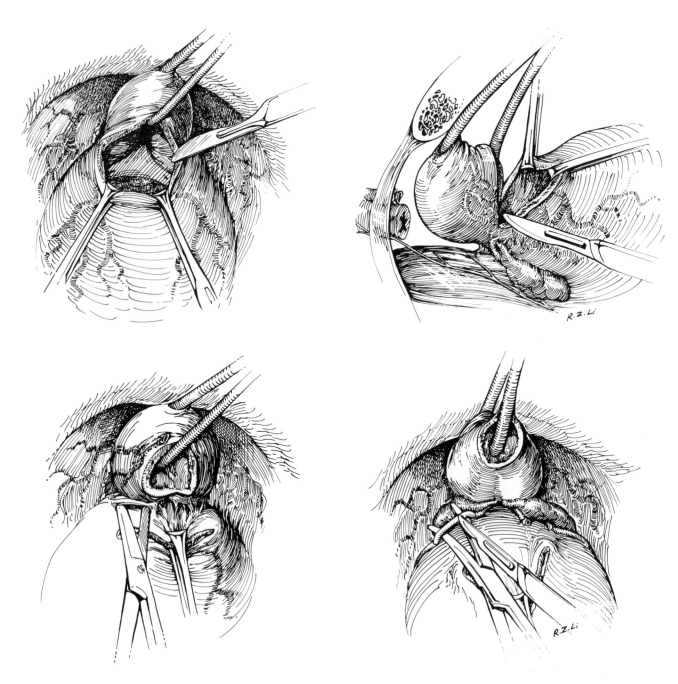

FIGURE 11.15
Transection of bladder outlet and dissection of vasa deferentia and seminal vesicles

the prostate has been amputated from the base of the bladder.

The bladder lumen is entered anteriorly with sharp dissection just above the palpable prostate (Figure 11.15). The tip of the Foley catheter is brought through this incision and clamped with the distal end to serve as a sling for subsequent retraction. Indigo carmine is administered intravenously to help identify the ureteral orifices, and the bladder mucosa 1 cm below the orifices is incised. The plane between the posterior bladder outlet and the seminal vesicles and vasa deferentia is exposed with upward retraction of the prostate. The posterior bladder outlet is transected with a scissors and the specimen is removed. If the vasa deferentia and seminal vesicles were not isolated earlier, a plane behind the bladder outlet is developed with scissors, and the vasa and vesicles are mobilized after dividing the bladder outlet.

The lumen of the bladder outlet is reduced as necessary to accommodate the small finger (Figure 11.16). Through-and-through heavy absorbable sutures are used to approximate the posterolateral margins in a tennis-racket manner. The ureteral orifices should be visualized during this maneuver to prevent entrapment.

We use a metal sound with grooves on the end to direct and stabilize needles during the placement of sutures in the urethral stump. An in-and-out movement of the sound also helps to expose the margins of the stump. Through-and-through heavy absorbable su-

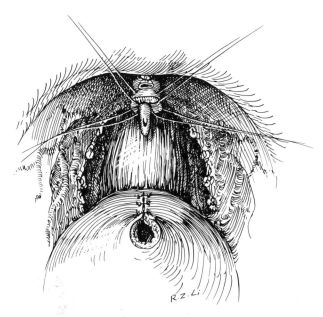

FIGURE 11.16
Reduction of bladder outlet and vesicourethral anastomosis

tures on $\frac{5}{8}$ tapered needles are placed at the 2 and 10 o'clock positions. Each suture is clamped with a marked hemostat for subsequent identification. Sutures are then placed at the 4 and 8 o'clock positions, taking care to avoid entrapment of the adjacent neurovascular bundle. The luminal end of each suture is then passed through the corresponding position of the bladder outlet. If the urethral suture was placed from the inside out, the needle is removed and the luminal end is rethreaded on another curved needle. When each of the anastomotic sutures is properly positioned, a 22 F Foley catheter with a tested 30-ml balloon is advanced through the urethra and into the bladder. To make tying of the anastomotic sutures easier, the balloon is not inflated. The center blade of the self-retaining retractor is removed to reduce tension on the anastomosis and the posterior sutures are tied. Care is taken to approximate the bladder outlet directly with the urethral stump. The two anterior sutures are then tied, the Foley balloon is inflated, and the catheter is placed on modest traction.

A large Penrose drain is positioned in each obturator fossa and brought out through the inferior angle of the incision.

POSTOPERATIVE CARE AND COMPLICATIONS The urethral catheter is maintained on modest traction for 1 to 2 days to support the vesicourethral anastomosis. If the catheter is removed accidentally, we make one attempt at gentle blind reinsertion. If unsuccessful, the catheter is replaced under direct vision with urethroscopy. The risks of accidental removal are reduced if the nursing staff and patient appreciate the importance of the catheter.

Hematuria is usually minimal, but drainage from the Penrose drains may be profuse for 1 or 2 days after surgery. This drainage consists primarily of lymphatic fluid rather than urine. The drains are generally removed on the fourth or fifth postoperative day. Parenteral antibiotics are continued for 5 days, and prophylactic oral antibiotics are taken until catheter removal. When convalescence is uneventful, the patient is discharged 7 to 10 days after surgery and returns 2 weeks later for a cystogram. The catheter is removed if extravasation of contrast material at the vesicourethral anastomosis is not observed. Antibiotics are continued for 2 additional weeks. The agent is selected on the basis of susceptibility testing if the urine is infected.

Some degree of urgency or stress incontinence is inevitable after catheter removal, but resolves usually within 1 to 2 weeks. Stress urinary incontinence persisting for longer than 3 months is often permanent but occurs in less than 5 percent of patients. Erectile function is preserved in about 75 percent of patients if one or both neurovascular bundles are not damaged.

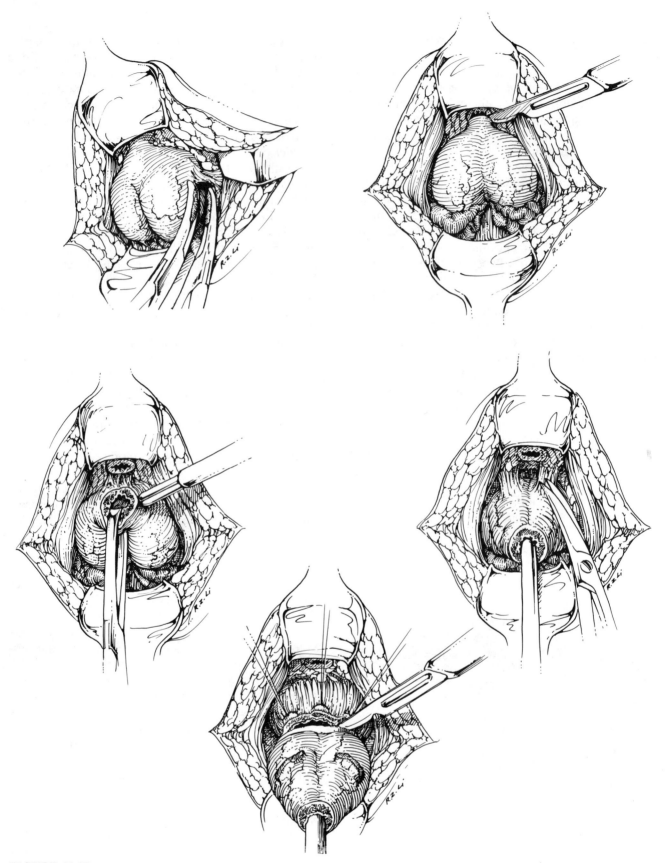

FIGURE 11.17
Transection of posterolateral vascular pedicles, urethra, puboprostatic ligaments, and anterior bladder outlet in radical perineal prostatectomy

However, erections that are suitable for satisfactory intercourse may not develop for 6 to 12 months.

Radical Perineal Prostatectomy

The perineal approach to radical prostatectomy is probably associated with less postoperative morbidity than the retropubic approach, and exposure of the urethrovesical anastomosis is superior.

OPERATIVE TECHNIQUE   The posterior surface of the prostate is approached through a perineal incision using the techniques described for subtotal perineal prostatectomy. However, the dissection must be carried more superiorly to expose the seminal vesicles (Figure 11.17). Denonvilliers' fascia is divided in the midline and swept laterally to expose the neurovascular bundles. The posterolateral vascular pedicles coursing superomedially from the bundles are then de-

veloped and divided immediately adjacent to the capsule. As with the radical retropubic prostatectomy, palpable induration adjacent to the pedicles mandates division more distant from the capsule and sacrifice of the neurovascular bundles. Some surgeons prefer to expose and divide the vascular pedicles after transection of the urethra and amputation of the prostate from the bladder outlet.

The curved Lowsley tractor is removed, and the urethra is transected at the apex of the prostate. Damage to the neurovascular bundles can be avoided if the fascia lying lateral to the apex is deliberately preserved. A straight Lowsley tractor or Foley catheter is then introduced through the apex of the prostate for retraction.

Anterior dissection of the prostate may proceed above or below the lateral pelvic fascia. If a plane is

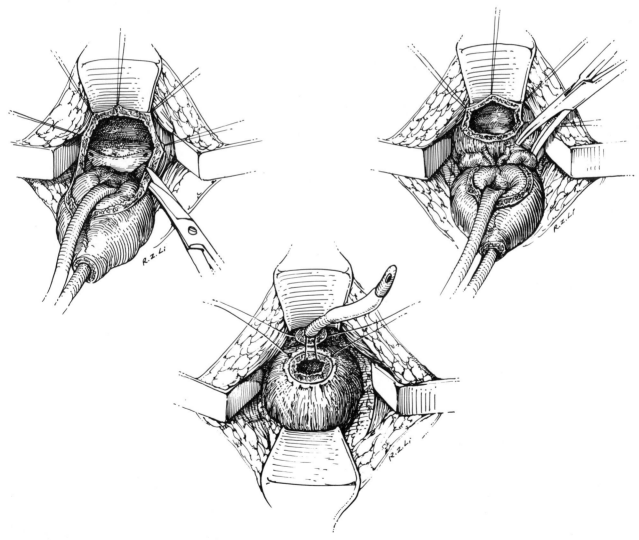

FIGURE 11.18
Division of posterior bladder outlet, dissection of seminal vesicles and vasa deferentia, and vesicourethral anastomosis

established below the fascia, the puboprostatic ligaments are not encountered, and the risk of injury to the dorsal venous complex is reduced. If a plane is developed above the fascia, as shown in Figure 11.17, the puboprostatic ligaments are transected, and the dorsal venous complex is secured with suture ligatures at the bladder outlet.

The bladder is entered above the anterior palpable prostate, and the incision is extended laterally to expose the ureteral orifices (Figure 11.18). The posterior bladder outlet is incised below the orifices and divided anterior to the seminal vesicles and vasa deferentia. If not done previously, the posterolateral vascular pedicles are developed and transected. Each vas deferens is isolated and transected between large hemostatic clips. The specimen is removed after the seminal vesicles are dissected from the posterior wall of the bladder and the adjacent Denonvilliers' fascia. Care is taken to ligate the apical vessels to the seminal vesicles.

The size of the bladder outlet is reduced as necessary with interrupted heavy absorbable sutures. A 22 F Foley catheter with a 30-ml balloon is introduced, and the bladder outlet is anastomosed with the urethra using six to eight interrupted through-and-through absorbable sutures.

A Penrose drain is positioned next to the anastomosis and brought out through a stab wound lateral to the perineal incision. The subcutaneous tissues and skin are closed with interrupted absorbable sutures.

The general postoperative care and complications parallel those for radical retropubic prostatectomy. The Penrose drainage is usually less, but the skin incision is more susceptible to breakdown.

IMPLANTATION OF RADIOACTIVE MATERIALS

Radiation therapy delivered from interstitial radioactive iodine or gold seeds provides excellent control of primary prostatic carcinomas and in some cases is curative. However, the best results are achieved with small tumors, and renewed interest in radical prostatectomy has dampened enthusiasm for these treatment modalities.

The radioactivity emanating from ^{125}I seeds is attenuated by surrounding tissues, and a homogeneous distribution of 25 to 50 seeds within the prostate is required for adequate dosimetry. The radioactivity of ^{198}Au seeds penetrates deeper, and implantation of a large number of seeds with a uniform distribution is not necessary. However, the half-life of this energy is less than 7 days, and supplemental external beam radiation therapy is required for tumoricidal treatment.

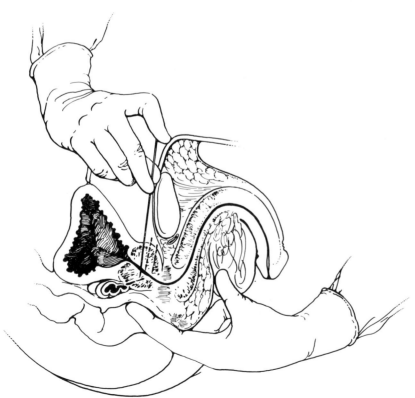

FIGURE 11.19
Implantation of prostate with ^{125}I seeds

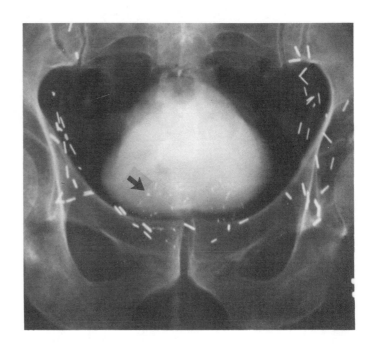

FIGURE 11.20
Radiographic appearance of prostate after implantation with ^{125}I seeds (arrow)

OPERATIVE TECHNIQUE   The patient is placed in a low lithotomy position, a sterile O'Connor sheath is inserted into the rectum, and a urethral catheter is introduced and left in the sterile field. A staging pelvic lymphadenectomy is generally performed before implantation of the prostate. The endopelvic fascia is then incised, and the anterolateral prostate is mobilized from the levator ani muscles. The anterior prostate is freed to the puboprostatic ligaments. With a finger in the rectum to define the posterior boundary of the implantation, the surgeon punctures the prostate with multiple hollow needles (Figure 11.19). Radioactive seeds are introduced into the needles and implanted with a Mich applicator. When ^{125}I is used, the needle is withdrawn 3 to 4 mm after placement of each seed until the entire tract is implanted. The radiographic appearance of the prostate after proper ^{125}I implantation is shown in Figure 11.20. Several hemostatic sutures applied to the prostatic capsule are generally necessary to control bleeding from puncture sites. A Penrose drain is positioned in each obturator fossa and brought out through the inferior angle of the incision.

POSTOPERATIVE CARE AND COMPLICATIONS   General postoperative care and complications parallel those following pelvic lymphadenectomy alone, but irritative and obstructive voiding symptoms are usually experienced for the first 2 to 4 weeks after surgery. Although urinary retention is not common, management with catheter drainage rather than transurethral resection of the prostate is advisable. The half-life of ^{125}I is 60 days, and operative intervention removes some of the seeds. In addition, healing of the prostatic fossa is compromised by continual radiation exposure.

CHAPTER 12

Surgery of the Seminal Vesicles

The seminal vesicles are thin-walled, septated structures approximately 6 cm in length. They secrete a gelatinous material that makes up a large portion of the ejaculate. The seminal vesicles are located anterior to Denonvilliers' fascia between the rectum and bladder. The ureters pass anterior to their superior aspects and the vasa deferentia lie medially (Figure 12.1). The distal end joins with the vas deferens to form the ejaculatory duct. This conduit traverses the prostate and enters into the posterior urethra lateral to the verumontanum. The vesicles are supplied by branches of the inferior vesicle artery and the artery of the vas deferens. Most of the venous drainage is to the periprostatic plexus. Blood vessels enter each vesicle at both the apex and base.

Primary disorders of the seminal vesicles are decidedly unusual and include cystic dilatation due to obstruction of the ejaculatory ducts, ectopic insertion of a ureter, infection, and on rare occasions, a primary neoplasm. Most are manifested by vague pelvic discomfort and produce palpable induration or enlargement. The lumen of a seminal vesicle can be opacified for radiographic study by antegrade injection of contrast medium through the vas deferens. Contrast can be introduced directly into large cystic masses by transperineal or transrectal puncture, or by transvesical puncture using endoscopic equipment. Cannulation of the ejaculatory ducts for the retrograde injection of contrast medium is usually quite difficult.

Transrectal ultrasonography, computed tomography, and magnetic resonance imaging can also define the nature and extent of seminal vesicle enlargement.

Seminal Vesiculectomy

The primary operative procedure of the seminal vesicles is excision. Infections generally respond to antimicrobial therapy, and abscessed seminal vesicles requiring incision and drainage are remarkably infrequent.

OPERATIVE TECHNIQUE   A perineal, transperitoneal, or transvesical approach may be used for removal of the seminal vesicles. However, exposure with the perineal approach is limited, and the alternatives should be used if there is marked enlargement. Catheterization of the ureters before surgery facilitates their intraoperative identification and reduces the risks of accidental injury.

The perineal approach parallels that described for radical perineal prostatectomy. Denonvilliers' fascia is incised and the vesicle is isolated by developing a plane along the adventitia with sharp dissection. The apical vessels are secured with a hemostatic clip, and the vesicle is delivered into the wound and transected next to the base of the prostate. The stump is secured with a suture ligature.

A lower abdominal incision is used for the transperitoneal and transvesical approach. With the transperitoneal procedure the peritoneum of the cul de sac is incised, and the ipsilateral posterolateral vascular pedicle to the bladder is developed and divided as described for a radical cystectomy. Satisfactory exposure may also necessitate transection of the anterolateral vascular pedicle. The bladder is retracted

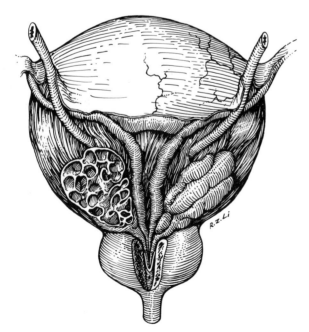

FIGURE 12.1
Relationships of seminal vesicles to bladder, ureters, vasa deferentia, and prostate (posterior view)

anteromedially and the apex of the vesicle is mobilized, taking care to secure the feeding vessels. The remainder of the vesicle is isolated by developing a plane on the adventitia. It is divided next to the base of the prostate, and the stump is secured with a suture ligature.

With the transvesical procedure the bladder is approached in an extraperitoneal fashion. A generous cystotomy is performed, and blade retractors are introduced to expose the trigone and posterior bladder wall. A vertical incision is made from the midtrigone to a point corresponding to the apex of the seminal vesicle. The margins of the bladder are retracted laterally with stay sutures or Allis clamps, and the vesicle is isolated and removed as described above. The posterior bladder incision and the anterior cystotomy are closed in the conventional manner. Drainage of the bladder with a suprapubic cystostomy is advisable.

POSTOPERATIVE CARE AND COMPLICATIONS Injury to the neurovascular bundles coursing lateral to the seminal vesicles may result in postoperative impotence. However, these bundles are preserved if the dissection is confined to the adventitia of the vesicles. Infertility is inevitable if both seminal vesicles are removed.

Surgery of the Penis

The penis comprises the paired corpora cavernosa, the ventral corpus spongiosum, and investing fascia and skin (Figure 13.1). The substance of each corpus cavernosum is a network of endothelial-lined spaces with intervening smooth muscle. Engorgement of the spaces with blood leads to penile erection. The crus, or proximal extent of each corpus cavernosum, is attached to the undersurface of the pubic arch and is covered by the ischiocavernosum muscle (Figure 13.2). The crura converge in the midline under the symphysis pubis and are separated by a septum as the corpora cavernosa extend to the glans penis.

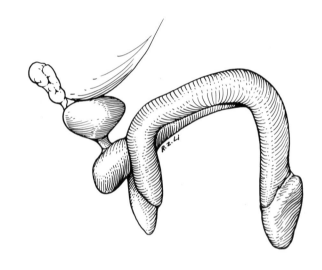

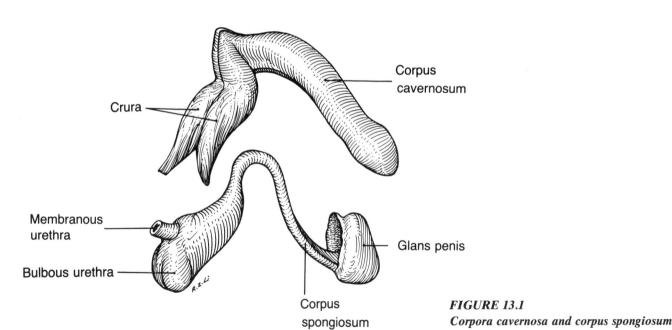

Crura

Corpus cavernosum

Membranous urethra

Bulbous urethra

Glans penis

Corpus spongiosum

FIGURE 13.1
Corpora cavernosa and corpus spongiosum

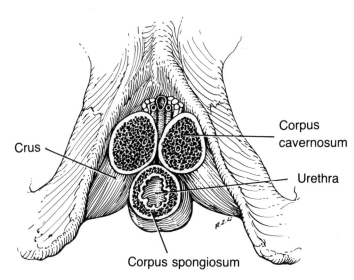

FIGURE 13.2
Cross-section of penis at pubic arch

The corpus spongiosum, situated in the midline below the corpora cavernosa, surrounds the urethra. The proximal end of the corpus is attached to the urogenital diaphragm. The segment lying between the urogenital diaphragm and the symphysis pubis is dilated, or bulbous, and is protected on the ventral surface by the bulbocavernosus muscle. The glans penis is a distal expansion of the corpus cavernosum that is pierced by the urethral meatus.

Beneath the skin of the penile shaft is the loosely adherent dartos fascia, an extension of Scarpa's fascia

that invests the three corporal bodies (Figure 13.3). Buck's fascia lies deep to the dartos fascia and superficial to the tunica albuginea. The latter is the tough fibrous wall of each corporal body. The penis is suspended from the symphysis pubis by the fundiform ligament, which is an extension of the linea alba, and the suspensory ligament. These stabilizing fibrous attachments fuse with Buck's fascia.

The blood supply of the penis is derived from the internal pudendal artery, which arises from the hypogastric artery. The first branch of the artery enters the bulbar corpus spongiosum and perfuses the spongiosum, glans penis, and urethra. The more distal pudendal artery divides to form the deep and the dorsal arteries of the penis. The former penetrates the crus and traverses the entire length of the corpus cavernosum as the cavernosus (profundus) artery. The dorsal artery runs lateral to the midline between Buck's fascia and the tunica albuginea. Terminal branches of the dorsal artery also supply the glans penis.

Venous drainage of the penis is rich and intercommunicating. The subcutaneous veins above Buck's fascia drain into the superficial dorsal vein of the penis, which in turn drains into the scrotal, saphenous, and femoral veins. Veins from the glans penis and corpora cavernosa enter into the midline deep dorsal vein lying between the tunica albuginea and Buck's fascia. This vein passes between the suspensory ligaments and through the urogenital diaphragm to communicate with the plexus anterior to the prostate gland. Veins from the anterior urethra communicate with the deep

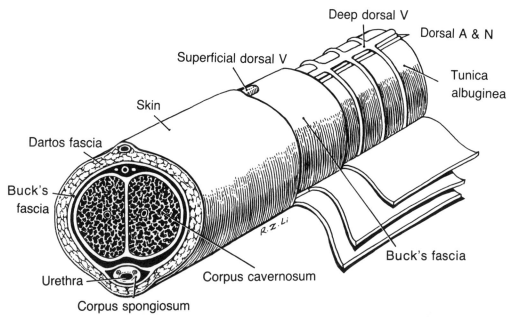

FIGURE 13.3
Cross-section of penile shaft

dorsal vein, and those of the bulbar corpus spongiosum join with veins from the posterior urethra to form the bulbar vein. The bulbar vein drains into the pudendal vein. The corpora cavernosa are drained also by the cavernosal veins, which exit from each crus to communicate with the pudendal vein.

The penis is innervated by branches of the pelvic plexus, which is derived from autonomic fibers of the S-2 through S-4 nerve roots and from branches of the hypogastric plexus. Superficial nerve fibers branch from the dorsal penile nerves. Nerves to the corpora cavernosa that are required for physiologic erection course posterolateral to the prostate and membranous urethra. Techniques for preservation of these bundles form the basis of the nerve-sparing radical retropubic prostatectomy.

The lymphatics of the penile skin and distal urethra drain to the inguinal lymph nodes, and those of the corpora cavernosa, corpus spongiosum, and proximal urethra drain to the pelvic lymph nodes.

PARTIAL PENECTOMY

Amputation of the penis distal to the suspensory ligament is performed usually for the treatment of squamous carcinomas. The operation is recommended only when there is 2 cm of uninvolved penile shaft between the suspensory ligament and the tumor. Mutilating traumatic injuries, invasive nonmalignant growths (e.g., Buschke-Löwenstein tumor), and invasive distal urethral carcinomas are also indications for partial penectomy.

OPERATIVE TECHNIQUE   The distal penis is covered with a rubber glove or the equivalent to prevent contamination of the wound by tumor cells or infecting bacteria (Figure 13.4). A tourniquet is applied to the base of the penis to limit bleeding during the amputation. The penile skin is incised circumferentially 2 cm proximal to the lesion. The dorsal neurovascular complex is isolated, secured with nonabsorbable sutures, and transected. The corpora cavernosa are transected, and the cavernosal arteries and veins are secured with suture ligatures. The corpus spongiosum is divided 1 cm beyond the level of the cavernosal transection to provide tissue for construction of a meatus.

The lateral margins of the tunica albuginea of the corpora cavernosa are approximated in the midline with interrupted heavy absorbable sutures. Each stitch should include the septum that separates the corporal bodies. The occlusive tourniquet is then removed and residual bleeders are fulgurated or ligated. The lateral edges of Buck's fascia and the skin are closed separately in the midline above the urethra using interrupted absorbable sutures. The dorsal aspect of the

corpora spongiosum is spatulated, and the urethral mucosa and corpus spongiosum are fixed to the adjacent skin edges with interrupted absorbable sutures. Urethral catheter drainage is advisable for 1 to 2 days.

TOTAL PENECTOMY

Total penectomy involves removal of both corpora cavernosa and the distal corpus spongiosum. A perineal urethrostomy is created with the bulbous urethra. This approach to the management of penile cancer is necessary if satisfactory surgical margins cannot be achieved with partial penectomy.

OPERATIVE TECHNIQUE   The lithotomy position is required for appropriate exposure. The distal penis is covered with a rubber glove and a circumferential incision is made at the base (Figure 13.5). The incision is extended in the midline superiorly and inferiorly to enhance exposure of the suspensory ligament and the crura and to facilitate wound closure. The suspensory ligament is divided on the undersurface of the symphysis, and the dorsal neurovascular complex is isolated, cross-clamped, transected, and ligated. The penis is retracted upward and the bulbocavernosus muscle is divided in the midline. The bulbar corpus spongiosum is then freed from the corpora cavernosa and transected. The crus of each corpus cavernosum is separated from the inferior border of the pubic arch, transected just proximal to the tip or excised completely, and the surgical specimen is removed. Branches of the internal pudendal artery and vein are encountered during this dissection and must be ligated.

A disc of skin and subcutaneous fat are removed from the midline of the perineum, and the proximal corpus spongiosum is brought through the defect. Redundant tissue is excised, the dorsal surface is spatulated, and the full thickness of the corpus spongiosum is fixed to the adjacent skin edges with interrupted absorbable sutures.

A Penrose drain is positioned under each pubic arch and brought through a stab wound in the anterior scrotal wall. The wound is closed by approximating anterior scrotal tissue in a vertical or transverse manner. The bladder is drained with a urethral catheter.

The drains and urethral catheter are generally removed after 2 to 3 days.

CIRCUMCISION

The prepuce forms a hood over the glans penis and is frequently removed in the neonatal period. Adults may request circumcision for cosmetic or hygienic reasons.

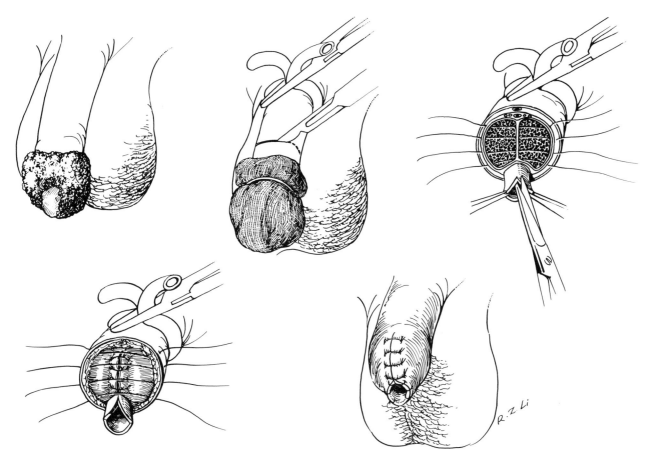

FIGURE 13.4
Partial penectomy

Medical indications for the procedure include local-ized squamous carcinomas, scarring of the foreskin (phimosis), or recurrent inflammation of the foreskin (posthitis) or of the glans penis (balanitis). Diabetes mellitus predisposes to the inflammatory conditions.

OPERATIVE TECHNIQUE At times a circumcision must be preceded by a dorsal slit procedure. An inability to retract the foreskin for instrumentation of the urethra and a paraphimosis that is not amenable to manual reduction (Figure 13.6) are the most common indica-tions. The penis is anesthetized by infiltration of the base with lidocaine (Figure 13.7). Two straight clamps are applied to the dorsal aspect of the foreskin on each side of the midline. The intervening tissue is incised to a point several millimeters distal to the coronal sul-cus, the clamps are removed, and the skin edges are sealed with a continuous absorbable suture.

The standard circumcision is performed also with local anesthesia. The foreskin is retracted over the shaft of the penis to break adhesions to the glans and to permit cleansing of the entire surgical field. The foreskin is then drawn over the glans and stabilized with hemostats applied at the 4 and 8 o'clock positions

(Figure 13.8). A straight crushing clamp is applied to the dorsal midline with the tips positioned several mil-limeters distal to the visible ridge created by the base of the glans penis. After several minutes the clamp is removed and the foreskin is divided in the resulting groove. This provides adequate exposure for amputation of the foreskin with a full thickness cir-cumferential incision.

A circumcision can be performed also by dissection of preputial skin from the penile shaft (Figure 13.9). The foreskin is retracted proximally, and a circumfer-ential skin incision is made several millimeters proxi-mal to the coronal sulcus. The foreskin is then drawn over the glans and incised several millimeters distal to the ridge formed by the base of the glans penis. A tongue of ventral skin should be preserved to facilitate wound closure. The two incisions are then connected on the dorsal aspect, and the foreskin is dissected sharply from loose areolar attachments.

Following either method of preputial amputation, the skin of the penile shaft is retracted to expose bleed-ing vessels in the bared areolar tissue. Prominent bleeders are secured with free ties of absorbable suture

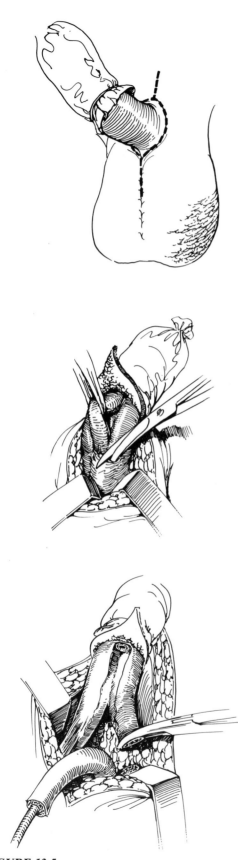

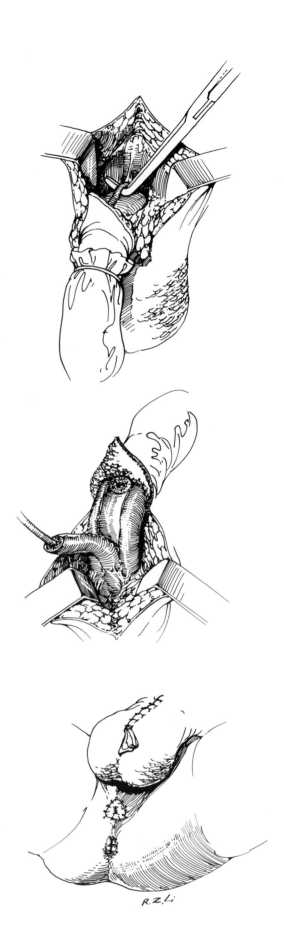

FIGURE 13.5
Total penectomy

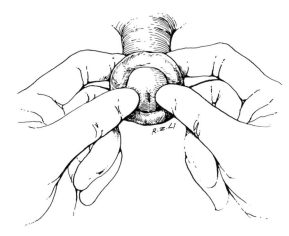

FIGURE 13.6
Manual reduction of paraphimosis

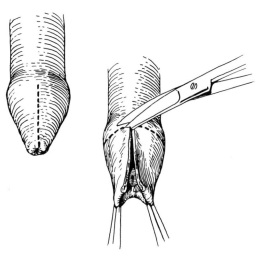

FIGURE 13.8
Circumcision by amputation of foreskin

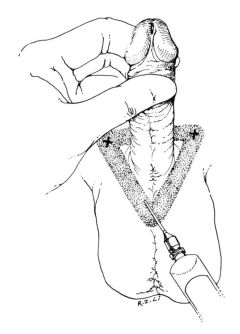

FIGURE 13.7
Penile block

material, and smaller vessels are managed with electrocautery. The opposing skin edges are then aligned with four absorbable sutures spaced at 90° intervals. A mattress suture may be used at the frenulum to help control bleeding that is characteristically brisk at this site. The intervening skin margins are approximated with interrupted absorbable sutures. For optimal hemostasis, every stitch should encompass a generous portion of the subcutaneous tissue. The wound is dressed with lubricated gauze.

POSTOPERATIVE CARE AND COMPLICATIONS The application of ice packs for 12 hours helps to reduce edema and discomfort. Intercourse is restricted until the

wound has healed completely. Severe pain is unusual and infection is remarkably uncommon, but ecchymosis of the distal penile shaft should be expected. Unsecured arterial bleeders may lead to hematoma formation. Evacuation of clot is occasionally necessary if the collection of blood is large. The use of interrupted sutures rather than a continuous suture for skin closure permits drainage without disruption of the entire suture line.

OPERATIONS FOR PENILE PROSTHESES

Prosthetic devices for the treatment of erectile impotence occupy each corpus cavernosum and are either nonhydraulic or inflatable in design. Nonhydraulic prostheses are made of silicone. A built-in hinge, malleable metal wire, or springlike mechanism permits downward positioning that helps to conceal the penis beneath the clothing.

Inflatable prostheses are of two general designs. The first inflatable prosthesis was composed of two cylinders linked by tubing with a fluid reservoir and an inflation-deflation device (Figure 13.10). The reservoir and inflation-deflation device are implanted outside the corporal bodies. Prostheses of this basic design, as well as newer adaptations in which the pump and reservoir are contained within a single unit, are available from several manufacturers. A cylindrical inflatable prosthesis with a built-in reservoir and inflation-deflation device that can be accommodated within each corporal body has also been introduced recently.

Patient selection criteria for penile prostheses in general, and for nonhydraulic and inflatable prostheses, are variable. It is important that both the

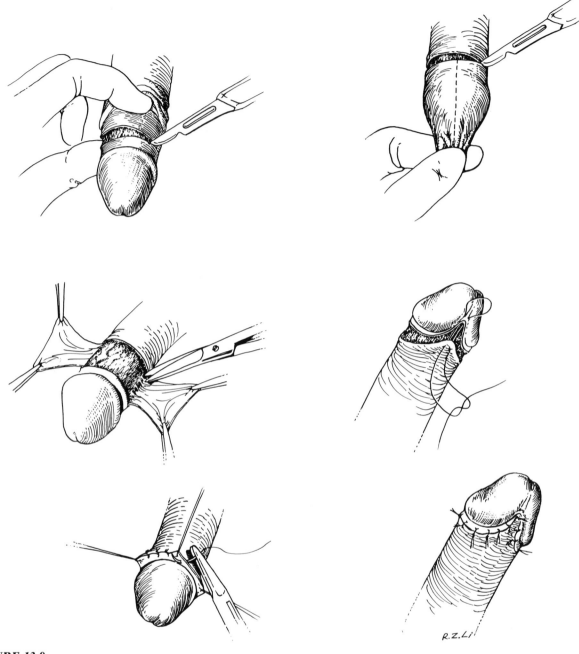

FIGURE 13.9
Circumcision by dissection of foreskin

patient and his partner understand the anticipated anatomic and functional outcomes of the operations. Individuals who request an inflatable device must accept the risk of mechanical failure and possess the manual dexterity for operation of the inflation-deflation pump.

OPERATIVE TECHNIQUE   The patient showers with an antiseptic solution the night before surgery, and parenteral antibiotics are administered in the perioperative period. Nonhydraulic prostheses or self-contained in-

flatable prostheses can be implanted with a suprapubic or a perineal approach.

With the suprapubic approach a transverse incision is made over the upper edge of the symphysis pubis, and the dorsal surfaces of the corpora cavernosa are exposed just distal to the suspensory ligament (Figure 13.11). A 2-cm longitudinal incision of the tunica albuginea is made between stay sutures. Care is taken to avoid injury to the medial neurovascular complex. A

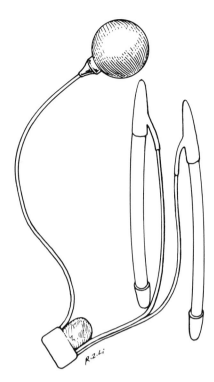

FIGURE 13.10
Inflatable penile prosthesis

tract within the corpus cavernosus extending to the glans penis and to the end of the crus is created with scissors. The tract is then dilated by the gentle insertion of No. 7-10 Hegar dilators. Forceful dilatation may cause perforation of the tunica albuginea.

Measuring devices are provided by the manufacturer for determining the appropriate length and width of the prosthesis. The prosthesis is introduced into the crus, bent, and manipulated into the distal corpus cavernosum. The fit should be sufficiently snug so that the prosthesis does not move to and fro within the tunica albuginea, but not so tight that the shaft of the penis becomes bent. The tunica albuginea is closed with a continuous nonabsorbable suture. The operative site is not drained, but a urethral catheter is advisable to prevent postoperative urinary retention.

The dorsal lithotomy position is required for prosthesis implantation with a perineal approach. A plastic adhesive drape or towel is secured to the perineum and buttocks to isolate the anus from the surgical field, and a urethral catheter is introduced to facilitate intraoperative identification of the corpus spongiosum. The bulbocavernosus muscle is exposed through a midline perineal incision, and the corpus cavernosum is entered through a 2-cm longitudinal incision in the more lateral crus (Figure 13.12). The development of the proximal and distal tracts within the

corpora cavernosa, placement of the prostheses, and closure of the tunica albuginea are accomplished as described for the suprapubic approach.

The three-piece inflatable prosthesis is implanted through a vertical or transverse suprapubic incision. The anterior rectus sheath is incised transversely for 4 cm. The rectus muscles are retracted laterally so that a preperitoneal space can be developed for the reservoir. The tubing of the reservoir is usually brought through the incision of the anterior rectus fascia. The reservoir is filled with saline or contrast material, and the fascia is closed with interrupted nonabsorbable sutures. The corpora cavernosa are exposed, incised, and dilated as described for the suprapubic placement of a nonhydraulic prosthesis. The sutures for closure of the tunica albuginea are positioned before the cylinders are implanted to prevent accidental puncture with a needlepoint. A cylinder of appropriate size is then introduced into each corpus cavernosum. The tubing is brought out through the suture line.

A pocket for the inflation-deflation pump is developed beneath the dartos muscle of the scrotum on the side of manual dominance. The tubing is connected with the tubing of the reservoir and the two inflatable cylinders. When the connections are completed, the cylinders are inflated to ensure proper function. A small suction drain is placed in the subcutaneous tissue before closure. Foley catheter drainage is advisable.

POSTOPERATIVE CARE AND COMPLICATIONS Most patients with nonhydraulic prostheses can be discharged on the day of surgery. A broad-spectrum oral antibiotic is taken for a minimum of 2 weeks.

After implantation of an inflatable prosthesis, the drain is removed on the first or second postoperative day. During convalescence the inflation-deflation device is periodically tugged into the dependent scrotum to maintain a proper position. Several weeks after leaving the hospital, the patient is instructed in the technique of prosthesis inflation and deflation. Intercourse should not be attempted until these maneuvers are mastered.

Infection of nonhydraulic and inflatable prostheses is unusual and is manifested by pain and erythema. In most cases the nonhydraulic prosthesis and all components of the hydraulic prosthesis must be removed to eradicate the infection.

Undersized nonhydraulic prostheses tend to slip away from the glans over time and result in a floppy distal penis. Oversized prostheses may cause pain or erode into the glans or urethra.

Leakage from the tubing or other components of inflatable prostheses, kinking of the tubing, and malfunction of the inflation-deflation mechanism have become less frequent with improved operative

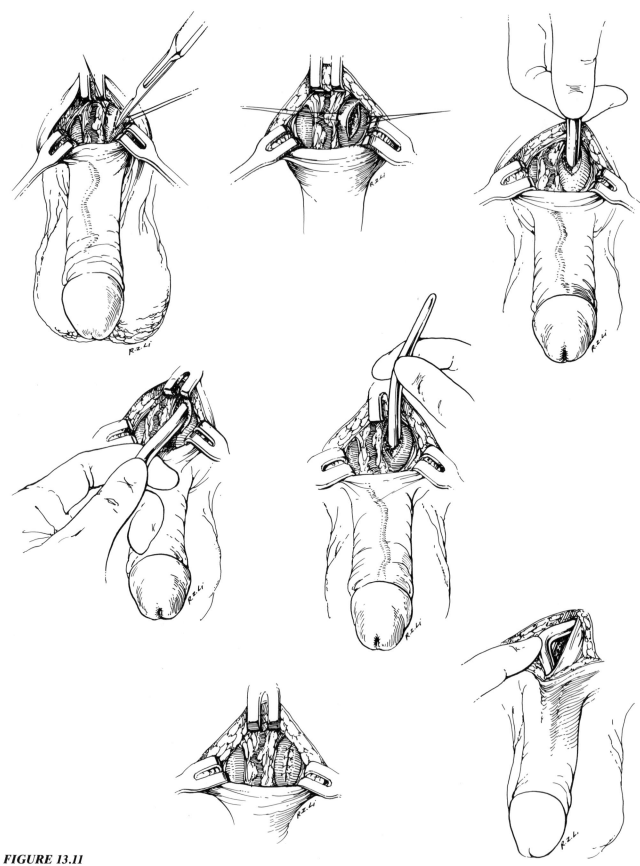

FIGURE 13.11
Suprapubic insertion of nonhydraulic penile prosthesis

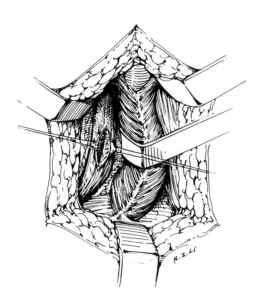 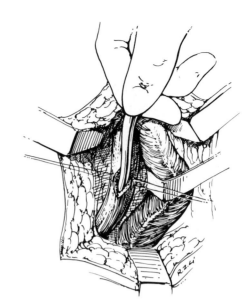

FIGURE 13.12
Perineal insertion of nonhydraulic penile prosthesis

techniques and design modifications. These complications, however, require operative intervention for repair. The risks of mechanical failure with self-contained inflatable prostheses are not well defined.

OPERATIONS FOR PEYRONIE'S DISEASE

Peyronie's disease refers to localized fibrosis and induration of the tunica albuginea of the corpora cavernosa (Figure 13.13). The palpable fibrous plaque is located usually on the dorsal surface and may produce pain and curvature of the penis during erections. The plaque may stabilize or regress in the absence of therapeutic intervention and responds occasionally to steroid injections or para-aminobenzoic acid.

Surgical treatments involve excision of the plaque and repair of the defect with a free graft of expansile autologous tissue. The results of operative interventions, however, are unpredictable and surgery is best reserved for patients with a 6- to 12-month history of unsatisfactory sexual function.

OPERATIVE TECHNIQUE A circumscribing incision is made proximal to the glans, and the skin of the penile shaft is retracted to expose the area of interest (Figure 13.14). An erection is created by applying a tourniquet to the base of the penis and injecting saline into the corpora cavernosa with a 20-gauge butterfly needle. This helps to delineate the extent of the fibrous process. The plaque is then excised just beyond the limits of palpable induration. If the plaque involves the dorsal midline, the neurovascular complex must be

carefully isolated before approaching the underlying fibrosis. A free graft of skin or tunica vaginalis is procured and trimmed to an appropriate size. It is positioned in the defect with four to six interrupted nonabsorbable sutures, and the intervening defects are sealed with continuous fine nonabsorbable sutures. The skin incision is closed with interrupted absorbable sutures.

If skin is used for the repair, a 1-mm full-thickness graft is obtained from a non-hair-bearing area. The epidermis is removed with a scalpel or dermatome, and the defatted subcutaneous surface is applied to the corporal tissues.

POSTOPERATIVE CARE AND COMPLICATIONS Erections during the postoperative period are discouraged and intercourse is restricted for 6 to 8 weeks. Impaired erectile function and loss of sensation distal to the

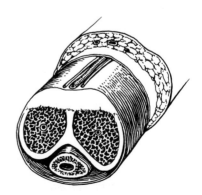

FIGURE 13.13
Peyronie's plaque

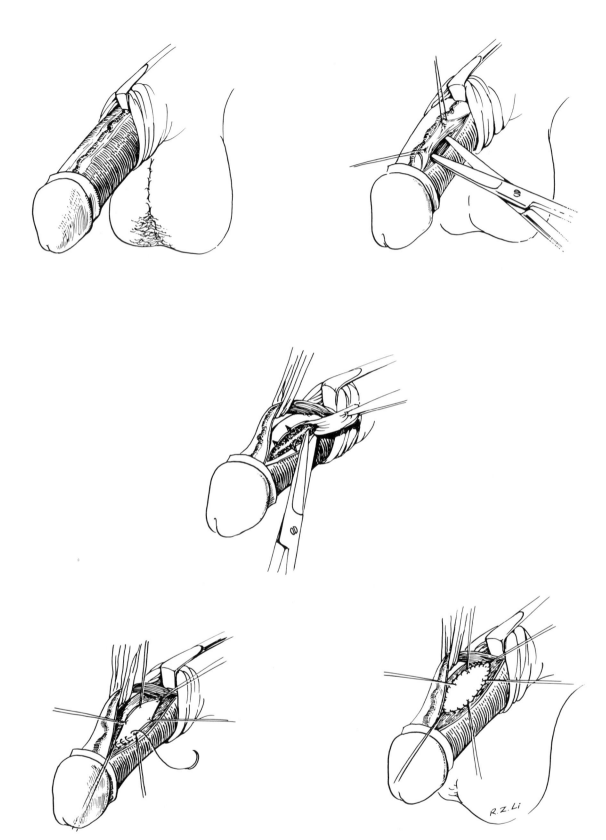

FIGURE 13.14
Excision and patch of Peyronie's plaque

plaque are inevitable if the dorsal penile nerves are damaged. Fibrosis of the graft leads to recurrent curvature and pain with erection.

REPAIR OF PENILE CURVATURE

Congenital curvature of the penis is caused by a disproportion in the length of the paired corpora cavernosa. The penis appears normal when flaccid but bends inferiorly or laterally with erection. Documentation of the curvature before surgery is mandatory, and intervention is recommended only if the deformity interferes with intercourse or is of excessive concern to the patient.

OPERATIVE TECHNIQUE The tunica albuginea of the corpora cavernosa is exposed with a circumferential incision proximal to the glans and retraction of the penile skin (Figure 13.15). An artificial erection is created as described above to delineate the magnitude and site of curvature. A wedge of tunica albuginea is removed from the convex border of the longer corpo-

ral body, and the defect is closed with nonabsorbable sutures with the knots tied inward. This process is repeated until the penis is straight while erect.

OPERATIONS FOR PRIAPISM

Priapism is a sustained erection that results from an abnormally high resistance to venous outflow from the corpora cavernosa. It is most common among men with sickle cell disease, but may also be associated with leukemia, neurologic or psychiatric disorders, pelvic tumors or trauma, and prolonged sexual stimulation. Priapism is a side effect of a variety of drugs, including the phenothiazines, antihypertensive agents, and marijuana.

Exchange transfusions in patients with sickle cell disease, leukophoresis in patients with leukemia, intracorporal injection of alpha-adrenergic agents, or irrigation of the corporal bodies with saline may lead to detumescence. However, operative intervention is advisable if the erection is unresponsive to conservative

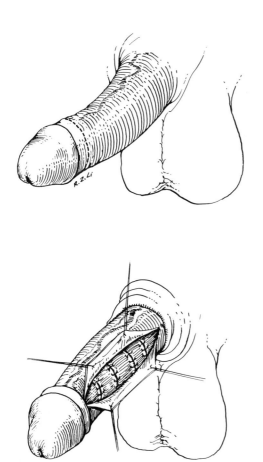

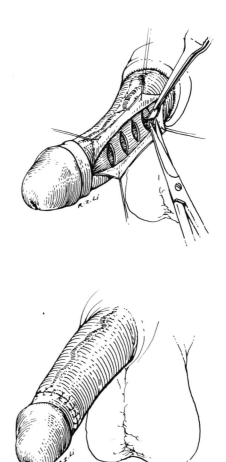

FIGURE 13.15
Correction of penile curvature

measures over an 8- to 12-hour period. Impotence due to fibrosis of the corpora cavernosa is not uncommon when the condition persists for more than 48 hours.

Urinary retention is not unusual and is preferably managed by percutaneous cystostomy rather than urethral catheterization. With the exception of the cavernosal-saphenous shunt, existing surgical procedures to treat priapism are designed to divert blood from the corpora cavernosa to the corpus spongiosum.

Winter Shunt

The Winter shunt is a reasonable initial surgical intervention that is generally performed with local anesthesia.

OPERATIVE TECHNIQUE   When the penis has been anesthetized, the glans is punctured superolateral to the meatus with a Tru-cut biopsy needle in the closed position (Figure 13.16). The obturator of the needle is extended into the tip of the corpus cavernosum, and the sheath is advanced over the obturator as would be done during biopsy of the prostate. The needle is then twisted and withdrawn to shear off a disc of tunica albuginea separating the glans and the corpus. Two defects should be made between each corpus and the glans. The puncture wounds in the glans are closed with simple nonabsorbable sutures.

El-Ghorab Shunt

The El-Ghorab shunt is an open procedure that creates larger tracts between the tips of the corpora cavernosa

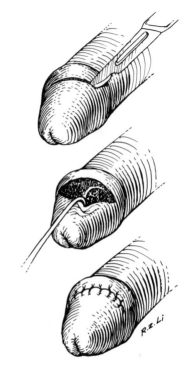

FIGURE 13.17
El-Ghorab shunt

and the glans than can be made with the Winter procedure.

OPERATIVE TECHNIQUE   The dorsal aspect of the glans penis is incised 1 cm distal to the coronal sulcus to expose the ends of the corpora cavernosa (Figure 13.17). A disc of the tunica albuginea $\frac{1}{2}$ cm in diameter is removed from each corpus, and thick venous blood is irrigated and evacuated. The incision in the glans is closed with a continuous fine nonabsorbable suture.

Cavernosal-Spongiosum Shunt

With this procedure shunts are made between the corpora cavernosa and the corpus spongiosum by direct anastomosis.

OPERATIVE TECHNIQUE   The urethra is catheterized to facilitate intraoperative identification of the corpus spongiosum. The corpus spongiosum and corpora cavernosa are exposed through two longitudinal skin incisions on the ventrolateral penile shaft just distal to the scrotum (Figure 13.18). Alternatively, the skin of the penile shaft can be retracted after making a circumferential incision proximal to the glans. Buck's fascia is opened, and the groove between the corpus spongiosum and the corpus cavernosum is developed toward the midline. To seal the back wall of the proposed shunt, the opposing tunica albuginea of the corporal bodies are approximated with a continuous nonabsorbable suture for a distance of about 2 cm.

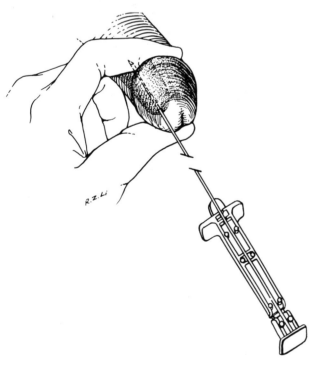

FIGURE 13.16
Winter shunt

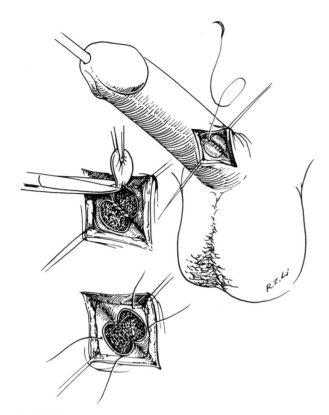

FIGURE 13.18
Cavernosal-spongiosum shunt

An oval disc of tunica albuginea is then excised from the adjacent surfaces of the corpus spongiosum and corpus cavernosum, and venous blood is evacuated from the corpus cavernosum. The lateral margins of the shunt are closed with a continuous nonabsorbable suture. Buck's fascia is approximated with a continuous absorbable suture, and the skin is closed with interrupted absorbable sutures.

A shunt between the contralateral corpus cavernosum and the corpus spongiosum is usually required for satisfactory detumescence. This shunt is positioned 2 cm proximal or distal to the first to reduce tension on the corpus spongiosum.

Cavernosal-Saphenous Shunt

The cavernosal-saphenous shunt for diversion of blood to the femoral vein has been replaced by the aforementioned procedures. It is a more extensive operation, and thrombosis of the shunt in the early postoperative period is common.

OPERATIVE TECHNIQUE The saphenous vein is approached through an incision in the groin and is isolated for 8 to 10 cm from the femoral vein. The distal aspect is ligated, the proximal segment is occluded with a vascular clamp, and the vessel is transected (Figure 13.19). An incision is then made at the lateral

base of the penis, and the saphenous vein is tunneled through the subcutaneous tissue. A 1-cm disc of tunica albuginea is excised from the side of the corpus cavernosum, and venous blood is evacuated. The spatulated saphenous vein is anastomosed with the defect in an end-to-side manner using a continuous fine nonabsorbable suture. Shunting of the contralateral corpus cavernosum using the same technique may be required for satisfactory detumescence.

POSTOPERATIVE CARE AND COMPLICATIONS
After all operative interventions for priapism, the flaccid penis is wrapped with an Ace bandage, bent onto the perineum, and secured with additional wraps. Alternatively, a pediatric blood-pressure cuff may be applied to the penis and inflated for 10 seconds every 15 to 20 minutes. Hourly surveillance by one observer is recommended so that recurrent engorgement can be identified and managed promptly. Even when an effective shunt has been created, the penis appears to be partially erect due to induration of the corporal bodies and edema of the penile skin. A true erection, however, is unmistakable and is managed in our practice with a cavernosal-spongiosum shunt if a Winter or El-Ghorab procedure was performed initially. Sitz baths are begun several days after surgery to promote the resolution of inflammation and edema.

Fibrosis of the corpora cavernosa leads to impotence in as great as one half of affected patients. However, shunts that do not close spontaneously over time are another cause for postoperative impotence. This possibility should be excluded by radiographic examinations during injection of the corpora cavernosa with contrast medium. Contrast immediately opacifies the corpus spongiosum if a shunt is patent, and potency may be restored by the simple process of shunt closure.

OPERATIONS FOR PENILE TRAUMA

The magnitude of injury following penile trauma varies widely and is usually evident by physical examination. A retrograde urethrogram is obtained if a urethral injury is suspected. Ruptures of the urethra are managed by methods described in the following chapter.

Lacerations of the penile skin are repaired by debridement and primary closure. Extensive avulsion injuries are treated by debridement and application of a split-thickness skin graft (Figure 13.20). When the avulsion is circumferential, residual skin distal to the injury and proximal to the glans should be excised. Otherwise, the disruption of more proximal lymphatic channels results in chronic disfiguring lymphedema.

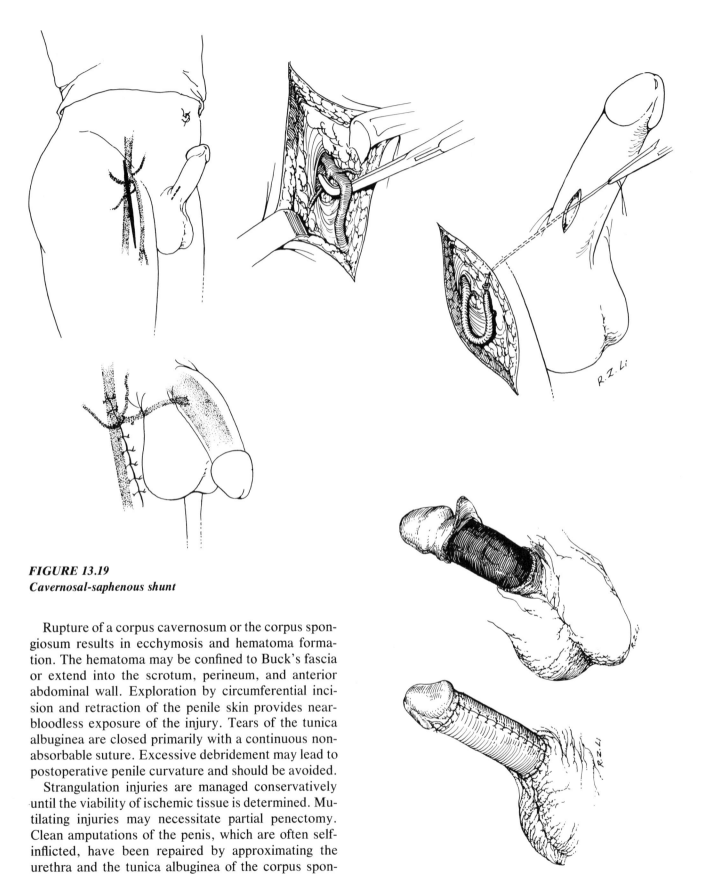

FIGURE 13.19
Cavernosal-saphenous shunt

Rupture of a corpus cavernosum or the corpus spongiosum results in ecchymosis and hematoma formation. The hematoma may be confined to Buck's fascia or extend into the scrotum, perineum, and anterior abdominal wall. Exploration by circumferential incision and retraction of the penile skin provides near-bloodless exposure of the injury. Tears of the tunica albuginea are closed primarily with a continuous nonabsorbable suture. Excessive debridement may lead to postoperative penile curvature and should be avoided.

Strangulation injuries are managed conservatively until the viability of ischemic tissue is determined. Mutilating injuries may necessitate partial penectomy. Clean amputations of the penis, which are often self-inflicted, have been repaired by approximating the urethra and the tunica albuginea of the corpus spongiosum and corpora cavernosa and microsurgical anastomosis of one or more dorsal arteries and veins.

FIGURE 13.20
Split-thickness skin graft of penile shaft

CHAPTER 14

Surgery of the Urethra

The urethra extends from the bladder outlet to the external meatus. The mucosa of the proximal urethra is transitional, and the mucosa of the distal urethra is squamous. There are four segments of anatomic, functional, and surgical relevance in males (Figure 14.1). The prostatic urethra traverses the prostate gland and is approximately 3 cm in length. The membranous urethra lies within the urogenital diaphragm and is 2 cm long. Both smooth and skeletal muscle surround the membranous urethra to create the external urinary sphincter. The bulbous urethra extends from the urogenital diaphragm to a point below the suspensory ligament of the penis and is encompassed by the wide bulbous portion of the corpus spongiosum. The caliber of the bulbous urethra is greater than that of the other urethral segments. The pendulous, or penile, urethra extends from the level of the suspensory ligament to the external meatus and is also encompassed by the corpus spongiosum. The blood supply and lymphatic drainage are summarized in Chapter 13.

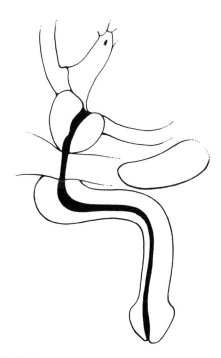

FIGURE 14.1
Male urethra

The female urethra is 3 to 5 cm in length and lies immediately anterior to the vagina and posterior to the symphysis pubis. Disorders of the urethra are substantially less frequent in females than in males.

URETHRECTOMY

Malignant tumors of the urethra or bladder are the primary indications for urethrectomy. Isolated urethral neoplasms are rare. Distal lesions may be treated by subtotal urethrectomy or partial penectomy. However, tumors arising from the mid- or proximal urethra or tumors at any site in the urethra associated with invasive bladder cancer are generally managed by urethrectomy combined with radical cystectomy.

In women, urethrectomy is a routine component of radical cystectomy for transitional cell carcinoma of the bladder. In men it is performed with cystectomy in the absence of urethral involvement when there is diffuse carcinoma in situ of the bladder or tumor invasion of the prostate. Tumor recurrence in the urethra is common in these situations.

Complete excision of the male urethra after cystectomy is hazardous because the most proximal membranous segment lies adjacent to adherent bowel in the pelvis. If a urethrectomy is not performed with a cystectomy for bladder cancer, it is advisable to dissect the proximal urethra from the urogenital diaphragm and to transect the urethra as distally as possible. This simplifies complete excision if required at a later date.

OPERATIVE TECHNIQUE Urethrectomy in men is carried out in an identical manner whether performed in conjunction with or after cystectomy. In the former situation the procedure is begun after the bladder is completely mobilized and the apex of the prostate has been exposed.

The patient is placed in the lithotomy position, and the bulbous urethra is approached through a midline or curvilinear transverse perineal incision (Figure 14.2). The bulbocavernosus muscle is divided in the midline to expose the corpus spongiosum. The indwelling urethral catheter used during cystectomy, or a urethral sound introduced during secondary procedures, helps to identify the correct planes of subsequent dissection.

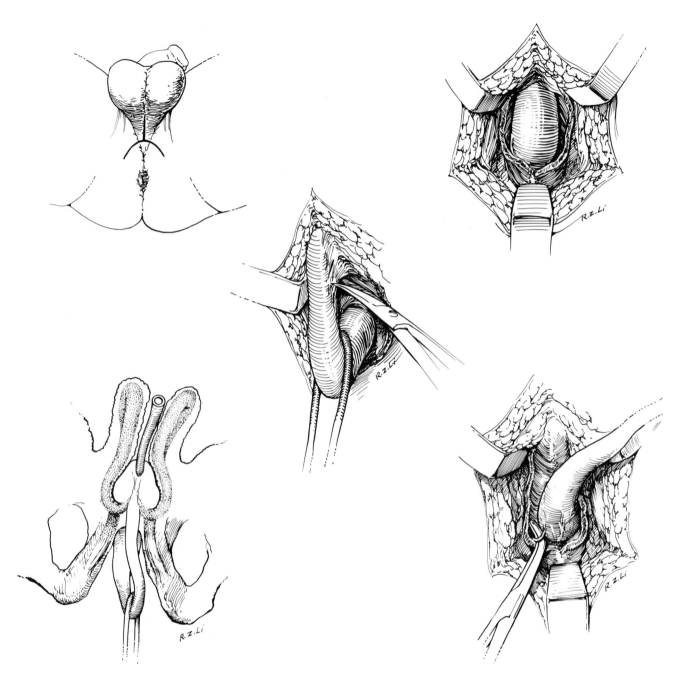

FIGURE 14.2
Urethrectomy in the male

The inferolateral groove between the corpus spongiosum and corpus cavernosum is incised on each side, the superomedial attachments are divided, and a Penrose drain is advanced through the defect for traction. As one works distally, the plane of dissection on the corpus spongiosum is remarkably easy to develop. Bleeding is minimal, but small communicating vessels in the midline of the corpora cavernosa require coagulation. As the urethra is retracted into the wound, the penis becomes inverted. When the glans is reached, one can transect the urethra and oversew the distal lumen. Alternatively, the inverted penis may be reduced to permit sharp excision of the most distal urethra from the ventral aspect of the glans (Figure 14.3). The urethra is then pulled into the perineal wound, and the defect in the glans is closed with interrupted absorbable sutures.

The proximal dissection to the urogenital diaphragm is done in the same manner as the distal dissection. Vessels supplying the bulbous urethra enter at the 4

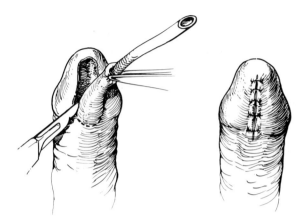

FIGURE 14.3
Excision of distal urethra in male urethrectomy

and 8 o'clock positions and are usually identifiable. Each pedicle is isolated, clamped, transected, and ligated. Avulsion of these vessels should be avoided because retraction from the operative field leads to troublesome bleeding. The membranous urethra is dissected from the urogenital diaphragm, and the specimen is removed if a cystectomy has already been performed. When urethrectomy is undertaken in conjunction with a cystectomy, the membranous urethra is mobilized with a combined pelvic and perineal approach. The urethra is drawn into the pelvis after the vascular pedicles of the prostate are divided, and it is removed en bloc with the surgical specimen.

A small Penrose drain is positioned in the fossa of the corpus spongiosum and brought out through a perineal stab wound. A mildly compressive circumferential dressing is applied to the penis. If Foley catheter drainage of the pelvis is to be used after cystectomy, the catheter is brought through the defect in the urogenital diaphragm and the perineal incision. The bulbocavernosus muscle is approximated in the midline with interrupted absorbable sutures, as are the subcutaneous tissues and the skin.

POSTOPERATIVE CARE AND COMPLICATIONS The Penrose drain is removed on the first postoperative day. Ecchymosis and edema of the penis are the rule, but usually resolve spontaneously within 1 to 2 weeks.

MEATOTOMY

Meatal stenosis is an uncommon cause of obstructive voiding symptoms but may cause spraying of the urinary stream. It is rare in females. Meatal stenosis in boys is caused usually by persistence of an epithelial membrane that occludes the ventral aspect of the meatus. Simple incision of the membrane with scissors

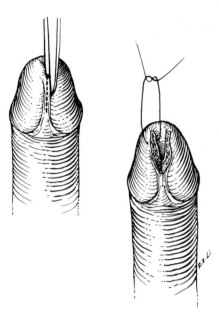

FIGURE 14.4
Meatotomy in men

under local anesthesia corrects the deformity. Bleeding is minimal, and sutures are rarely necessary if the membrane is crushed with a clamp before incision. The child's mother is instructed to spread the meatus several times a day to prevent adherence of the incision lines and to intermittently apply an antibiotic ointment.

Meatal stenosis in men generally results from urethral instrumentation or inflammation of the glans penis. The meatotomy is performed by sharply dividing fibrotic tissue ventral to the meatus (Figure 14.4). The edges of the urethra and skin are then approximated with interrupted absorbable sutures. An antimicrobial ointment is applied liberally during the healing phase, and the meatus is intermittently calibrated by the patient to prevent recurrent narrowing.

OPERATIONS FOR URETHRAL STRICTURES

Urethral strictures result from trauma, inflammation, or infection. They are rare in women, but are the most common surgical disorder of the urethra in men. Most patients present with obstructive voiding symptoms or urinary retention. The diagnosis is made by retrograde urethrography. The proximal extent of the stricture is delineated with a voiding cystourethrogram. Treatments are dictated by the location, length, and density of the fibrotic process and include dilatation, internal urethrotomy, and open repair.

Urethral Dilatation

The gradual stretching of urethral strictures may be sufficient for the management of short lesions that are not dense. Patience must be exercised during the process. After diagnosis the stricture is gently dilated with soft urethral catheters, urethral sounds, filiforms and followers, or filiforms and Council catheters (Figure 14.5). The stricture is dilated every week with an instrument 2 F larger than that used the previous week until a caliber of 24 F to 26 F is established. The frequency of dilatation is then decreased. Should dilatation ultimately be required more often than every 3 to 6 months, alternative forms of management are usually advisable.

Internal Urethrotomy

Internal urethrotomy, or incision of a urethral stricture under direct endoscopic vision, is favored by many urologists as the initial treatment for a stricture, or as a secondary treatment if a reasonable caliber is not maintained by dilatation. One incision through the thickness of the stricture is made at the 12 o'clock position with a blade that is attached to the working element of a resectoscope (Figure 14.6). Before incision, a ureteral catheter is advanced through the stricture to serve as a guide should bleeding impair visibility. After internal urethrotomy, the urethra should accept a 24 F catheter without undue force.

Excision

Strictures measuring 2 cm or less located anywhere in the bulbous or pendulous urethra are usually amenable to excision and primary anastomosis.

OPERATIVE TECHNIQUE   Strictures of the pendulous urethra are exposed by circumferential incision and retraction of the penile skin. Those of the bulbous urethra are approached through a perineal incision. The corpus spongiosum surrounding the strictured urethra and corpus spongiosum 1 cm proximal and distal to the area of disease is freed from the corpora cavernosa as described for urethrectomy. The fibrotic segment is excised, and the ends of the normal urethra are

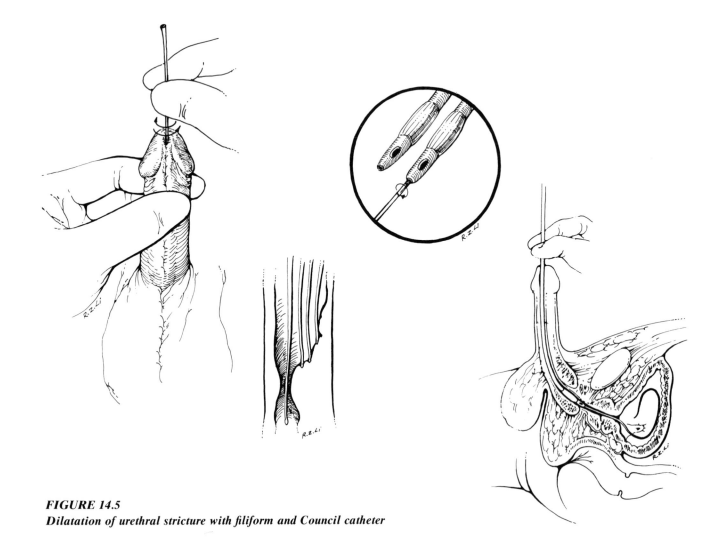

FIGURE 14.5
Dilatation of urethral stricture with filiform and Council catheter

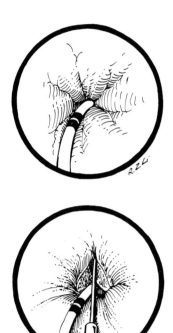

FIGURE 14.6
Endoscopic incision of urethral stricture

spatulated on opposing surfaces. The anastomosis is performed with interrupted absorbable sutures that encompass the urethral mucosa as well as the full thickness of the corpus spongiosum. Additional mobilization of the proximal or distal urethra may be required for a tension-free anastomosis. However, extensive mobilization of the pendulous urethra may lead to ventral curvature of the penis.

Marsupialization Procedures

These techniques for stricture repair require two operations but are useful if excision and a primary anastomosis is not feasible, or if there is a coexisting fistula or abscess.

OPERATIVE TECHNIQUE Strictures of the pendulous urethra are approached through a ventral midline incision. The corpus spongiosum overlying the stricture and the adjacent 1 cm of normal urethra is incised in a longitudinal manner. The full thickness of the corpus spongiosum is then fixed to the skin edges with interrupted absorbable sutures.

For strictures of the bulbous or membranous urethra, skin for anastomosis with the incised corpus spongiosum and also for the secondary repair is made available with a scrotal inlay. The stricture is approached through a curvilinear transverse or midline perineal incision, and the affected urethra and 1 cm of proximal and distal normal urethra are opened (Figure 14.7). A second midline incision is then made more

anteriorly in the scrotum. The scrotum is retracted toward the perineum, and the skin edges of the second incision are sutured to the full thickness of the corpus spongiosum. The initial incision is closed in two layers with interrupted absorbable sutures after a Penrose drain is positioned in the subcutaneous space.

The second stage of the marsupialization procedure is performed after 3 to 6 months. During the interval, hair on a scrotal inlay is epilated and intermittent dilatation of the proximal and distal lumens is performed to prevent stenosis. The urethra is closed by circumscribing the adjacent skin and undermining the corpus spongiosum medially (Figure 14.8). The skin edges are then approximated over a 24 F catheter. The laterally displaced bulbocavernosus muscles are also mobilized and sutured over the urethra to reinforce the closure, and the subcutaneous tissue and skin are closed with interrupted absorbable sutures.

Skin Grafts

Full-thickness skin grafts can be used as a patch to increase the caliber of the strictured urethra or to form a tube to replace an entire segment of the urethra. Properly applied grafts rapidly develop a new blood supply from the recipient bed. These techniques are quite versatile and are applicable for the repair of strictures at any location and of any length.

OPERATIVE TECHNIQUE Strictures of the pendulous urethra are exposed by circumferential incision and retraction of the penile skin; those of the bulbous urethra are exposed through a perineal incision. The stricture and 1 cm of adjacent normal urethra are opened, and a patch is used if the fibrosis is not exceedingly dense or irregular (Figure 14.9). The size of a graft required for loose coverage over a 24 F catheter is measured. A full-thickness skin graft of appropriate dimensions is procured from the penis or other non-hair-bearing sites, and the subcutaneous tissue is excised with scissors.

The graft is positioned with the epithelial surface on the luminal side and fixed to the urethral mucosa and corpus spongiosum at four or more points with absorbable sutures. The intervening margins are then closed with continuous absorbable sutures. The bulbocavernosus muscle, if present, is approximated in the midline, and the subcutaneous tissue and skin are closed with absorbable sutures.

If the stricture appears too dense or irregular for a patch and excision with primary anastomosis is not feasible, a tubularized graft is used to replace the diseased segment (Figure 14.10). The strictured urethra and surrounding corpus cavernosum are excised. Healthy corpus spongiosum, however, provides an excellent bed for the graft and should be preserved. The ends of the normal urethra are spatulated, and a graft

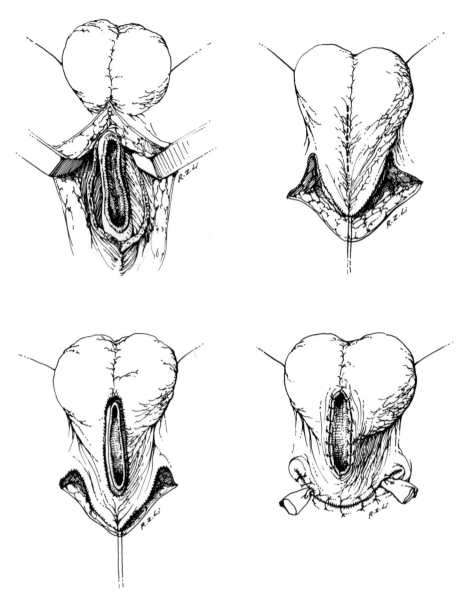

FIGURE 14.7
Marsupialization of bulbous urethral stricture

of appropriate length that can be tabularized over a 24 F catheter is laid in the defect and anastomosed to the urethral mucosa with interrupted absorbable sutures. A 24 F catheter is introduced, and the graft is closed longitudinally with a continuous fine absorbable suture.

To reduce the risks of postoperative fistulas, the longitudinal suture line of the graft can be positioned dorsally. This is done by tubularizing the graft over a 24 F catheter before it is positioned between the ends of the urethra. The proximal and distal anastomoses are then performed with interrupted absorbable sutures.

Vascularization of the graft is impeded by bleeding, infection, and application to avascular fibrous tissue. Special precautions that help to prevent shifting of the graft from underlying tissues include bedrest for 5 to 7 days and the prevention of erections.

Vascularized Skin Flaps

Skin flaps with vascular pedicles have been popularized recently for repairs of strictures and hypospadias. As with skin-graft procedures, the technique requires only one operation. The viability of the flap, however, is not dependent on the acquisition of a new blood supply.

OPERATIVE TECHNIQUE   The scrotal flap procedure for repair of bulbous urethral strictures is shown in Figure 14.11. A curved perineal incision extending into the posterior scrotum is made, and a flap of scrotal and perineal skin that includes the dartos muscle and a generous thickness of perineal subcutaneous tissue is

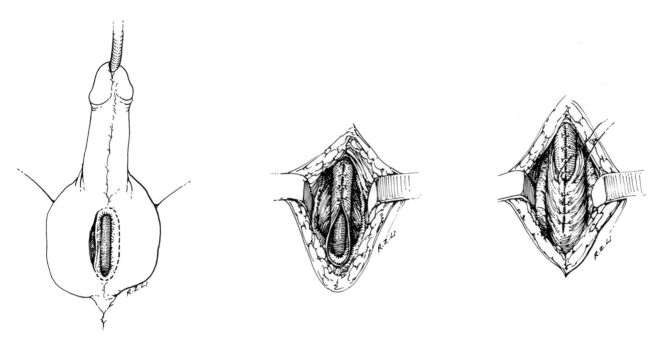

FIGURE 14.8
Closure of marsupialized bulbous urethral stricture

developed with sharp dissection. To create the vascular pedicle, the skin is incised below the apex of the flap and a plane is established between the skin and dartos muscle, working toward the perineum.

The stricture and adjacent normal urethra are opened, and the apex of the flap is sutured to the proximal urethrotomy. The graft is trimmed to an appropriate size and attached with several additional

absorbable sutures to ensure proper fit. The edges of the flap and a full thickness of the corpus spongiosum are then approximated with continuous absorbable sutures. Care must be taken to avoid undue tension or twisting of the pedicle. The bulbocavernosus muscle is closed loosely over the flap, and the subcutaneous tissue and skin are approximated in two separate layers.

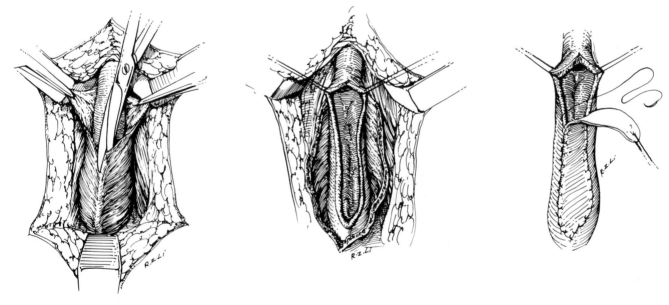

FIGURE 14.9
Repair of bulbous urethral stricture with full-thickness skin graft

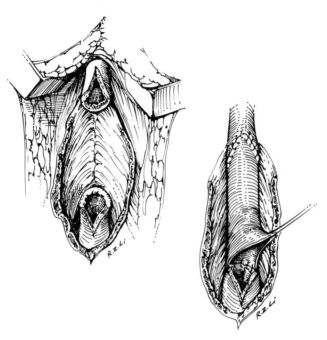

FIGURE 14.10
Replacement of strictured urethra with tubularized full-thickness skin graft

Operations for Posttraumatic Membranous Strictures

Posttraumatic strictures of the membranous urethra are caused usually by pelvic fracture and avulsion of the prostate from the urogenital diaphragm. The strictures often obliterate the entire lumen, may extend for 2 or 3 cm, and are characteristically dense and fibrotic (Figure 14.12). For these reasons, and because exposure can be troublesome, restoration of urethral continuity is always a challenge. Each of the foregoing techniques for stricture repair may be employed, and perineal exposure is usually adequate. However, satisfactory exposure may necessitate a combined perineal and retropubic approach with partial or complete removal of the symphysis pubis.

OPERATIVE TECHNIQUE An initial perineal approach is recommended. The patient is placed in an exaggerated lithotomy position, and the bulbous urethra is exposed through a generous midline or combined midline and curvilinear transverse perineal incision. The bulbocavernosus muscle is divided, and the bulbous cor-

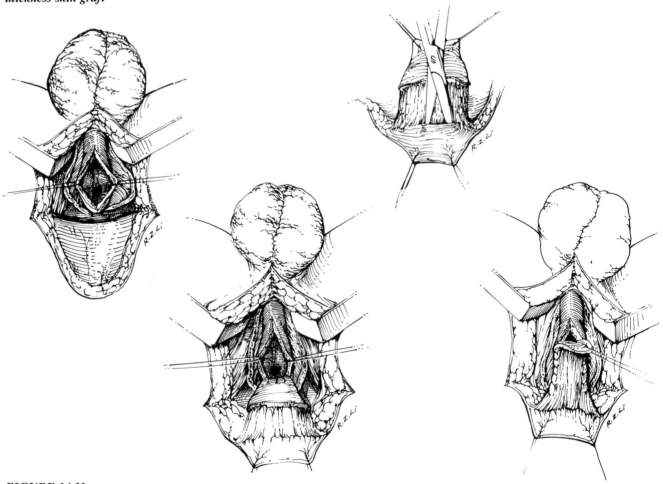

FIGURE 14.11
Repair of urethral stricture with vascularized skin flap

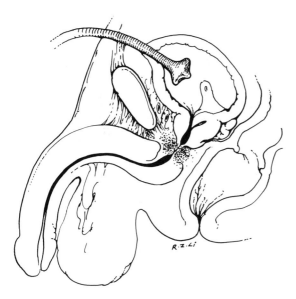

FIGURE 14.12
Dense stricture of membranous urethra resulting from traumatic avulsion of the prostate

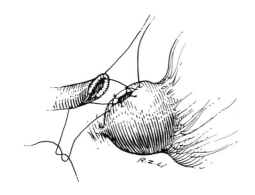

FIGURE 14.13
Anastomosis of bulbous urethra with anterior prostate

pus spongiosum is mobilized to the urogenital diaphragm and transected. A metal sound is introduced through the preexisting suprapubic cystostomy tract and manipulated into the prostatic urethra. Fibrous tissue is excised from the anterior aspect of the urogenital diaphragm and prostate overlying the tip of the sound, and the instrument is advanced into the wound. The spatulated proximal bulbous urethra, if patent and supple, may be amenable to direct anastomosis with the prostate using interrupted absorbable sutures (Figure 14.13). The dorsal sutures are placed first, a urethral catheter is introduced, and the ventral anastomosis is completed. When the most proximal lumen of the bulbous urethra is fibrotic or obliterated, the dorsal aspect may be incised just beyond the diseased segment and anastomosed with the prostate (Figure 14.14).

When a tension-free anastomosis cannot be achieved, the corpus spongiosum is mobilized from the corpora cavernosa as far as the glans penis. This can add 4 to 5 cm to the length of the urethra. Arteries entering the bulbous urethra must be transected, but ischemia is unusual because the blood supply to the corpus spongiosum is derived also from vessels that enter the glans penis.

If a satisfactory anastomosis remains impossible, the following maneuvers are recommended to reduce the distance between the proximal uninvolved urethra and the prostate and to bypass the stricture. The patient's legs are adjusted to a low lithotomy position, and the retropubic space and anterior symphysis pubis are exposed through a low midline incision. The prostate is freed from the posterior symphysis, and the suspensory ligament of the penis is transected. Dissection with the scalpel and a heavy scissors is generally required because dense fibrosis and obliterated tissue

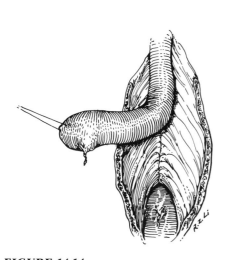
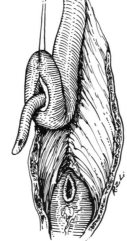
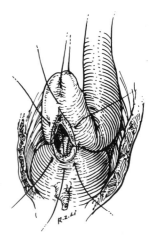

FIGURE 14.14
Anastomosis of dorsal bulbous urethra with anterior prostate

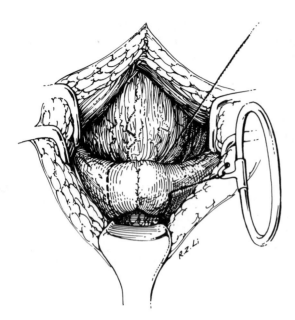

FIGURE 14.15
Transpubic approach to membranous urethral stricture

planes are the rule. A wedge of the symphysis is removed with the Gigli saw to expose the anterior prostate (Figure 14.15). Preservation of the periosteum provides tissue to close the bony defect.

A tunnel is then made between the diverging crura of the penis. The corpus spongiosum is drawn through the defect, spatulated on the ventral surface, and anastomosed to the anterior aspect of the prostate with interrupted absorbable sutures (Figure 14.16). Mobilization of the prostate in a downward direction to reduce tension on the suture line is ill-advised and in most cases impossible.

POSTOPERATIVE CARE AND COMPLICATIONS

The optimal duration of urethral catheter drainage after internal urethrotomy or open urethral stricture repairs depends on the nature of the repair and on the philosophy of the urologist. The catheter prevents urinary extravasation at the site of repair and stabilizes circumferential suture lines. On the other hand, inflammation and infection are inevitable if the catheter is maintained for longer than 5 to 7 days. We prefer to insert a percutaneous cystostomy at the time of urethroplasty and to remove the urethral catheter after 5 to 7 days. A voiding cystourethrogram is performed, and the suprapubic tube is clamped if there is no extravasation. This cystourethrogram also serves as a baseline for follow-up contrast studies should obstructive symptoms recur. The voiding study is repeated one week later, and the suprapubic tube is removed if the suture line remains watertight. The urethra is inter-

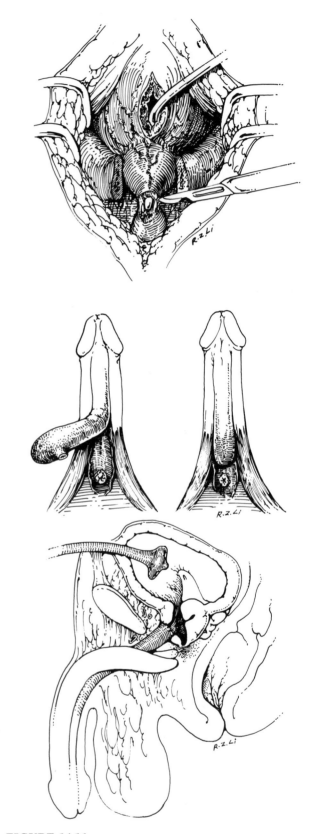

FIGURE 14.16
Anterior transposition of bulbous urethra and anastomosis with prostate

mittently calibrated for 3 to 6 months after surgery to prevent narrowing at the operative site.

Complications inherent to all procedures include fistulas, diverticula, periurethral abscess, and recurrent stricture formation.

After repair of membranous urethral strictures, continence is maintained by the bladder outlet only. However, if the original injury resulted in functional damage to the bladder outlet, or if transurethral resection of the prostate is performed at a later date, incontinence is not unusual. Impotence is a possible complication of the operation, but is often preexisting as a result of the original injury. For medical-legal reasons, it is important to document clearly the status of erectile function before surgery. Finally, extensive mobilization of the corpus spongiosum may lead to ventral curvature of the penis.

URETHRAL DIVERTICULECTOMY

Diverticula of the male urethra are either congenital or result from trauma or urethral surgery. They almost always arise from the ventral aspect of the urethra. If a diverticulum is large, urine collects during micturition and causes postvoid dribbling. When the outlet is narrow, the urine stagnates and predisposes to infection or abscess. Coexisting distal urethral strictures promote expansion of diverticula and are repaired before or during a diverticulectomy. The site and extent of a diverticulum, as well as the presence or absence of urethral strictures, are documented by retrograde and antegrade urethrography.

The repair of all but the most massive diverticula is usually straightforward. Diverticula located in the pendulous urethra are exposed by circumferential incision and retraction of the penile skin. Those arising from the bulbous urethra are approached through a perineal incision. A urethral catheter serves as a useful landmark during the operation. The diverticulum is dissected from surrounding areolar tissue and transected flush with the urethra if the mouth is narrow. The urethra is closed with interrupted absorbable sutures. If the mouth of the diverticulum is capacious, one preserves the wall just beyond the urethra to provide tissue to close the defect.

Most urethral diverticula in women are thought to result from inflammation of the periurethral glands. They are usually smaller than those in men, and the outlet is characteristically narrow. Most arise from the ventral urethra. Voiding disturbances or a urethral discharge, dyspareunia, and vaginal pain are common presenting complaints. Some diverticula are palpable on pelvic examination. The diagnosis is made by voiding urethrography and cystoscopy.

A urethral catheter is introduced, and a transverse incision is made in the anterior vagina below the meatus. The diverticulum is exposed by dissecting the vaginal wall from the urethra and bladder outlet. It is then isolated and transected flush with the urethra. If the diverticulum is located near the bladder outlet, the plane of dissection must be confined to the wall of the outpocketing. This reduces the risks of injury to the sphincteric musculature and postoperative incontinence. The urethral defect is closed with interrupted absorbable sutures, and the anterior vaginal wall is repositioned over the urethra and closed with a continuous absorbable suture.

Drainage of the bladder with a urethral catheter for 3 to 5 days is advisable after diverticulectomy in men and women.

OPERATIONS FOR HYPOSPADIAS

The congenital defect hypospadias results from incomplete development of the distal corpus spongiosum and urethra. It may be associated with testicular maldescent and inguinal hernias as well as anomalies of the urinary and extraurinary systems. Severe hypospadias is often seen in intersex states.

Hypospadias is characterized grossly by a urethral opening in the ventral midline at or proximal to the coronal sulcus, a persistent groove in the ventral glans penis, and a hooded foreskin caused by the underdevelopment of ventral preputial tissue (Figure 14.17). Ventral curvature of the penis, or chordee, is produced by fibrous tissues adjacent and distal to the underdeveloped urethra. The urethral meatus of most affected patients is situated in the distal third of the penile shaft. In approximately 10 to 20 percent of cases it is in the middle third of the shaft, and in

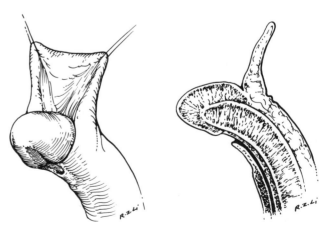

FIGURE 14.17
Appearance of hypospadias

approximately 10 to 20 percent it lies between the perineum and the middle third of the shaft. The degree of chordee correlates directly with the extent of proximal malposition of the meatus.

Hypospadias repair is preferentially undertaken between 6 and 18 months of age. The objectives of the operation are threefold. The chordee, if present, is corrected by mobilization of the distal urethra and excision of ventral fibrous bands at and distal to the meatus. Intraoperative simulation of an erection by compression of the penile base with a tourniquet and injection of saline into the corpus cavernosum helps to document the adequacy of the straightening procedure. Correction of the chordee results usually in a more proximal location of the meatus on the penile shaft. Construction of the distal urethra and creation of a meatus at or near the apex of the glans penis are the other objectives of the operation.

Magnification of the operative field and the use of fine microsurgical instruments facilitate the repair of hypospadias. Compression of the base of the penis with a tourniquet or local infiltration of the area of dissection with a dilute epinephrine solution helps to maintain a bloodless field. The appropriate method of repair is dictated primarily by the presence or absence of chordee and the site of the meatus after correction of the chordee. However, these parameters cannot be predicted with absolute certainty before surgery, and the urologist who undertakes the procedure must be well versed in the details of numerous techniques and maneuvers. Moreover, expendable penile skin is used in most repairs and is of limited availability if revisionary surgery is required. Repair of all but the most distal hypospadias, therefore, should be left to surgeons with interest and expertise in the field.

This section addresses one-stage repairs for distal, middle, and proximal hypospadias. The reader is encouraged to consult texts on pediatric urologic surgery for more detailed discussions as well as for descriptions of other operative techniques.

Meatoplasty and Glanuloplasty

Hypospadias deformities with the meatus at or just proximal to the coronal sulcus are amenable to meatoplasty and glanuloplasty if there is no complicating chordee. Introduced by Dr. John Duckett and called the MAGPI procedure, the technique advances the meatus to the apex of the glans and corrects the congenital groove.

OPERATIVE TECHNIQUE A circumferential incision is made about 6 to 8 mm proximal to the glans and the meatus (Figure 14.18). Skin is dissected from the penile shaft, taking care to avoid injury to the fragile urethra. A longitudinal incision is made in the glanular groove and is closed transversely with interrupted sutures. The ventral skin lying just proximal to the meatus is then drawn distally. The more lateral skin edges that are brought to the midline with this maneuver are then sutured together to maintain the meatal advancement. The circumferential penile incision is closed with interrupted sutures.

Hodgson II Procedure

If the meatus is too proximal for the MAGPI operation and there is no chordee, the distal urethra may be constructed by the onlay of transposed vascularized preputial skin.

OPERATIVE TECHNIQUE The penile skin is circumscribed proximal to the meatus and retracted, and a buttonhole is made for ventral transposition of the prepuce (Figure 14.19). The length of preputial skin beyond the buttonhole should correspond to the distance between the meatus and the apex of the glans penis. The lateral margins of the onlay are incised and dissected medially, and skin on each side of the glanular groove is excised. The edge of the onlay is sutured to the edge of the groove and to the skin surrounding the meatus. The preputial skin superficial to the onlay is fixed to the lateral margin of the glanular skin. The dorsolateral circumferential skin incision and the defect on the ventral shaft are closed primarily. The meatus is now located at the apex of the glans, but the ventral glans is covered with penile rather than glanular epithelium.

Mathieu Procedure

The Mathieu procedure is an alternative to the Hodgson II operation for distal hypospadias without chordee.

OPERATIVE TECHNIQUE The dorsolateral preputial skin is incised proximal to the glans. On the ventral surface the incision is extended proximally to outline the margins of a flap that corresponds in length to the distance between the meatus and the apex of the glans (Figure 14.20). The glans is then incised on each side of the groove and undermined laterally. The flap is dissected from the urethra, rotated distally, and fixed to the medial edges of the glanular incision. The lateral glanular flaps are sutured in the midline to cover the skin flap, and dorsal preputial skin is tranposed to repair the ventral epithelial defect.

Mustarde Procedure

This repair is suitable for midpenile hypospadias associated with chordee. If the glans has a conical configuration the neourethra can be tunneled to the apex.

OPERATIVE TECHNIQUE The penile skin is circumscribed distal to the meatus, and fibrous bands between the meatus and the glans are removed to correct the chordee (Figure 14.21). A flap of appropriate length is

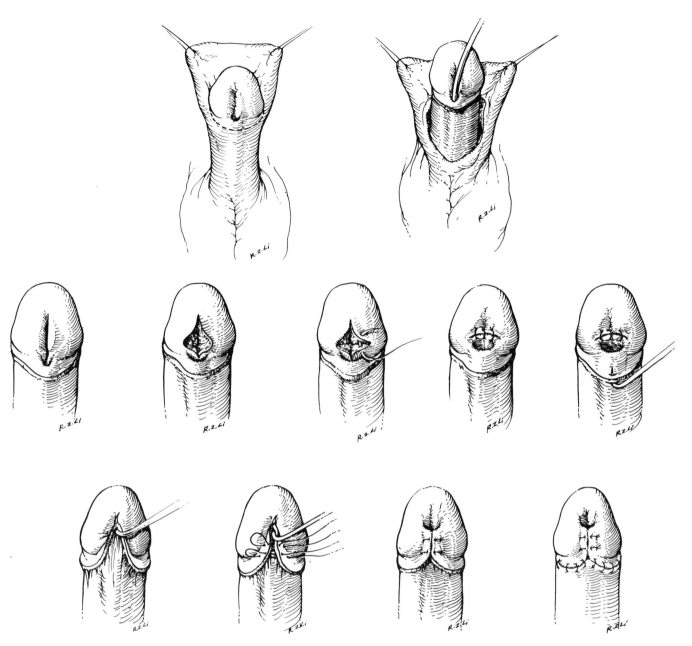

FIGURE 14.18
MAGPI repair of distal hypospadias without chordee

developed from skin overlying the urethra, taking care to preserve vascular subcutaneous tissues. The flap is then tubularized over a 10 or 12 F catheter with interrupted absorbable sutures. Using scissors, a channel 16 to 18 F in caliber is made in the glans to a point above the ventral groove. The tubularized flap is then drawn through the tunnel, and the margins of the lumen are fixed to skin of the glans. The epithelial defect on the ventral shaft is covered with preputial skin that is transposed with the buttonhole technique.

Hodgson III Procedure

The Hodgson III operation is used to repair proximal hypospadias with or without chordee. Preputial skin and skin of the proximal penile shaft are transposed in a manner analogous to the Hodgson II onlay procedure. However, a tubularized neourethra must be created because skin between the meatus and the glans is necessarily sacrificed while correcting the chordee.

OPERATIVE TECHNIQUE   The penile skin proximal to the glans is incised circumferentially and the chordee

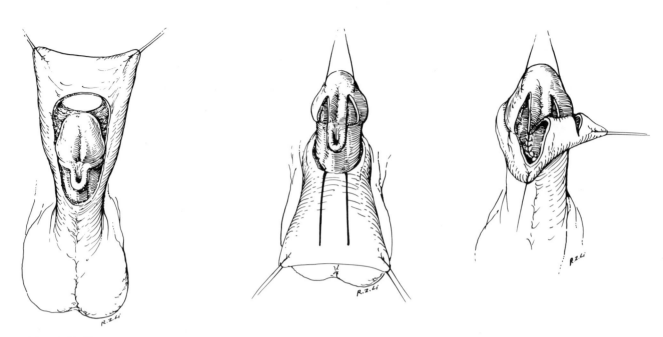

FIGURE 14.19
Hodgson II repair of distal hypospadias without chordee

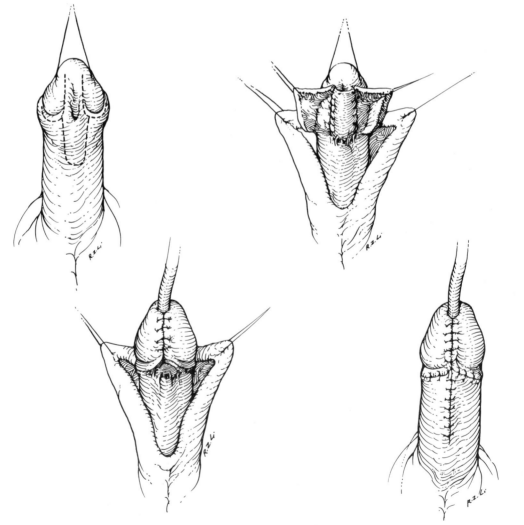

FIGURE 14.20
Mathieu repair of distal hypospadias without chordee

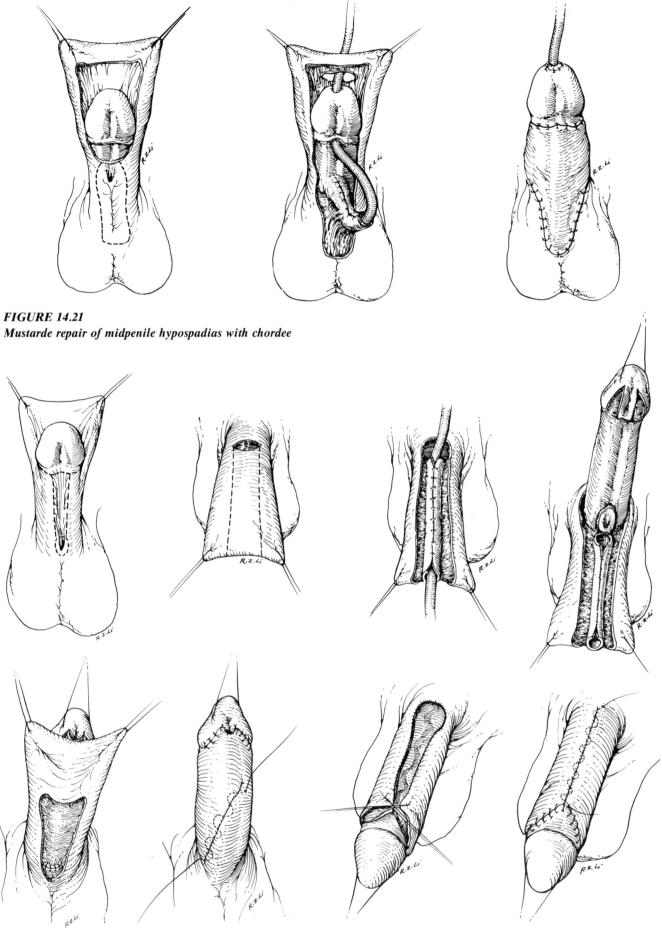

FIGURE 14.21
Mustarde repair of midpenile hypospadias with chordee

FIGURE 14.22
Hodgson III repair of proximal hypospadias with chordee

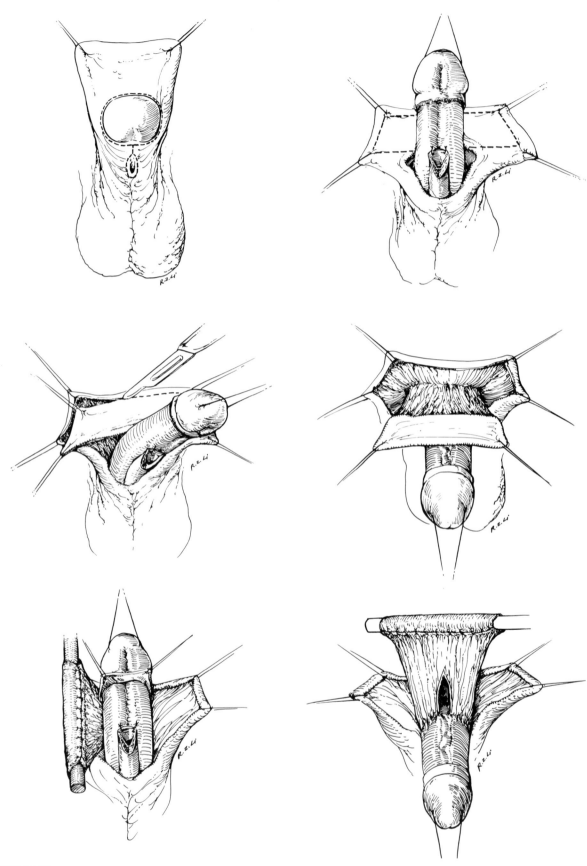

FIGURE 14.23
Island flap repair of proximal hypospadias with chordee

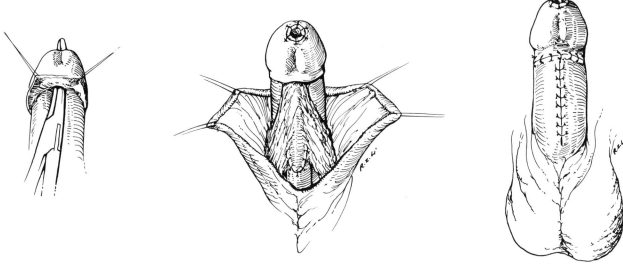

FIGURE 14.23
Island flap repair of proximal hypospadias with chordee (continued)

is corrected (Figure 14.22). Preputial skin and skin of the dorsal penile shaft of an appropriate length and width for construction of the neourethra are then outlined. The lateral margins of the skin are incised and undermined medially, and the flap is tubularized over a 10 or 12 F catheter. The suture line should not extend to the ends of the flap. This creates a spatulation for the anastomosis with the meatus and permits an onlay technique for construction of the new meatus.

The tubularized flap and adjacent penile and preputial skin are transposed ventrally with the buttonhole technique, and the lumen of the proximal neourethra is anastomosed with the meatus. The epithelium is excised adjacent to the glanular groove, and a meatus is constructed as described for the Hodgson II onlay procedure. The epithelial defect on the ventral shaft is covered with redundant preputial skin. There is also a defect on the dorsal shaft because penile skin as well as preputial skin was transposed ventrally. This defect can usually be closed primarily.

Island Flap Procedure

The island flap procedure is reminiscent of the Hodgson III operation, but the blood supply to the tubularized neourethra is derived from a vascular pedicle of subcutaneous tissue.

OPERATIVE TECHNIQUE The penile skin proximal to the glans is incised circumferentially and the chordee is corrected. The margins of a transverse flap of appropriate length and width for construction of a neourethra are incised on the inner preputial membrane (Figure 14.23). The vascular pedicle is developed by undermining the skin away from the flap, taking

care to preserve the subcutaneous tissue. The flap is tubularized over a 10 or 12 F catheter and rotated around the lateral aspect of the penile shaft. Alternatively, the pedicle may be divided in the midline to allow ventral transposition of the tube in a buttonhole manner.

A channel in the glans is then formed as described for the Mathieu repair. The proximal neourethra is anastomosed with the meatus, and the distal end is drawn through the tunnel in the glans and fixed to the skin. The denuded shaft and neourethra are covered with redundant penile and preputial skin.

POSTOPERATIVE CARE AND COMPLICATIONS

After all but the most distal hypospadias repairs, the penis is dressed with lubricated gauze and immobilized with fluff dressings and elastic tape. The dressings are removed after 5 to 7 days. Opinions concerning the advisability and duration of suprapubic urinary diversion and urethral stenting are variable. Each prevents the extravasation of urine through suture lines and promotes healing. However, bladder spasms induced by the tubes can be troublesome in small children. Oral antimicrobial therapy during bladder drainage prevents or delays bacteriuria.

After the initial healing phase, the meatus is intermittently probed with a small plastic tip to prevent adhesion of the healing edges and obliteration of the lumen from encrustations. Close observation during the first 3 months is important to ensure proper attention to wound care.

Wound infection is rare. However, partial necrosis of the skin flaps is not unusual and urethrocutaneous fistulas develop in 10 to 20 percent of patients. Fistulas can be closed by a number of techniques when the operative site has healed completely. Residual chordee, meatal stenosis, and urethral strictures or diverticula are additional late complications.

OPERATIONS FOR URETHRAL TRAUMA

Rupture of the urethra from blunt, penetrating, or iatrogenic trauma is the principal injury of surgical concern. Tears of the urethral mucosa during instrumentation are managed by transurethral or suprapubic bladder drainage for 3 to 5 days. Most heal spontaneously without stricture formation.

Traumatic rupture of the urethra is manifested usually by an inability to void, blood at the urethral meatus, and perineal or penile hematomas. The site of injury is delineated with a retrograde urethrogram. If a urethral catheter has been introduced before investiga-

tion, contrast medium is injected around the catheter. A cystogram and an intravenous pyelogram are performed to rule out coexisting injuries to the bladder and upper urinary tract.

The etiology and management of traumatic urethral ruptures above and below the urogenital diaphragm differ substantially. Rupture of the bulbous or pendulous urethra results from penetrating wounds or direct perineal trauma. The site of injury is exposed by circumferential incision and retraction of the penile skin or through a perineal incision (Figure 14.24). Primary end-to-end anastomosis of the debrided urethra is usually feasible. A suprapubic cystostomy and stenting urethral catheter are advisable. The catheter is removed after 5 to 7 days, and a voiding urethrogram is obtained to document a watertight closure.

If a tension-free primary anastomosis is not possible, the patient is unstable, or the rupture is associated with periurethral infection or abscess, a urethrostomy is performed proximal to or at the site of injury. Ure-

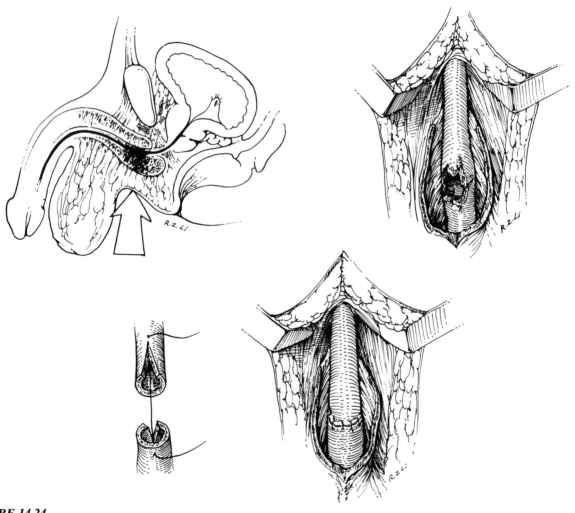

FIGURE 14.24
Primary repair of bulbous urethral rupture

thral continuity is restored after 3 to 6 months when inflammation has resolved completely. The techniques described for the repair of urethral strictures are employed for the secondary procedure.

Urethral rupture at or above the urogenital diaphragm is associated usually with pelvic fracture. Potentially lethal injuries at other sites are not uncommon. The mechanism of urethral disruption typically involves avulsion of the prostate from the urogenital diaphragm. On rectal examination the prostate is often displaced superiorly. Retrograde urethrography demonstrates extravasation of contrast medium into the pelvis, and elevation and compression of the bladder by pelvic hematoma is seen on the intravenous pyelogram. The optimal approach to initial management remains unsettled and is dependent partly on the overall condition of the patient.

A suprapubic cystostomy only may be performed. If the rupture is incomplete, urethral continuity is usually restored with resolution of the pelvic hematoma (Figure 14.25). However, with complete disruptions a space develops between the prostatic and membranous urethral segments, and the urethral lumen is obliterated after the hematoma resolves (Figure 14.26). Advocates of this strategy believe that the risks of pelvic abscess, incontinence, and impotence are less than with primary intervention to realign the urethra.

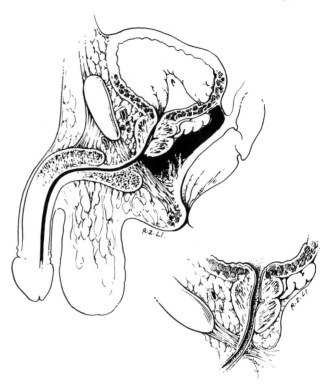

FIGURE 14.25
Incomplete rupture of membranous urethra and healing without stricture

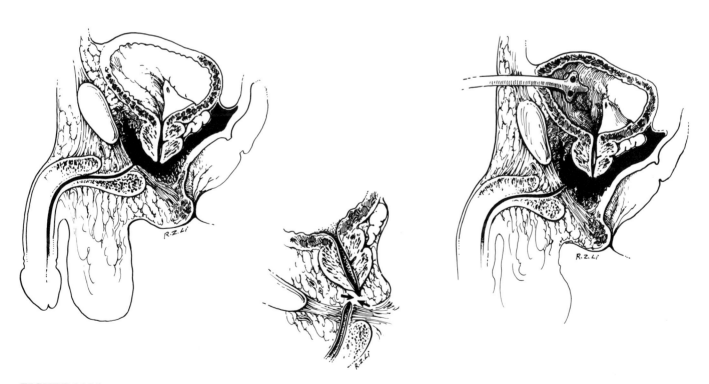

FIGURE 14.26
Complete rupture of membranous urethra treated by suprapubic cystostomy with subsequent formation of dense urethral stricture

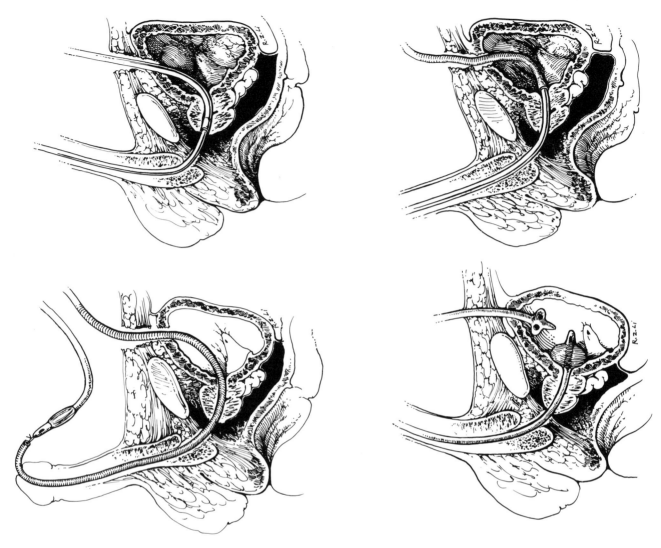

FIGURE 14.27
Realignment of ruptured membranous urethra with interlocking sounds

In addition, this approach precludes the conversion of partial disruptions to complete disruptions by instrumentation and obviates a major operation in patients who are often unstable.

Some urologists recommend realignment of the urethra as soon as possible after injury. This is done by exposing the apex of the prostate through a lower abdominal incision and introducing a urethral catheter into the bladder under direct vision. Alternatively, a catheter can be manipulated through the defect with interlocking sounds (Figure 14.27). Intact pubopros-

tatic ligaments are transected so that traction on the catheter will approximate the apex of the prostate with the urogenital diaphragm. If technically feasible, the urethra is anastomosed to the prostate under direct vision.

Regardless of initial management, pelvic abscesses, incontinence, and impotence are recognized complications of membranous urethral ruptures. Varying degrees of stricture formation should be anticipated and reconstructive procedures 3 to 6 months after injury are often necessary.

Surgery of the Scrotal Contents

The scrotal sac holds the testes, their adnexa, and the proximal spermatic cords in two separate compartments formed by a medial septum. The wall of the sac is composed primarily of the dartos muscle. This muscle is adherent to the overlying skin and gives the scrotum a wrinkled appearance. Remnants of the external spermatic fascia, cremasteric muscle, and internal spermatic fascia lie between the dartos and the parietal tunica vaginalis. The latter is derived from the parietal peritoneum and creates a nonadherent envelope for the testis. Posterior to the epididymis the parietal tunica vaginalis fuses and then reflects over the epididymis and testes as the visceral tunica vaginalis (Figure 15.1). A small quantity of fluid separates the mucosal surfaces of the visceral and parietal tunics and accounts partly for the mobility of the testes within the scrotum.

The blood supply of the scrotum is derived from branches of the external and internal pudendal arteries and from the cremasteric and testicular arteries. The scrotum is innervated by branches of the ilioinguinal, genitofemoral, pudendal, and posterior femoral cutaneous nerves. Lymphatic vessels drain to the superficial inguinal lymph nodes.

The testis has a tough fibrous capsule (the tunica albuginea) from which multiple septa arise to divide the parenchyma into hundreds of small compartments (Figure 15.2). Each compartment contains convoluted seminiferous tubules. Sperm from the germinal epithelium of the tubules course into 10 to 20 ducts situated in the superior aspect of the testis. These ducts, or rete testis, connect with the efferent ductules, which extend from the testis to the head of the epididymis. The superior component of the epididymis (the head) is composed of convoluted extensions of the efferent ductules. The ductules coalesce to form one tubule (the body of the epididymis), which traverses the posterior aspect of the testis. At the inferior pole of the testis, the epididymis forms the vas deferens, a muscular duct that travels within the spermatic cord to the pelvis.

The appendix testis, a remnant of the Mullerian duct, is a fleshy, 1- to 2-mm appendage arising from the tunica albuginea below the head of the epididymis. The appendix epididymis is a structure of similar size

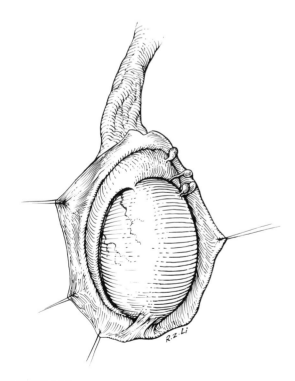

FIGURE 15.1
Testis and adnexa within parietal tunica vaginalis

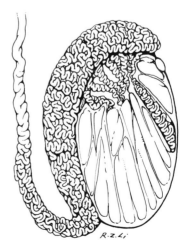

FIGURE 15.2
Intratesticular anatomy

and consistency attached to the tunica albuginea just next to the head of the epididymis. The appendix epididymis is a remnant of the wolffian duct. The fibrous gubernaculum attaches the testis to the dependent scrotal sac.

The spermatic cord contains the vas deferens, the gonadal artery, a plexus of gonadal veins, lymphatics from the testis and epididymis, and a branch of the genitofemoral nerve. It travels from the posterosuperior aspect of the testis to the internal inguinal ring and is loosely invested by the internal spermatic, cremasteric, and external spermatic fasciae. The gonadal artery branches from the infrarenal aorta and accompanies the gonadal veins to the internal inguinal ring. The plexus of gonadal veins within the spermatic cord coalesces into two or three veins at the internal inguinal ring and drains into the infrarenal vena cava on the right and the renal vein on the left. The lymphatic channels from the spermatic cord traverse the retroperitoneum with the gonadal vessels. Drainage on the right is to nodes situated between the infrarenal aorta and vena cava; drainage on the left is to nodes located anterolateral to the aorta at or below the takeoff of the renal arteries.

The scrotal contents are approached through a scrotal or inguinal incision. When a tumor of the intrascrotal contents is suspected, one always uses the inguinal incision. The scrotal incision is preferably transverse to parallel the course of subcutaneous blood vessels. It is closed by approximation of the dartos muscle with a continuous absorbable suture. This helps to secure bleeding vessels, which predominate in the dartos. The skin is closed with interrupted sutures of the same material.

Because of the relatively loose nature of the scrotal tissues, postoperative edema is usually disproportionate to the magnitude of the surgery, and small unsecured vessels may result in the formation of large hematomas. Drainage with a ¼-in Penrose drain exiting through a stab wound in the dependent scrotum is advisable after some surgical procedures. Ice packs are applied to the scrotum for 12 to 24 hours after surgery to reduce swelling. An athletic supporter helps to relieve discomfort and holds dressings over the incision.

TESTICULAR BIOPSY

Biopsy of the testis is an integral diagnostic test in the evaluation of azoospermia. Histologic examination of the testicular parenchyma differentiates between duc-

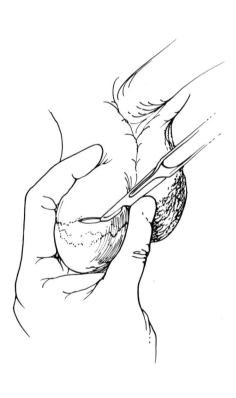

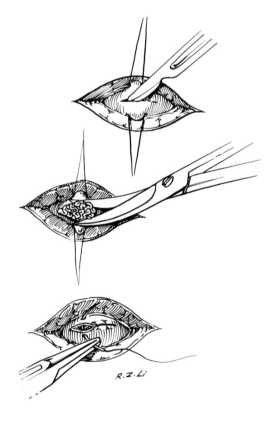

FIGURE 15.3
Biopsy of the testis

tal obstruction, which may be reversible, and sperma-
togenic failure, which is generally not treatable.
Among infertile men with identifiable sperm in the
ejaculate, the results of a biopsy can have prognostic
significance, but the therapeutic relevance is limited.
Biopsies of both testes in infertile men and biopsy of
parenchymal abnormalities to rule out carcinoma are
almost never indicated.

OPERATIVE TECHNIQUE   Biopsy of the testis is an outpatient procedure performed with local or regional anesthesia. The testis is grasped firmly between the
thumb and forefinger with the epididymis located posteriorly (Figure 15.3). A 1-cm transverse incision is
made through the skin and the dartos muscle, and the
parietal tunica vaginalis is opened. The testis is stabilized with two stay sutures applied to the tunica albuginea, and an ellipse of the fibrous capsule is
incised between the sutures. Seminiferous tissue attached to the tunica is squeezed into the wound and
sheared with a knife or a scissors. Zenker's or Bouin's
fixative is preferable to formalin for preservation of the
germinal epithelium and should be available in the operating room before a biopsy.

SIMPLE ORCHIECTOMY

Simple scrotal orchiectomy refers to the removal of
the testis and epididymis only and is generally performed with local anesthesia. Epididymo-orchitis and
testicular abscesses that are refractory to antimicrobial therapy are the most common indications for unilateral procedures. Bilateral simple orchiectomy is
done almost exclusively as a means of androgen deprivation therapy in patients with advanced carcinoma of
the prostate.

OPERATIVE TECHNIQUE   The spermatic cord is infiltrated with 25 ml of lidocaine where it crosses the
pubic tubercle, and the scrotal skin is infiltrated for a
transverse incision. The skin, dartos muscle, and parietal tunica vaginalis are incised (Figure 15.4), and the
testis and cord are delivered into the wound. The fascia of the spermatic cord is opened just above the
testis, and the vas deferens is separated from the remaining cord structures. Each of the bundles is separately cross-clamped, transected, and secured with
nonabsorbable suture ligatures. When the orchiectomy
is not performed for an inflammatory disorder, a testicular prosthesis may be inserted if requested by the
patient. After bilateral orchiectomy the scrotum is
wrapped with an Elastoplast dressing to reduce the
risks of hematoma formation.

Preservation of the epididymis or evacuation of the
testicular parenchyma from the tunica albuginea (subcapsular orchiectomy) are alternatives to the standard

simple orchiectomy in patients with prostate cancer.
However, these maneuvers complicate an otherwise
simple procedure and are of minimal cosmetic benefit.

INGUINAL (RADICAL) ORCHIECTOMY

Inguinal orchiectomy is the en bloc removal of the
contents of a hemiscrotum, the investing parietal
tunica vaginalis, and the entire spermatic cord. It is
necessarily performed through an inguinal incision and
is done usually for the diagnosis and treatment of testicular neoplasms.

OPERATIVE TECHNIQUE   A standard inguinal incision
is used to expose the external oblique fascia. The fascia is incised in the direction of its fibers from the
external ring to a point above the internal ring (Figure

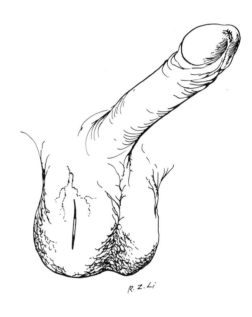

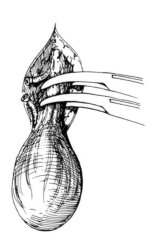

FIGURE 15.4
Simple orchiectomy

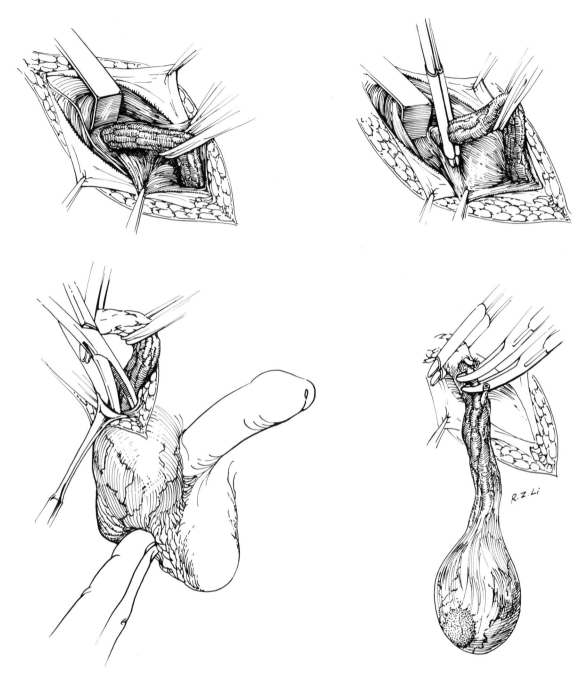

FIGURE 15.5
Inguinal orchiectomy

15.5). The ilioinguinal nerve is teased from the spermatic fascia and retracted inferiorly, and the spermatic
cord is mobilized by blunt dissection at the level of the
pubic tubercle. When a malignancy is suspected, the
cord is occluded with a rubber-shod clamp or encircling Penrose drain to prevent the theoretical possibility of tumor dissemination during manipulation of the
testis.

The testis and enveloping parietal tunica vaginalis
are delivered into the wound by pushing the hemiscrotum and its contents upward and bluntly dissecting the
tunics from loosely adherent areolar tissue. The
hemiscrotum is packed with a sponge, and the cord is
mobilized to the level of the internal ring. The vas
deferens is separated from the remaining cord structures at the internal ring, and both bundles are individually clamped, transected, and secured with nonabsorbable suture ligatures. The ligature on the gonadal

vessels is cut long so that the distal extent of the vessels can be identified during subsequent retroperitoneal lymphadenectomy.

The pack is removed from the hemiscrotum, and its interior is invaginated into the wound to permit fulguration of bleeding vessels under direct vision. A testicular prosthesis may be implanted if requested by the patient. The scrotum is not drained, but an Elastoplast dressing is applied loosely to facilitate hemostasis.

POSTOPERATIVE CARE AND COMPLICATIONS Despite meticulous attention to hemostasis, small hematomas in the empty hemiscrotum are common. The masses resolve over 1 to 2 months but can be worrisome if the orchiectomy was performed for a neoplasm. The incidence of local tumor recurrence following a properly performed inguinal orchiectomy, however, is negligible. Germ cell tumors of the testis metastasize through the lymphatics, but the initial site of spread is to the retroperitoneal rather than the pelvic or inguinal lymph nodes. For this reason, excision of accessible lymph nodes adjacent to the inguinal canal is not warranted during radical orchiectomy for tumor.

ORCHIOPEXY

Orchiopexy is a procedure for positioning the cryptorchid testis into the scrotal sac. Cryptorchid testes are located within the inguinal canal, in subcutaneous tissue distal to the inguinal canal, or in the retroperitoneum proximal to the inguinal canal. It is important to differentiate retractile testes, which can be manipulated into the scrotal sac, from cryptorchid testes. Retractile testes are managed initially with human chorionic gonadotropin injections.

An orchiopexy is usually performed during early childhood. It creates a normal appearance to the external genitalia, improves spermatogenesis, reduces the incidence, or at least increases the detectability, of testicular cancer, decreases the risks of torsion, and allows repair of inguinal hernias resulting from the usually patent processus vaginalis. The rationale for orchiopexy as opposed to orchiectomy is arguable in men.

The fundamental maneuvers of orchiopexy include mobilization of the spermatic vessels to permit tension-free placement of the testis to the hemiscrotum, fixation of the testis in the hemiscrotum, and repair of the associated hernia.

OPERATIVE TECHNIQUE An inguinal incision is made in the skin crease, the external oblique fascia overlying the inguinal canal is incised to the external ring, and the cremasteric muscle is divided (Figure 15.6). If the testis is found in the inguinal canal, the gubernaculum is transected, and the spermatic cord with the adherent processus vaginalis are mobilized to the internal ring. The processus vaginalis, which extends along the superomedial aspect of the cord, is dissected from the spermatic fascia just distal to the internal ring. It is then transected, ligated with a fine nonabsorbable suture, and allowed to retract through the internal ring.

In most cases these maneuvers permit tension-free positioning of the testis into the hemiscrotum. The dartos pouch is preferred for fixation and is created using the following techniques. The skin of the dependent is incised, and a plane is developed between the skin and dartos muscle. A defect is created in the dartos muscle at the superior aspect of the pouch and the testis is pulled into the pouch. It is then fixed to the dartos muscle with fine nonabsorbable sutures. Drainage of the hemiscrotum is not necessary, and the scrotal and inguinal wounds are closed in the conventional manner.

An inability to position the testis in the scrotum without undue tension results from inadequate length of the gonadal vessels rather than of the vas deferens. Mobilization of the vessels from retroperitoneal attachments usually rectifies the problem. In addition, a more direct path for the gonadal vessels from the retroperitoneum to the scrotum can be developed by incising the floor of the inguinal canal and dividing the inferior epigastric artery and vein. The spermatic cord is then repositioned medially, and the internal ring and lateral inguinal canal are closed with interrupted nonabsorbable sutures.

Transection of the gonadal artery and vein above the internal ring should be considered when satisfactory relocation of the testis remains impossible despite the maneuvers detailed above. The blood supply from collateral vessels of the vas deferens is usually adequate to prevent testicular infarction. The contribution of these collaterals to testicular perfusion is determined by clamping the gonadal vessels for 5 minutes and incising the tunica albuginea of the testis. Brisk bleeding suggests adequate blood flow from the collaterals.

If the testis cannot be located through the inguinal approach, the retroperitoneum is explored through a midline incision. Testes located high in the retroperitoneum may be implanted into the scrotum after transection of the gonadal vessels. Care must be taken to avoid injury to the vasculature of the vas deferens. Microsurgical anastomosis of the gonadal vessels with the inferior epigastric vessels is an alternative approach to this situation. Atrophic testes in the retroperitoneum should be removed.

POSTOPERATIVE CARE AND COMPLICATIONS Most patients do not require hospitalization after a straightforward orchiopexy. Migration of the testis from the dartos pouch may occur in the postoperative period if the

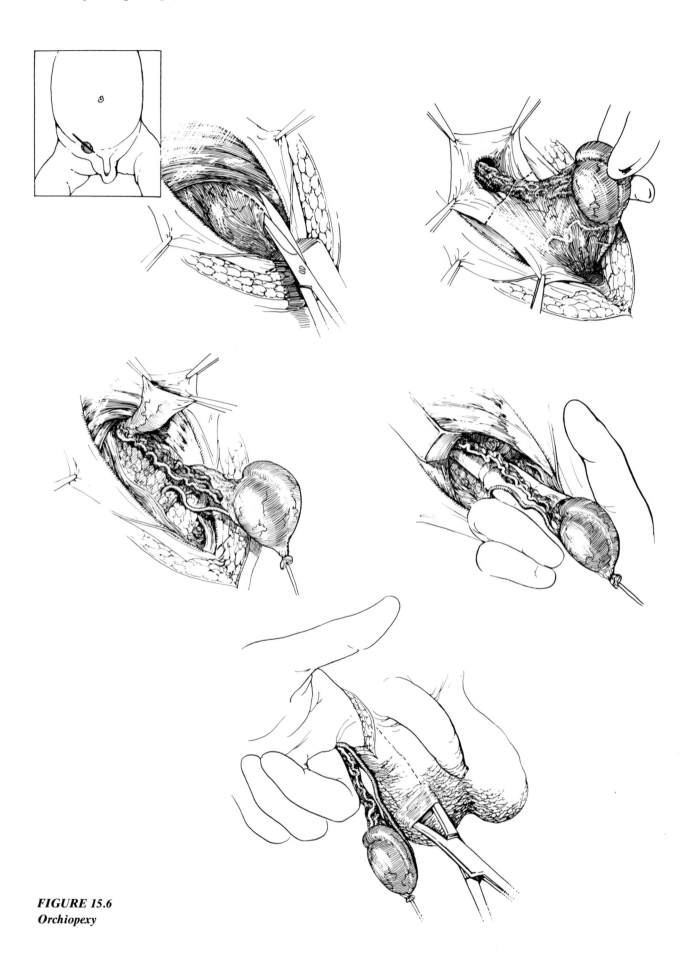

FIGURE 15.6
Orchiopexy

spermatic cord is unduly taut. Late complications include testicular atrophy due to vascular compromise and obstruction of the vas deferens due to intraoperative trauma or devascularization.

OPERATIONS FOR TESTICULAR TRAUMA

Severe testicular injuries result usually in distention of the hemiscrotum with blood. Exploration is advisable for evacuation of clot and, if present, repair of disruptions of the tunica albuginea or gonadal vessels.

OPERATIVE TECHNIQUE The testis is approached through a transcrotal incision. Hematoma is evacuated, and the scrotal contents are delivered into the wound. Tears of the tunica albuginea are debrided and closed with a continuous nonabsorbable suture. Bleeding veins in the spermatic cord are ligated. Injury to the gonadal artery is unusual unless the spermatic cord has been completely avulsed. Penrose drainage is recommended.

OPERATIONS FOR TESTICULAR TORSION

Testicular torsion results from a rotation of the spermatic cord immediately adjacent to the testis and causes occlusion of the gonadal vessels. In most cases an abnormally loose attachment between the epididymis and testis predisposes to the condition.

The process produces acute scrotal pain and, in some cases, nausea and vomiting. Characteristic physical findings include a firm, tender testis that is displaced high in the scrotum and induration of the spermatic cord immediately above the testis. The epididymis is frequently positioned anteriorly. The contralateral testis and epididymis usually have the same abnormal attachment as the torsed testis, and the testis has a horizontal rather than a vertical orientation.

Emergent intervention is necessary to prevent testicular infarction. Differentiation between torsion and epididymo-orchitis may be difficult by physical examination alone. Pyuria suggests inflammation rather than torsion. Radionuclide scans reveal impaired perfusion with torsion, but a similar result is often seen with epididymo-orchitis owing to compression of the distal ramifications of the gonadal artery.

Testicular torsion in neonates results from twisting of the spermatic cord proximal to the tunica vaginalis. The testis is rarely viable and orchiectomy is generally necessary.

OPERATIVE TECHNIQUE If the patient is seen soon after the onset of pain, the spermatic cord is infiltrated with lidocaine and manual detorsion of the testis is attempted. When successful there is prompt relief of severe pain.

Regardless of the outcome of preoperative manipulations, the testis is always explored through a transscrotal incision as soon as feasible. The testis is delivered into the wound and the cord is untwisted under direct vision (Figure 15.7). It is then replaced in

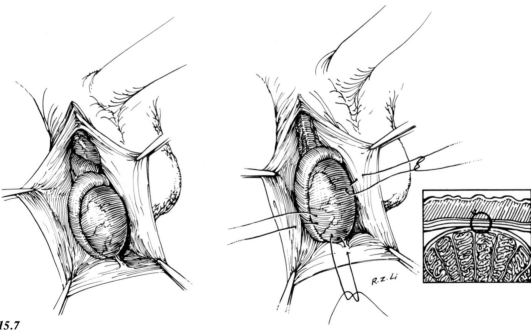

FIGURE 15.7
Repair of testicular torsion

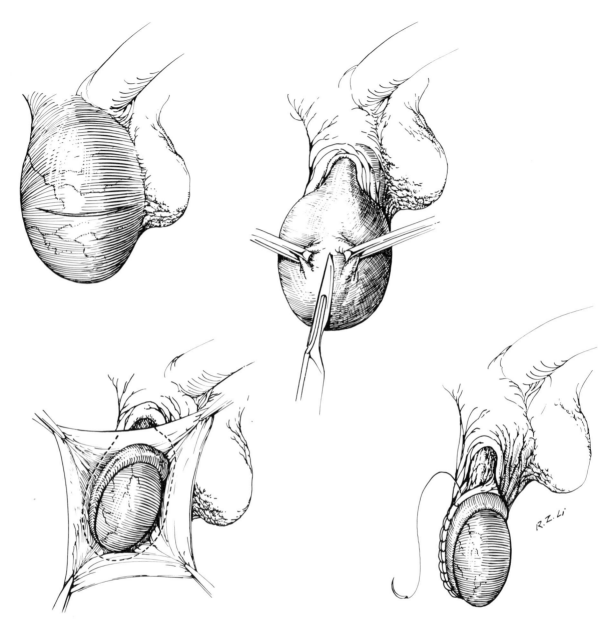

FIGURE 15.8
Hydrocelectomy

the scrotal sac, and the tunica albuginea is anchored to the dartos muscle with nonabsorbable sutures. The sutures are placed on the lateral aspects of the testis as well as at the inferior margin to prevent subsequent rotation in any direction. Because the anatomic abnormality predisposing to torsion is usually bilateral, the contralateral testis is exposed through a second transscrotal incision and attached to the dartos muscle with three sutures. Drainage of the scrotum is generally not necessary.

Not infrequently the viability of the testis is indeterminant at the time of surgery. However, preservation of the gonad is always advisable unless frank necrosis is encountered.

HYDROCELECTOMY

A hydrocele is the accumulation of abnormal amounts of fluid between the membranes of the parietal and visceral tunica vaginalis. The fluid collection does not usually cause pain. However, hydroceles may reach large, and at times enormous, proportions that warrant operative intervention. Aspiration of fluid is generally futile as rapid reaccumulation is the rule.

OPERATIVE TECHNIQUE A hydrocele is approached through an inguinal or transverse scrotal incision. The former is recommended if the fluid collection extends to the external inguinal ring or if a coexisting testicular tumor is at all suspect. The scrotum is incised to but

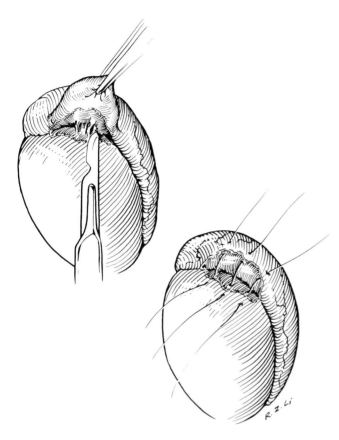

FIGURE 15.9
Spermatocelectomy

not through the parietal tunics, as decompression of the hydrocele usually makes the subsequent dissection more difficult. A plane is established between the tunics and the aerolar tissue of the scrotal wall, and the entire mass is delivered into the wound (Figure 15.8). Two Allis clamps are applied to the fluid-filled sac at a site opposite the epididymis, the hydrocele is incised between the two clamps, and the fluid is aspirated. Small concretions are often seen floating in the fluid.

The opening of the parietal tunica vaginalis is extended superiorly and inferiorly, and the testis and epididymis are carefully inspected and palpated to rule out parenchymal abnormalities. The redundant parietal tunica vaginalis is then partially excised leaving a 1- to 2-cm border attached to the epididymis and the spermatic cord. The margins of the tunics are swung posterior to the epididymis and cord and approximated with a continuous absorbable hemostatic suture. The testis is replaced in the hemiscrotum and anchored to the dartos with three nonabsorbable sutures. This prevents torsion of the testis within the distended hemiscrotum. A Penrose drain is brought out through the dependent scrotum, and the wound is closed in the conventional manner.

POSTOPERATIVE CARE AND COMPLICATIONS The Penrose drain is removed on the first postoperative day.

Swelling of the scrotal wall and intrascrotal contents is inevitable and usually requires 1 to 2 months for complete resolution. The recurrence of a fluid collection is uncommon if the mucosal surfaces of the residual tunics are not opposed.

SPERMATOCELECTOMY

Spermatoceles are cystic dilatations of the efferent ductules located between the epididymis and the parenchyma of the testis. The cyst contains fluid and sperm and can usually be transilluminated. Pain, cosmetic considerations, and diagnostic uncertainty are reasonable indications for spermatocelectomy.

OPERATIVE TECHNIQUE The scrotum and parietal tunica vaginalis are opened with a transverse incision,

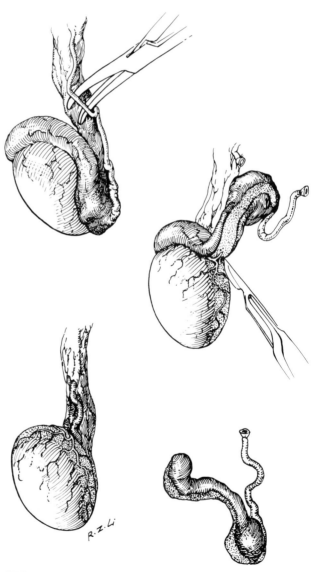

FIGURE 15.10
Epididymectomy

and the scrotal contents are delivered into the wound. An avascular plane separates the spermatocele from the adjacent testis and epididymis, and enucleation is usually straightforward (Figure 15.9). The tunic of the epididymis is then sutured to the tunica albuginea of the testis to cover the denuded fossa. Drainage of the scrotum is advisable if the spermatocele is large.

EPIDIDYMECTOMY

Removal of the epididymis is occasionally indicated for the eradication of focal infections that are resistant to antimicrobial therapy or for symptomatic chronic inflammation. Tumors of the epididymis are extremely rare and should be treated by radical orchiectomy.

OPERATIVE TECHNIQUE The testis is approached through a transverse scrotal incision and delivered into the wound. The proximal vas deferens is isolated, transected, and ligated, and the epididymis is freed from the inferolateral testis with sharp dissection (Figure 15.10). The gonadal artery and vein are encountered just below the head of the epididymis. Branches to the epididymis are transected and ligated, taking care to avoid injury to the testicular ramifications. The head of the epididymis is then dissected from the tunica albuginea, and the specimen is removed. Small bleeding vessels on the denuded tunica albuginea are controlled with electrocautery. The point of exit of the efferent ductules from the superior pole of the testis is oversewn with a figure-of-eight absorbable suture. Drainage of the hemiscrotum is usually advisable.

REMOVAL OF THE TESTICULAR APPENDAGES

Torsion of the appendix epididymis or appendix testis is unusual but may occur at any age. The resultant ischemia leads to well-localized pain and palpable swelling of the appendage. Spontaneous resolution of discomfort is not uncommon, but surgical exploration is mandatory if the appropriate diagnosis is at all questionable.

OPERATIVE TECHNIQUE The hemiscrotum is explored as for torsion of the testis. The twisted appendix is amputated flush with the tunica albuginea and the base is fulgurated. Removal of the companion appendix on the same testis is recommended, but prophylactic excision of the appendages of the contralateral testis is not warranted.

VASECTOMY

Vasectomy is a procedure for obstruction of the vas deferens that is done almost exclusively to produce permanent sterility. Psychosocial stability is a prerequisite because the outcome of the operation is often irreversible. Vasectomy before prostatectomy is recommended by some authorities to reduce the incidence of postoperative epididymitis.

OPERATIVE TECHNIQUE A vasectomy is performed with local anesthesia in the outpatient setting unless there are coexisting intrascrotal abnormalities that require correction or that make the procedure difficult.

The vas is grasped with the thumb and index finger at a point midway between the epididymis and external inguinal ring. It is then separated from the adjacent cord structures and worked to the anterolateral aspect of the scrotum (Figure 15.11). The skin and dartos muscle are anesthetized with lidocaine, and a 1-cm incision is made at right angles to the course of the vas. The tips of a towel clip are introduced into the wound to grasp the vas and the investing fascia. The fascia is incised for 1 cm in a longitudinal direction to expose the adventitia, and the vas is secured with a second towel clip. The first clip is removed, and a 2- to 3-cm loop of the vas is delivered into the wound. Residual fibrous attachments between the opposed vasal segments are divided bluntly by spreading a hemostat under the loop.

The proximal and distal ends of the vas are secured with hemostats, and the intervening segment is excised and sent for pathologic examination. The lumens are then fulgurated for 1 cm with a needle-point electrode, and each end is ligated with a nonabsorbable suture. Perivasal fascia is sutured over the proximal or distal lumen to form a barrier between the two segments.

An identical procedure is then done on the contralateral side. If the first incision is located in the midline, the contralateral vas can usually be manipulated medially and grasped with a towel clip through the same incision.

Excessive traction on the vas may produce lower abdominal discomfort or nausea and should be avoided throughout the procedure. The vas is remarkably mobile, and transection of one vas at two different sites is possible if the intrascrotal anatomy is not clearly delineated. At the conclusion of the operation a defect should be palpable in each vas.

POSTOPERATIVE CARE AND COMPLICATIONS Ecchymosis next to the incision is inevitable, and in most cases a nodule of about 1 cm in diameter is palpable for 2 to 4 weeks after surgery. However, the patient is always instructed to contact the physician if there is more pronounced intrascrotal swelling. Bleeding and hema-

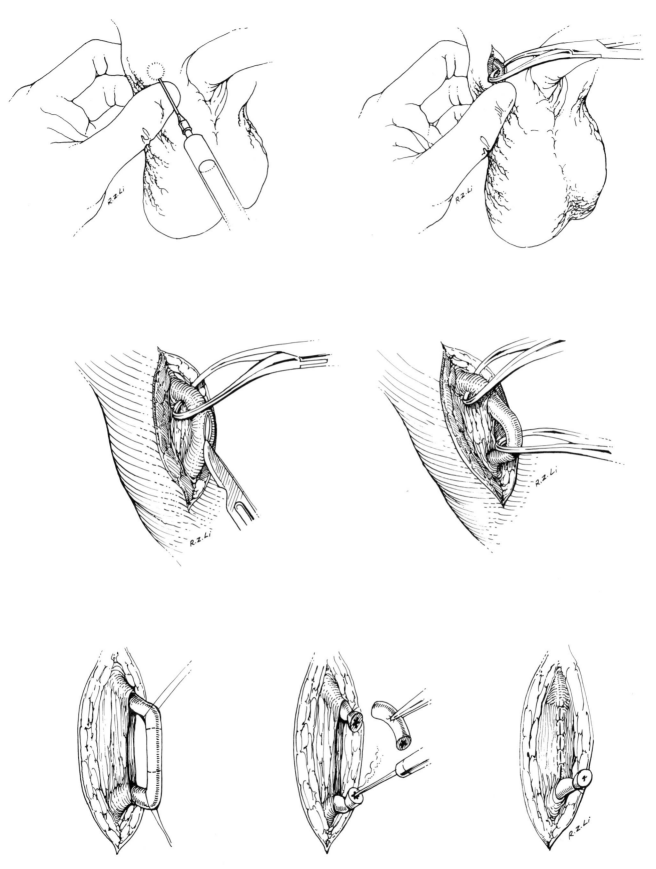

FIGURE 15.11
Vasectomy

toma formation due to unrecognized injury of vessels adjacent to the adventitia of the vas or oozing from the dartos muscle are the causes of this complication. Large hematomas are managed by exploration, evacuation of clot, ligation of the bleeder, and the placement of drains.

Intermittent scrotal pain is a recognized late complication of vasectomy, which results apparently from increased pressure within the epididymis. When debilitating, a vasovasostomy or epididymectomy should be considered.

The patient must understand that sterility is not assured until a semen analysis reveals no residual sperm. This usually requires 10 to 15 ejaculations or 1 to 2 months. Recanalization, which results from leakage of sperm from the proximal vas, occurs in less than 1 percent of cases but is clinically unrecognizable unless intermittent semen analyses are performed. All patients who choose vasectomy as a method of contraception must accept the remote possibility of an unexpected pregnancy.

VASOGRAPHY

Injection of contrast medium into the vas deferens is done to localize suspected obstruction of the vas deferens and to delineate the lumen of the seminal vesicles. Cannulation of the ejaculatory ducts for retrograde injection of contrast medium is difficult if not impossible.

OPERATIVE TECHNIQUE   The vas deferens is isolated as described for vasectomy. Contrast medium can be introduced on occasion by puncture of the vasal lumen with a 25-gauge needle. In most cases, however, it is preferable to expose the lumen with a transverse incision (Figure 15.12). A blunt needle is then inserted into the lumen under direct vision and contrast is gently injected in an antegrade direction. Retrograde injection to opacify the proximal vas deferens and epididymis is rarely warranted and may result in a chemical epididymitis. The incision in the vas is closed in two layers using the techniques described for vasovasostomy. The mucosa is approximated with two fine nylon sutures, and the anastomosis is reinforced with several seromuscular sutures of the same material.

Patency of the vas can be documented also by the antegrade injection of methylene blue. The bladder is catheterized before the procedure, and the appearance of discolored urine indicates that the vas is patent.

VASOVASOSTOMY

Vasovasostomy is performed primarily as a means for reversing a vasectomy. Congenital, postinflammatory,

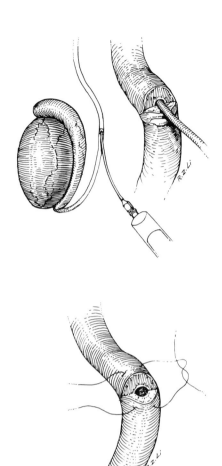

FIGURE 15.12
Vasography

or posttraumatic obstructions of the vas deferens are also indications for the operation. Most urologists with a clinical interest in male infertility use loupes or the operating microscope for intraoperative magnification. The benefits of a precise two-layer anastomosis of the mucosa and muscularis compared with a full-thickness anastomosis and supporting seromuscular sutures are unsettled.

OPERATIVE TECHNIQUE   The site of obstruction is approached by delivering the entire contents of the hemiscrotum through a transscrotal incision or by incision of the scrotum over the palpable vasal defect (Figure 15.13). The scarred segment is isolated and excised, and the proximal vas is sequentially transected until fluid appears in the lumen. This material is collected with a sterile capillary pipette and examined microscopically. The presence of sperm has important prognostic implications. Patency of the distal vas is demonstrated by antegrade passage of a 00 nylon suture or with vasography.

The ends of the vas are secured in a vas deferens approximation clip and each lumen is gently dilated.

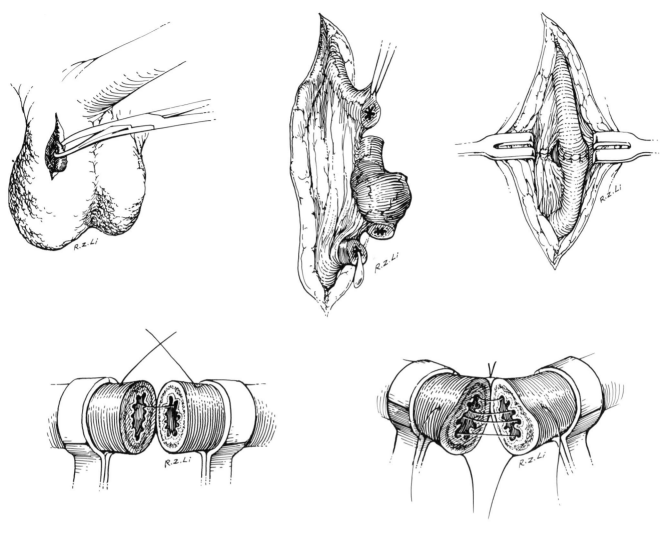

FIGURE 15.13
Vasovasostomy with one-layer anastomosis

The most straightforward method of anastomosis involves placement of 10-0 nylon sutures through the full thickness of the vasal wall at four quadrants. The bites should include a generous portion of the muscularis but the edge of the luminal mucosa only. It is advisable to position the last two sutures before they are tied. Four to six sutures of 8-0 nylon that encompass the muscularis and serosa are then applied to strengthen and seal the anastomosis. Perivasal fascia and areolar tissue are sutured over the anastomosis for added support, and the wound is closed without drainage. If indicated, the procedure is then performed on the contralateral side.

With the two-layer closure the luminal mucosa is anastomosed with six to eight interrupted sutures of 10-0 nylon. The seromuscular layer is closed with six to eight sutures of 8-0 nylon (Figure 15.14).

In the era before microsurgical techniques were applied to vasovasostomy, some authorities recommended stenting of the anastomosis with a wire. The wire was positioned across the repair and brought out through a puncture wound in the distal vas and overlying scrotal wall. The necessity for this maneuver when microscopic watertight anastomoses are performed, however, is questionable.

POSTOPERATIVE CARE AND COMPLICATIONS Intercourse is restricted for 1 month, and a semen analysis is performed after 1 to 2 months. The motility of ejaculated sperm at this time is often suboptimal, but improvement over the ensuing 5 months is the rule.

Persistent infertility despite technically successful anastomoses is the most common complication of vasovasostomy. Although most patients develop near-normal seminal parameters, conception is achieved in only 50 percent of cases. The reasons for this phenomenon are multifactorial and generally untreatable.

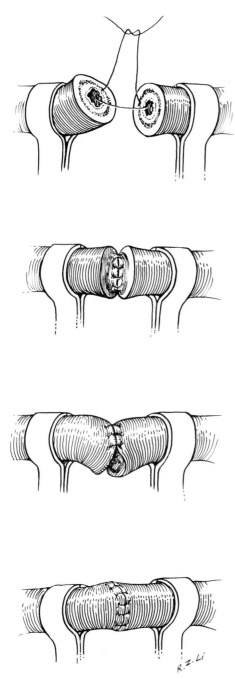

FIGURE 15.14
Two-layered anastomosis for vasovasostomy

VASOEPIDIDYMOSTOMY

Obstruction of the epididymal lumen results most often from vasectomy, but may also be postinflammatory or congenital. Identification of the appropriate convoluted tubule of the epididymis for anastomosis with the vas and performance of the anastomosis require microsurgical instrumentation and techniques.

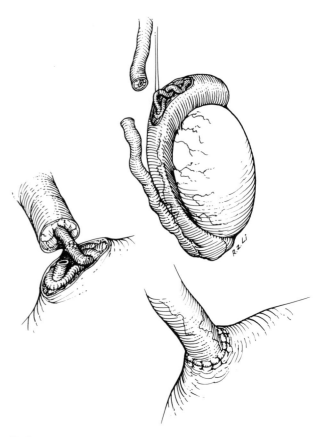

FIGURE 15.15
Vasoepididymostomy

OPERATIVE TECHNIQUE   The contents of the hemiscrotum are exposed through a transverse scrotal incision, and a vasogram is obtained to assess patency of the distal vas deferens. The vas is then transected distal to the convoluted segment, and the visceral tunic of the epididymis is opened (Figure 15.15). Dilated tubules proximal to the epididymal obstruction are visualized with the aid of the operating microscope. A tubule located as far as possible from the head of the epididymis is transected and the fluid is assessed microscopically. If whole sperm are not visualized, a more proximal tubule is transected. The appropriate tubule and the vas are then secured in a vas deferens approximation clip. The mucosa is anastomosed with four to six interrupted sutures of 10-0 nylon, and the muscularis of the vas and the tunic of the epididymis are approximated with supporting sutures of 8-0 nylon. An end-to-side rather than an end-to-end anastomosis is at times more convenient.

When a dilated tubule of the epididymis is not identifiable, the epididymis is serially transected in a transverse fashion from the tail toward the head until fluid is visualized in a tubular lumen. An end-to-end anastomosis between the vas and the tubule is performed as described earlier. The prospects of fertility are reduced as the anastomosis approaches the head of the epididymis because the epididymal environment is required for normal sperm maturation.

Postoperative care and complications parallel those of vasovasostomy. However, the likelihood of fertility is not as great.

SPERMATIC VEIN LIGATION

A varicocele consists of dilated spermatic veins within the scrotum. The condition results usually from incompetent valves in the spermatic vein and retrograde blood flow. Ligation of the spermatic vein interrupts the aberrant venous blood flow and decompresses the varicocele.

Varicoceles are distinctly more common on the left side than on the right. They may reach large proportions and require treatment for cosmetic reasons or, on

occasion, pain. Varicoceles have an unfavorable impact on spermatogenesis apparently because the temperature of the testicular parenchyma increases. Ligation of the spermatic vein may improve the quality of semen of affected men who are infertile.

The spermatic vein can be exposed in the retroperitoneum above the internal inguinal ring or in the inguinal canal. With the former approach only two to three veins are encountered, isolation of the gonadal artery is generally not difficult, and injury to the vas deferens is unlikely. With the inguinal approach the veins are more numerous, and injury to the vas deferens or gonadal artery is probably more common. However, the risk of missing a communicating vein at the internal inguinal ring is less.

OPERATIVE TECHNIQUE For both approaches the patient is placed in the reverse Trendelenburg position. This increases venous distention and facilitates intraoperative identification of the veins.

The retroperitoneal spermatic vein is approached

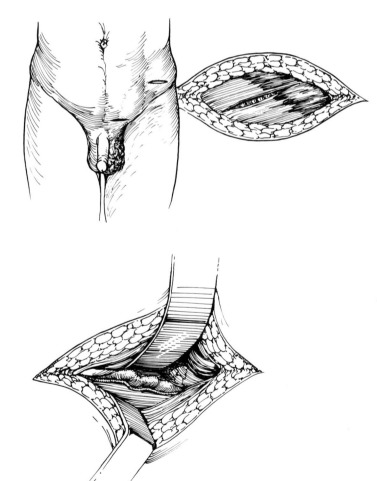
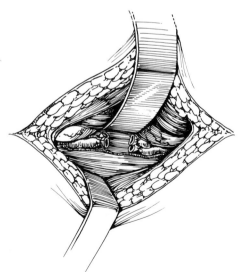

FIGURE 15.16
Spermatic vein ligation (retroperitoneal approach)

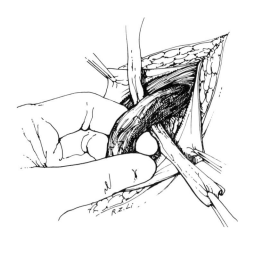

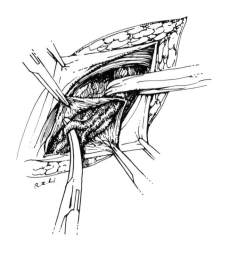

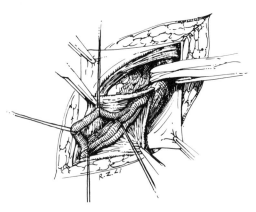

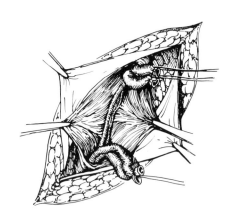

FIGURE 15.17
Spermatic vein ligation (inguinal approach)

through a transverse incision medial to the anterior superior iliac spine and above the internal ring (Figure 15.16). The external and internal oblique muscles are divided in the direction of their fibers and retracted apart. The filmy transversalis fascia is incised, and the peritoneum is swept medially to expose the veins. The spermatic artery is identified next to the veins and retracted if necessary. The vas deferens is usually visualized below the area of dissection. Each vein is doubly ligated, and the intervening segment is excised and sent for pathologic examination. The muscle layers are approximated with interrupted absorbable sutures. Drains are not necessary.

With the inguinal approach the spermatic cord is exposed as described for an inguinal orchiectomy. The spermatic fascia is incised, and the vas deferens and gonadal artery are isolated and retracted away from the veins (Figure 15.17). Each vein is doubly ligated, and the intervening segment is excised and sent to pathology for examination.

Surgery of the Adrenal Glands

The adrenal glands are yellowish pyramid structures situated superomedial to the kidneys. Each gland is invested by Gerota's fascia and anchored by multiple fibrous attachments. The right adrenal gland lies below the liver and lateral to the inferior vena cava. The left adrenal lies behind the pancreas and lateral to the aorta. It is more inferomedial in position than the right and is closer to the renal vessels.

The arterial supply is abundant and is derived from the aorta and the renal and inferior phrenic arteries (Figure 16.1). Each major artery divides into numerous small branches before entering the parenchyma. The venous drainage is more ordered. The main right adrenal vein is short and drains into the vena cava. The main left adrenal vein merges with the inferior phrenic vein to drain into the left renal vein. Lymphatic drainage is to the para-aortic nodal chains.

ADRENALECTOMY

Adrenalectomy is the only primary operation of the adrenal glands. Benign and malignant tumors arising from the cortex or medulla are the usual indications for surgery. Many tumors secrete steroids or catecholamines, and systemic manifestations of hormonal excess are often the first indication of the disease. The nature of hormonal synthesis and secretion, which provides information about the histology of the tumor, is determined by assays of the urine and serum. The site of the tumor is usually established with computed tomography or magnetic resonance imaging.

A detailed discussion of diagnostic methods to characterize hormonally active tumors, management of the systemic manifestations of steroid or catecholamine hypersecretion, and perioperative steroidal

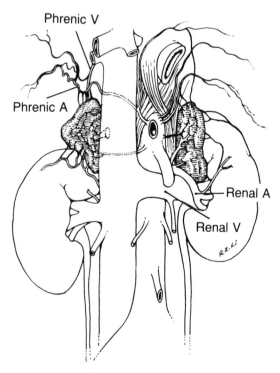

FIGURE 16.1
Location and vascular supply of the adrenal glands

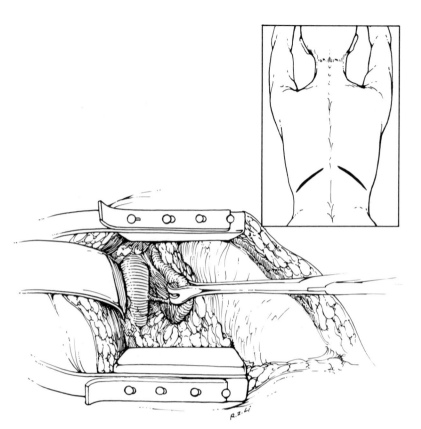

FIGURE 16.2
Bilateral posterior transcostal approach to the adrenal glands

replacement are beyond the scope of this text. Suffice to say that surgeons and anesthesiologists must have a working knowledge of these matters to properly prepare the patient for surgery and to prevent potentially lethal complications during and after surgery.

Adrenalectomy is at times advisable for management of such benign and hormonally inactive lesions as cysts and hamartomas. These masses may be impossible to differentiate from malignant tumors and can produce local symptoms if large. Bilateral adrenalectomy for the treatment of prostate or breast cancer is of historical interest only.

OPERATIVE TECHNIQUE   The operative approach to the adrenal gland is dictated largely by the nature of the disorder and the size of mass lesions. For example, generous transabdominal exposure is recommended for removal of pheochromocytomas. Approximately 10 percent of these tumors are multifocal, and secondary lesions may be discovered by palpation only. When the laterality of a hormonally active adrenal tumor cannot be delineated before surgery, or if a bilateral adrenalectomy is necessary, access to both adrenal glands through two posterior transcostal incisions (Figure 16.2) or a transabdominal incision is advisable. A standard tenth or eleventh rib transcostal flank incision may be sufficient when exposure of only one adrenal gland is required. Large adrenal tumors are best approached with a thoracoabdominal incision.

The basic techniques of adrenalectomy are as follows. Gerota's fascia is opened and perinephric fat is freed from the superior pole of the kidney. The kidney is retracted downward, and fibrous attachments to the lateral, anterior, and posterior surfaces of the adrenal gland are transected. Feeding vessels encountered during this dissection are less numerous than during inferior, medial, and superior dissection, but require suture ligation or control with hemostatic clips.

The dissection then proceeds inferomedially. On the right the vena cava is exposed, and the adrenal gland is mobilized to the level of the main adrenal vein (Figure 16.3). This vessel is doubly clamped, transected, and ligated. The superior aspect of the gland is then freed from fibrovascular attachments and the specimen is removed.

On the left the main adrenal vein is exposed as the inferior margin of the gland is mobilized (Figure 16.4). This vessel is also doubly clamped, transected, and ligated. The aorta is then exposed and fibrovascular medial attachments are secured and transected. Attachments to the superior aspect of the gland are handled in a similar fashion and the specimen is removed.

Because of the multiplicity of small adrenal vessels, liberal irrigation and meticulous inspection of the fossa are required to identify residual bleeders. A Penrose drain is positioned in the fossa, and Gerota's fascia is secured over the upper pole of the kidney.

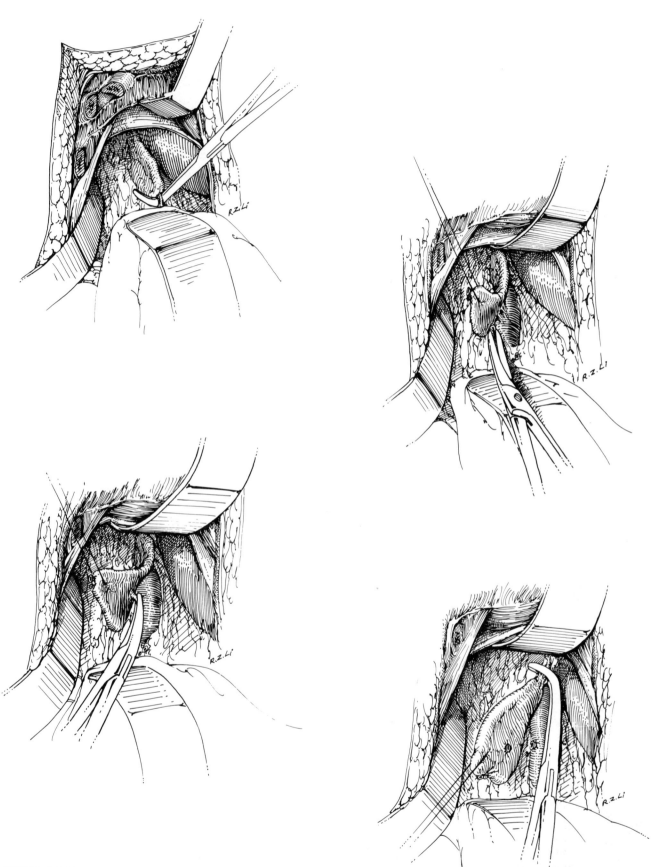

FIGURE 16.3
Right adrenalectomy performed through a transabdominal incision

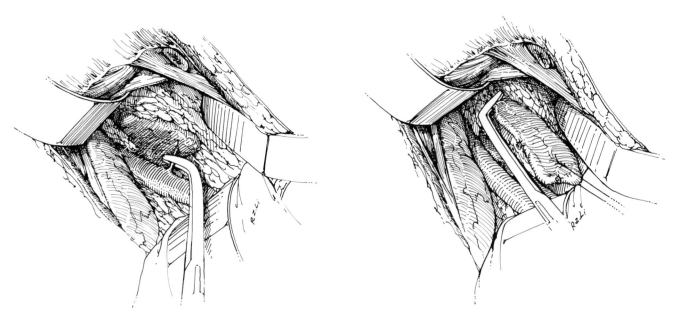

FIGURE 16.4
Left adrenalectomy performed through a transabdominal incision

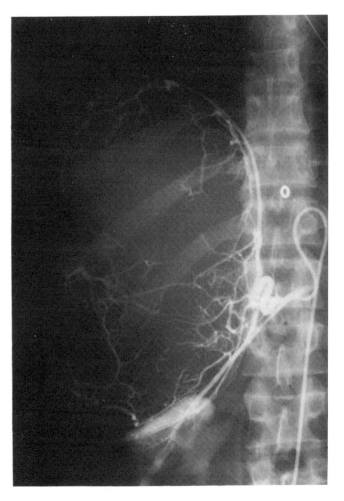

FIGURE 16.5
Arteriogram demonstrating large right adrenal cortical carcinoma

Large adrenal masses, such as that shown in Figure 16.5, may be impossible to separate from the kidney. When malignant, the mass is always removed en bloc with the kidney using the techniques described for a radical nephrectomy.

POSTOPERATIVE CARE AND COMPLICATIONS Bleeding from unsecured adrenal vessels is the most common postoperative complication and may require reexploration. Hemodynamic disturbances following the removal of lesions that secrete catecholamines and steroidal insufficiency after bilateral adrenalectomy or excision of a steroid secreting tumor can be avoided by compulsive perioperative management.

CHAPTER 17

Surgery of the Lymphatics

Lymphadenectomy is the removal of all lymphatic tissue within defined anatomic boundaries. It is performed usually to document the presence or absence of lymph node metastases from malignant tumors. This information may influence treatment strategies and objectives. For some urologic neoplasms (e.g., testicular and penile cancer) the removal of lymphatic metastases may be curative.

Lymph nodes and intervening lymphatic vessels are generally situated adjacent to major arteries and veins. They intermingle with fibroareolar tissues, and the peripheral margins are not well demarcated. As such, a critical component of a lymphadenectomy is accurate delineation of the boundaries of the lymphatic tissue to be removed. The tissue is then dissected from the adventitia of the blood vessels and removed en bloc in a systematic manner.

PELVIC LYMPHADENECTOMY

Pelvic lymphadenectomy is the removal of lymphatic tissue surrounding the common and external iliac arteries and veins and of the lymphatic tissue lying in the obturator fossa between the obturator nerve and external iliac vein (Figure 17.1). A small number of pelvic lymph nodes also lie between the sacrum and the rectum, but their location is inconsistent and the frequency of metastatic involvement is poorly defined. Excision of these nodes during pelvic lymphadenectomy is not warranted.

The initial lymphatic spread of malignant tumors arising in the posterior urethra, bladder, and prostate usually involves the pelvic lymph nodes. Tumors of the penis, scrotum, and distal urethra metastasize to the inguinal lymphatics before disseminating to the pelvic nodes. Testicular neoplasms rarely metastasize to the pelvic nodes unless the normal lymphatic channels have been obstructed by orchiopexy, prior pelvic operations, or massive retroperitoneal tumor deposits. Genitourinary cancers associated with pelvic lymph node metastases are usually incurable with surgery alone.

The anatomic boundaries of a pelvic lymphadenectomy include the muscular pelvic side wall laterally, the pelvic peritoneum and vesical fascia medially, the genitofemoral nerve superiorly, the obturator nerve inferiorly, and the femoral canal distally. The proximal limits vary according to the intent of the operation and the philosophy of the surgeon. However, the initial lymphatic spread of genitourinary tumors usually involves nodes situated below the bifurcation of the common iliac artery, and removal of lymphatics above the bifurcation rarely uncovers disease that is not identified in the more distal nodes.

The thoughtful surgeon should always bear in mind the rationale for pelvic lymphadenectomy. If documentation of metastatic disease has little impact on subsequent treatment or overall treatment outcome, heroic attempts to perform a thorough lymphadenectomy are ill-advised when difficulties are encountered during the dissection.

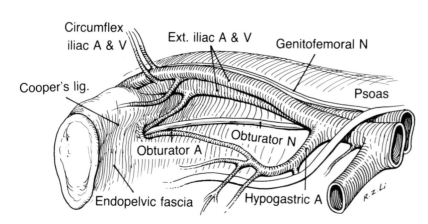

FIGURE 17.1
Anatomy of pelvic side wall

OPERATIVE TECHNIQUE A urethral catheter is introduced to decompress the bladder and facilitate access to the lateral pelvis. When done as a staging procedure, as a component of ilioinguinal lymphadenectomy, or before an anticipated radical prostatectomy, the area of dissection is exposed in an extraperitoneal manner. A lower midline incision extending from the umbilicus to the superior border of the symphysis pubis is recommended. A small opening in the peritoneum is made if there is a compelling indication for palpation of the intraperitoneal viscera. The defect is closed with a continuous absorbable suture before the lymphadenectomy is begun.

Incision of the filmy transversalis fascia is critical for development of the proper plane of dissection between the peritoneum and lateral pelvic lymphatics and blood vessels. Dissection beneath the transversalis fascia also protects against injury to the inferior epigastric vessels on the posterior surface of the rectus muscles. With medial retraction of the peritoneal envelope and bladder with the hand, and lateral retraction of the rectus muscle with a Richardson retractor, the external iliac vessels and obturator fossa can be exposed with remarkable ease. In the female the round ligament is encountered and is transected and ligated at the internal inguinal ring. In the male the vas deferens and gonadal vessels are encountered. An 8- to 10-cm segment of the vas is isolated and excised, and the ends are secured with free ties. The gonadal vessels are separated from the adherent peritoneum for a distance of 10 to 15 cm and retracted superolaterally. If the vessels are injured or compromise exposure, excision of the segment is advisable. Testicular atrophy or pain is an unusual sequela.

The contralateral pelvis is then developed in an identical manner to allow placement of a self-retaining retractor. The pelvic side wall is exposed throughout the operation by lateral retraction of the rectus muscle above the femoral canal with a Richardson retractor, superomedial retraction of the peritoneal envelope with a wide blade retractor, and medial retraction of the bladder with the hand or a wide blade retractor.

The medial limits of the dissection are defined with the foregoing maneuvers. The superior limit is established by incision of areolar tissue lateral to the external iliac artery and medial to the genitofemoral nerve (Figure 17.2). The external iliac vessels and surrounding lymphatics and the lymphatics in the obturator fossa are then mobilized en bloc from the psoas and obturator internus muscles. This maneuver develops the lateral constraints of the lymphadenectomy and simplifies the subsequent dissection.

The external iliac artery is identified by palpation, and lymphatic tissue on the superior surface is divided longitudinally from the bifurcation of the common iliac artery to the femoral canal (Figure 17.3). The incision may be extended superiorly along the common iliac artery if desired. A plane between the adventitia of the artery and the lymphatics is easily established with a scissors or a right-angle clamp, and all lymphatic tissue is freed in a circumferential manner. Lymphatic trunks at the proximal and distal extents of the dissection are cross-clamped, transected, and ligated. This allows inferomedial retraction of the surgical specimen. The external iliac artery is then pulled medially or laterally with a vein retractor to expose the vein. The lymphatics are incised in a longitudinal fashion on the superolateral surface of the vein, all tissue is freed from the adventitia in a circumferential manner, and the surgical specimen is retracted inferomedially (Figure 17.4).

The obturator nerve is identified and isolated at this juncture (Figure 17.5). Avulsion of the obturator vessels, which generally lie beneath the nerve, is a potential source of troublesome bleeding. Retraction of the nerve prevents injury during control of unexpected hemorrhage and helps to expose the bleeding vessels. If the distal obturator artery or vein is disrupted, the stump may retract into the obturator foramen and preclude control with sutures or hemostatic clips. In this situation the obturator canal is packed with Gelfoam and a figure-of-eight suture is applied over the foramen. The bleeding generally subsides with this maneuver, but a transient obturator nerve palsy is a possible sequela.

The external iliac vein and obturator nerve are retracted superolaterally and the distal ramifications of the lymphatic trunks are worked into a bundle just proximal to the femoral canal (Figure 17.5). This compartmentalization of lymphatic channels medial to the vein is facilitated by pushing tissue on the medial aspect of Cooper's ligament in a lateral direction and on the lateral aspect of Cooper's ligament in a medial direction. The bundle is then clamped just beyond to the node of Cloquet, ligated distal to the clamp, and transected proximal to the tie. This step occludes the pelvic lymphatics emanating from the femoral canal and obviates the application of multiple hemostatic clips.

Adherent lymphatics are then freed from the musculature above the obturator foramen. The obturator artery and vein may be left intact. Alternatively, they can be ligated and transected adjacent to the foramen and removed with the surgical specimen. The packet of lymphatics in the obturator fossa is teased from the perirectal fat deep to the obturator nerve (Figure 17.6), and the entire surgical specimen is retracted proximally to the bifurcation of the common iliac artery. Here the tissue is also worked into a discrete bundle or bundles, cross-clamped, transected, and ligated. The

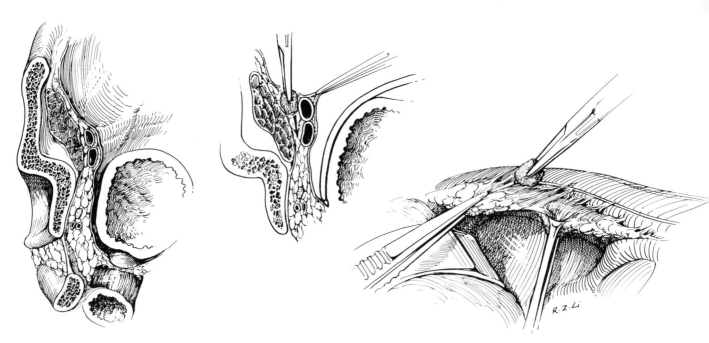

FIGURE 17.2
Mobilization of external iliac vessels and surrounding lymphatics from muscular pelvic side wall in pelvic lymphadenectomy

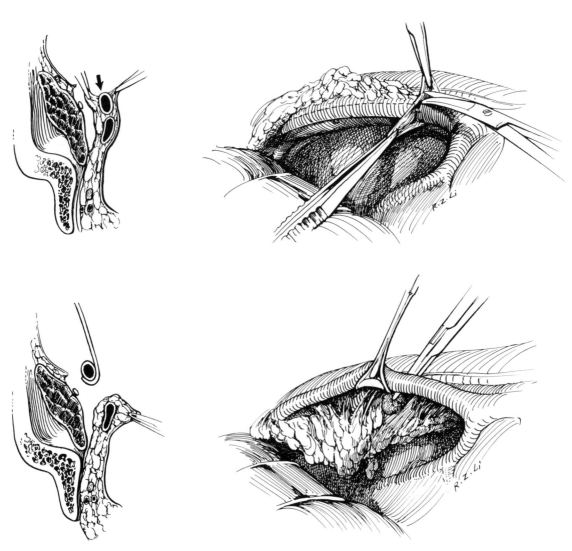

FIGURE 17.3
Dissection of lymphatics from external iliac artery

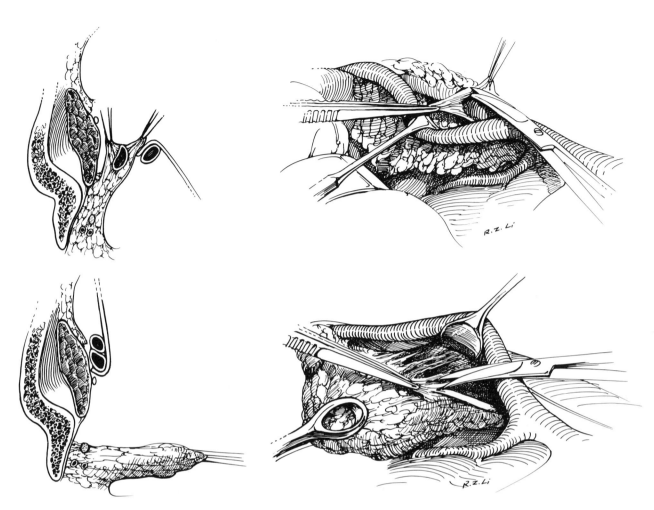

FIGURE 17.4
Dissection of lymphatics from external iliac vein

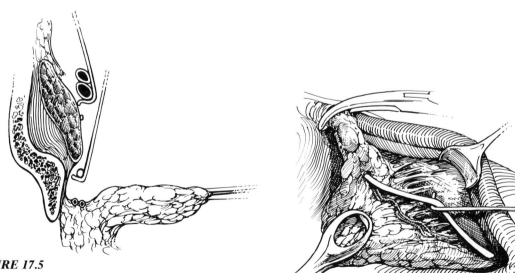

FIGURE 17.5
Mobilization of obturator nerve and transection of lymphatic bundle medial to external iliac vein at femoral canal

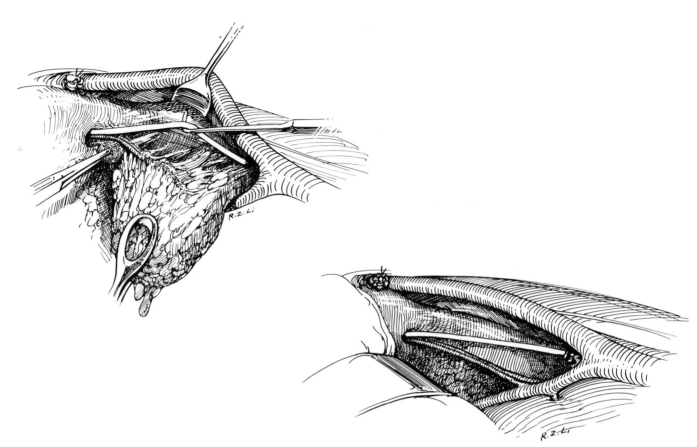

FIGURE 17.6
Teasing of lymphatics from obturator vessels and transection of proximal lymphatic bundle at bifurcation of common iliac artery

obturator artery and vein, if included in the specimen, are also secured with these ligatures. Hemostatic clips are rarely required.

The pelvis is liberally irrigated with sterile water and carefully inspected for bleeding. In contrast to saline, water lyses erythrocytes, and bleeding sites under the irrigant are easily visualized. The lateral pelvis is packed with small opened sponges, and the retractors are repositioned in the contralateral pelvis.

The operative field is always drained after an extra-peritoneal lymphadenectomy. The accumulation of lymphatic fluid in the undrained pelvis is inevitable, even when all transected lymphatic channels are meticulously secured. Suction drains positioned in the obturator fossae and brought out through separate stab wounds are favored by some surgeons. We prefer to place a large Penrose drain in each obturator fossa. The drains are brought out through a defect in the lower angle of the incision that is sufficiently large to accommodate two fingers. This allows adequate drainage of lymph as well as bedside access to the area of dissection should a lymphocele develop.

Prostatic cancer usually metastasizes to the obtura-tor lymph nodes first, and a staging pelvic lympha-denectomy performed before a radical retropubic prostatectomy is frequently limited to tissue in the ob-turator fossa. With this modified dissection, lymphatic tissue is incised along the medial border of the external iliac vein without disturbing lymphatics surrounding the external iliac artery (Figure 17.7). The tissue is then freed from the undersurface of the vein, the vein is retracted superolaterally, and the lymphatics adja-cent to the lateral border of the vein are incised. The surgical specimen is separated from the obturator in-ternus muscle, and the remainder of the procedure is performed as described above.

POSTOPERATIVE CARE AND COMPLICATIONS The drain-age of lymph during the first 1 to 2 postoperative days is often profuse, and the pelvic drains are not removed until the volume is less than 25 to 50 ml every 8 hours. Sterile appliances applied to the drainage site facilitate optimal nursing care and quantitation of the fluid.

Early complications include pelvic cellulitis or ab-scess and lymphocele formation. Lymphoceles are al-ways confined to the obturator fossa and are manifested usually by inordinate pelvic discomfort

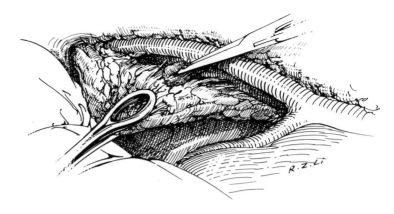

FIGURE 17.7
Dissection of lymphatics from external iliac vein in obturator lymphadenectomy

and, in some cases, an obturator nerve palsy. If drains are brought through the inferior angle of the incision, one can evacuate a lymphocele at the bedside by inserting a sterile, gloved index finger through the drain site. The obturator fossa is entered by hugging the posterolateral aspect of the pubic arch.

Manipulation of the external iliac veins predisposes to venous thrombosis and embolism. However, minidose heparin or alternative forms of anticoagulation do not appear to decrease the risks of these events. Transient edema of the external genitalia is common and responds usually to elevation with a pillow. Persistent edema of the genitalia or lower extremities is remarkably infrequent unless radiation therapy is administered after surgery.

Intraoperative injury to the obturator nerve results in difficulty with adduction of the ipsilateral leg. Unless the nerve has been completely transected, the neurologic deficit is usually short-lived. Ureteral injury is unusual if the lymphadenectomy is not carried above the bifurcation of the iliac vessels, or if the ureter is identified and mobilized medially before dissection of the common iliac artery.

RETROPERITONEAL LYMPHADENECTOMY

In urologic surgery, retroperitoneal lymphadenectomy is performed almost exclusively for the staging and treatment of nonseminomatous germ cell tumors of the testes. It is an extensive procedure but well tolerated because of the relative youth of most affected patients. With resectable retroperitoneal lymph node metastases and no evidence of tumor at other sites, cure can be achieved with surgery alone in approximately 50 percent of cases. When adjuvant chemotherapy is administered after surgery, the cure rate approaches 100 percent. Patients with "pure" seminomas but elevation in the serum alpha-fetoprotein level (a tumor marker secreted by nonseminomatous tumors only)

and patients with seminomas and residual retroperitoneal masses after radiation therapy or chemotherapy may also be candidates for retroperitoneal lymphadenectomy.

Bulky retroperitoneal disease is treated with combination chemotherapy before surgery to reduce tumor volume and facilitate complete resection of the metastases. Bleomycin is a component of most chemotherapeutic regimens and produces an interstitial fibrosis. Severe hypoxia may occur during surgery if the inspired oxygen exceeds 24 percent and the intravascular volume is expanded. The anesthesiologist must be aware of these hazards.

Opinions concerning the optimal extent of lymphadenectomy vary. The classic bilateral retroperitoneal lymphadenectomy involves removal of all lymphatic tissue in a field bordered by the superior aspect of the renal arteries, the ureters, the bifurcation of the common iliac artery on the ipsilateral side, and the mid-common iliac artery on the contralateral side (Figure 17.8). For practical purposes, modifications designed to limit the extent of the dissection to sites where metastases are most common do little to reduce the magnitude of the procedure or associated complications. However, preservation of the lumbar sympathetic nerves, which are necessary for seminal emission, greatly reduces the incidence of postoperative infertility. The procedure involves the preservation of both the paravertebral chain and the nerve fibers that course behind the vena cava and in front of the aorta below the inferior mesenteric artery. Preservation of the lumbar sympathetic nerves should be considered only if it does not compromise the completeness of the lymphadenectomy.

OPERATIVE TECHNIQUE A thorough mechanical bowel preparation and intravenous hydration the night before surgery are mandatory. Perioperative prophylactic antimicrobial therapy is recommended. The urine output during the operation is monitored by catheter drainage.

A midline transperitoneal incision extending from

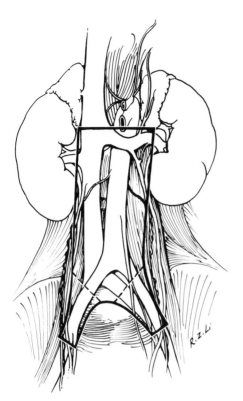

FIGURE 17.8
Constraints of bilateral retroperitoneal lymphadenectomy

In addition, the inferior mesenteric vein may be transected without adverse sequelae to increase exposure of the upper left retroperitoneum.

Each ureter is mobilized with the surrounding fibrofatty tissue and retracted laterally with vessel loops. The superior limits of the dissection are delineated by excising the flimsy areolar tissue on the superior aspect of the renal veins and on the intervening vena cava. This tissue contains several lymphatic vessels and must be secured with nonabsorbable sutures or hemostatic clips. The adrenal, lumbar, and spermatic veins branching from the left renal vein are ligated and transected. The spermatic vein is mobilized to the internal inguinal ring if the primary tumor arose in the left testis. Peritoneum lateral to the sigmoid colon must be incised and reflected to the interal ring to expose the distal vein. The vessel is then teased from the inguinal ring and removed.

Systematic excision of the lymphatics surrounding the aorta and the vena cava requires longitudinal division of tissues on the anterior and posterior surfaces of each vessel, and transection of the lumbar arteries and veins arising between the renal vessels and the bifurcations (Figure 17.11). Lymphatic tissue overlying the vena cava is divided from the renal veins to the mid-

the xiphoid to a point midway between the umbilicus and the symphysis, or a thoracoabdominal incision, provides the necessary exposure. The thoracoabdominal approach is preferable if bulky metastases are seen with computed tomography. The omentum and transverse colon are draped on the chest in moist towels, and the intra-abdominal and retroperitoneal structures are examined to identify unsuspected visceral metastases and to estimate the extent of retroperitoneal disease.

Exposure of the right retroperitoneum is achieved by incision of the posterior peritoneum medial to the inferior mesenteric vein from the cecum to the ligament of Treitz (Figure 17.9). The ligament is divided and the sweep of the duodenum is reflected laterally. The incision is then extended around the cecum and up the right gutter to the hepatic flexure. The cecum and ascending colon are mobilized superiorly, placed on the chest with the mesenteric small bowel, and stabilized with a wide blade retractor. The left retroperitoneum is exposed by freeing the mesentery of the descending colon from underlying lymphatic tissue to a point lateral to the ureter. Appropriate lateral retraction of the mesentery requires skeletonization of the inferior mesenteric artery for 5 cm from the aorta (Figure 17.10). The artery is divided just proximal to its major branches if the retroperitoneal disease is bulky.

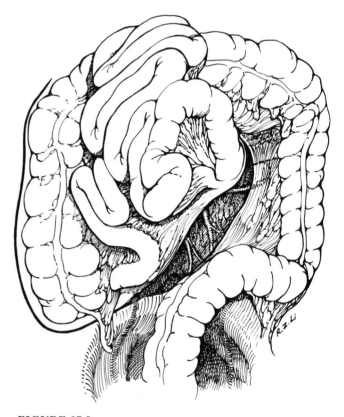

FIGURE 17.9
Mobilization of ascending colon and small intestine for exposure of retroperitoneum

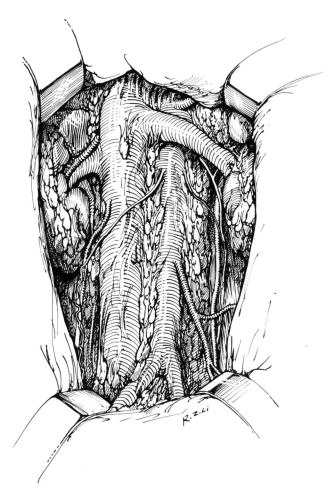

FIGURE 17.10
Exposure of retroperitoneum for lymphadenectomy

right common iliac vein (Figure 17.12). Lymphatics overlying the aorta are incised from the renal arteries to the bifurcation of the common iliac artery on the ipsilateral side, and to the midcommon iliac artery on the contralateral side. The gonadal arteries are encountered during this maneuver and are ligated flush with the aorta and transected. A subadventitial hematoma of the aorta often develops when a gonadal artery is avulsed. Control of this troublesome bleeding is achieved with a figure-of-eight suture encompassing the takeoff of the artery and the muscularis of the aorta.

The para-aortic lymphatics are located anterolateral, lateral, and posterolateral to the aorta and are removed first (Figure 17.13). The anterolateral and lateral tissues are cleared from the adventitia, and the aorta is retracted medially with two vein retractors to expose the lateral lumbar arteries. Each vessel is isolated for 1 to 2 cm from the aorta, ligated flush with the aorta and at 1 to 2 cm distal to the aorta, and transected. Lymphatic tissue between the aorta and the anterior spinal ligament is then divided in a longitudinal manner from the renal artery to the aortic bifurcation. The tissue along the anterolateral and lateral aspects of the left common iliac artery are mobilized, and the distal ramifications are worked into a bundle, doubly clamped, transected, and secured with nonabsorbable sutures. The para-aortic specimen is freed from the psoas muscle and the notch between the psoas muscle and the vertebral bodies, working toward the renal artery. The left renal vein is then retracted superiorly, and the mass of unattached lymphatic tissue is retracted inferiorly. Lymphatics coursing anterior and posterior to the left renal artery are freed from the adventitia and worked into two separate bundles. Each bundle is clamped, divided, and secured with a nonabsorbable suture, and the para-aortic specimen is removed.

The interaortocaval lymphatics between the aorta and vena cava are approached next. Tissue is dissected from the anteromedial and medial aspect of each vessel, and the lumbar arteries and veins are exposed by lateral retraction of the aorta and vena cava, respectively. After the vessels are ligated and transected, tissue between the vena cava and anterior spinal ligament is divided from the level of the right renal artery to the bifurcation of the vena cava.

Attention is then turned to the lymphatic trunks coursing anterior and posterior to the right renal artery between the aorta and the vena cava. These channels are numerous and drain into the cisterna chyli. The left renal vein is retracted superiorly and the lymphatics are pulled inferiorly (Figure 17.14); tissues anterior and posterior to the artery are worked into two separate bundles, clamped, transected, and secured with nonabsorbable sutures. The aorta and vena cava are both retracted laterally, and the lymphatics are separated sharply from the midline of the anterior spinal ligament, working away from the right renal artery (Figure 17.15). Tissue is then dissected from the lateral border of the right common iliac artery, worked into a bundle at the appropriate level, transected, and ligated. The interaortocaval specimen is then removed.

The paracaval lymphatics lying anterolateral, lateral, and posterolateral to the vena cava are substantially less pronounced than the para-aortic lymphatics but are removed using the same techniques (Figure 17.16). The paracaval lymphatics end just proximal to the right common iliac artery, as lymphatics surrounding this vessel had been removed previously with the interaortocaval specimen. The right gonadal vein is encountered while mobilizing tissue from the vena cava and is ligated flush with the great vessel. With right-sided testicular tumors the gonadal vein is freed to the internal inguinal ring and removed intact.

At this point the only lymphatic tissue remaining in

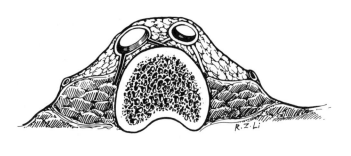

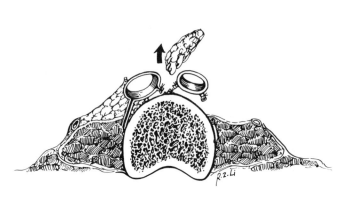

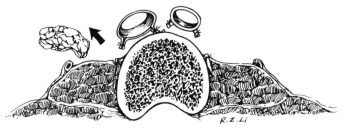

FIGURE 17.11
Technique for removal of lymphatics surrounding aorta and vena cava

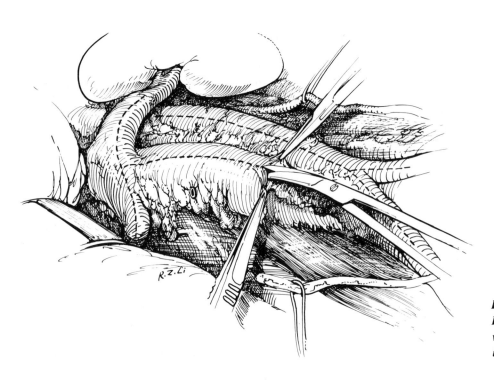

FIGURE 17.12
Division of lymphatics overlying vena cava, aorta, renal veins, and iliac arteries

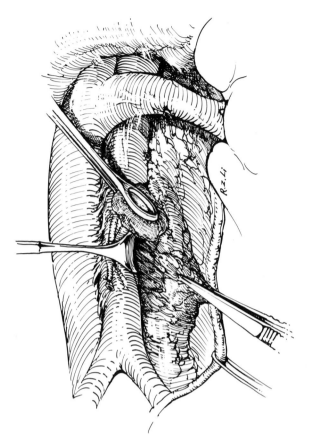

FIGURE 17.13
Dissection of lymphatics from anterolateral, lateral, and posterolateral aorta

the field of dissection is located below the aortic bifurcation. It is freed from the medial aspect of the common iliac arteries and from the intervening left common iliac vein. Lymphatics at the bifurcation of the common iliac artery on the side of the primary tumor and at the midcommon iliac artery on the contralateral side are worked into bundles, clamped, transected, and secured with nonabsorbable sutures.

Lymphatic tissue situated between the takeoff of the superior mesenteric artery and the renal arteries is not removed unless enlarged nodes are palpable, or bulky metastases are encountered below the renal arteries.

The retroperitoneum is irrigated with sterile water and all residual bleeders are secured. The posterior peritoneum is closed from the ligament of Treitz to the cecum with interrupted nonabsorbable sutures spaced at 1- to 2-cm intervals. A continuous suture is not used because lymphocele formation is inevitable when lymph cannot drain into the peritoneal cavity. The right colic gutter is closed with interrupted sutures and an appendectomy is performed as necessary. The retroperitoneum is not drained.

With massive retroperitoneal metastases, it is usu-

ally advisable to remove the tumor and the left colonic mesentery en bloc (Figure 17.17). Exposure is enhanced by dividing the peritoneum lateral to the splenic flexure and descending colon and retraction of the bowel medially. Should the mass extend above the renal vessels, the peritoneum lateral and superior to the spleen is incised and the splenic flexure, spleen, and pancreatic tail are reflected medially. Division of the inferior mesenteric artery at its takeoff from the aorta is invariably required for complete excision of large masses.

During retroperitoneal lymphadenectomy, the bowel is periodically inspected to identify vascular compromise. Excessive traction on the superior mesenteric artery and pancreas should be avoided. The central venous pressure and urinary output must be monitored closely. Lymphatic fluid and transudate accumulate in the operative field throughout the operation and require intermittent aspiration. Fluid that collects in the wall and lumen of the intestine also depletes the intravascular volume. In addition, manipulation of the renal artery leads to vascular spasm and decreased renal perfusion.

POSTOPERATIVE CARE AND COMPLICATIONS Proper fluid management during the first and second postoperative days requires serial hematocrit determinations

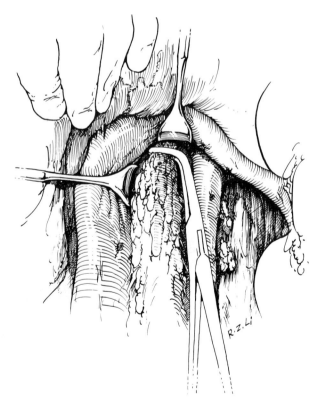

FIGURE 17.14
Dissection of lymphatics from proximal right renal artery

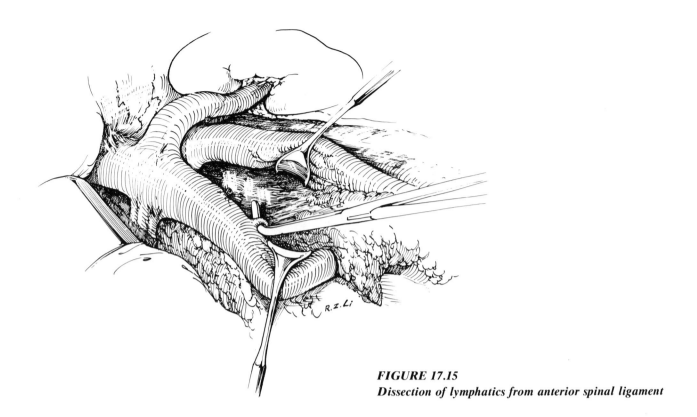

FIGURE 17.15
Dissection of lymphatics from anterior spinal ligament

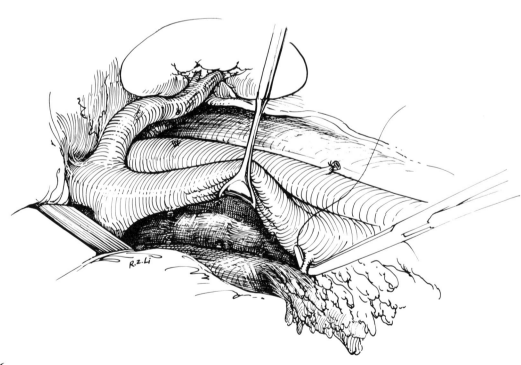

FIGURE 17.16
Dissection of lymphatics from anterolateral, lateral, and posterolateral vena cava

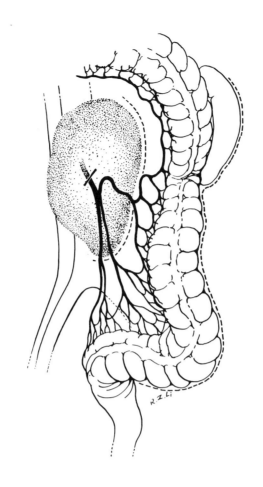

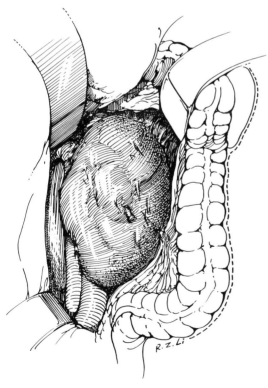

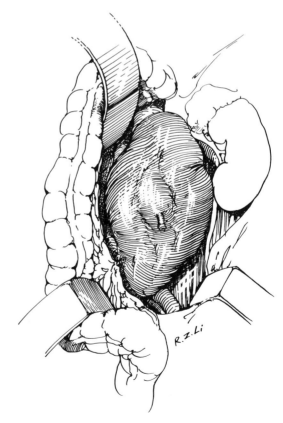

FIGURE 17.17
Exposure of large retroperitoneal mass

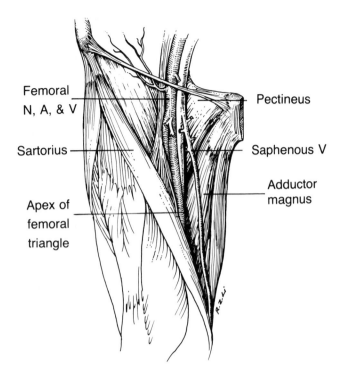

FIGURE 17.18
Anatomy of femoral triangle

and monitoring of the urinary output and central venous pressure. The urethral catheter permits hourly quantitation of urinary excretion and is left indwelling for 24 to 48 hours. A paralytic ileus of 3 to 4 days duration is the rule, and nasogastric suction is essential.

Pancreatitis from overzealous retraction, chylous ascites, and lymphocele formation are recognized but unusual complications. Most patients experience an absence of seminal emission unless disruption of the lumbar sympathetic chain lying adjacent to the vertebral bodies and sympathetic nerves that course anterior to the aorta below the inferior mesenteric artery is deliberately avoided.

INGUINAL LYMPHADENECTOMY

Inguinal lymphadenectomy is the removal of lymphatic tissue lying superficial to the fascia lata and the external oblique aponeurosis of the groin, as well as tissue lying deep to the fascia lata in the femoral triangle (Figure 17.18). The lymphatic metastases of penile, distal urethral, and scrotal tumors usually involve the inguinal nodes before spreading to the pelvic lymph nodes. Whether a lymphadenectomy should be performed in the absence of documented inguinal metastases, or when there are pelvic lymph node metastases and seemingly incurable disease, is controversial. Also

unsettled is the advisability of contralateral inguinal lymphadenectomy in the absence of documented metastases when there is known involvement of the other side. Inguinal lymphadenectomy is at times advisable for the palliative management of bulky nodal metastases or metastases that ulcerate through the skin, and to prevent tumor invasion into the femoral vessels.

Excision of the "sentinel node" at the time of partial or total penectomy for carcinoma provides useful information about the status of the inguinal nodes. The initial nodal metastases of penile carcinoma usually involve one or two superficial lymph nodes adjacent to the junction of the saphenous and femoral veins and superior to the superficial external pudendal vein (Figure 17.19). A 5-cm incision made two fingerbreadths lateral and inferior to the pubic tubercle provides adequate exposure. After identification of the saphenous vein and the medially branching superficial external pudendal vein, the appropriate nodes are removed. Closure requires approximation of subcutaneous tissue and skin only, and drains are not required.

OPERATIVE TECHNIQUE   A broad-spectrum antibiotic and minidose heparin are administered the day before surgery. For the procedure the patient is placed in the supine position and the ipsilateral leg is abducted, flexed, and externally rotated. Sandbags are placed under the calf and knee for support. The bladder is catheterized and the scrotum is taped superiorly.

A variety of incisions provide satisfactory exposure to the area of interest. We prefer an incision that extends from a point several centimeters below the pubic tubercle to a point several centimeters above the ante-

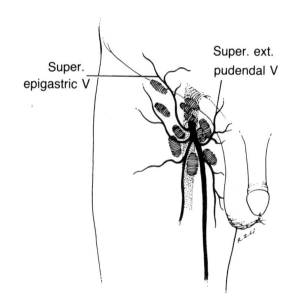

FIGURE 17.19
Location of "sentinel node" superior to superficial external pudendal vein

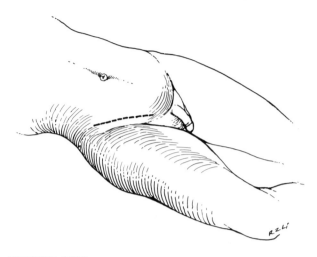

FIGURE 17.20
Incision for inguinal lymphadenectomy. The incision may be elliptical to encompass superficial nodal metastases

rior superior iliac spine (Figure 17.20). It is modified to an elliptical configuration to encompass bulging superficial or ulcerative nodes. The initial incision is made approximately 4 mm deep, and skin flaps of progressively increasing thickness are developed superiorly and inferiorly to isolate node-bearing subcutaneous tissue.

The upper skin edge is grasped with multiple Ader clamps or towel clips and pulled superiorly (Figure 17.21). The flap is developed with a scalpel to a point 4 cm above the inguinal ligament and is extended in a curvilinear manner to the anterior superior iliac spine laterally and to the pubic tubercle medially. The spermatic cord leaving the external inguinal ring should be identified but not disturbed. Subcutaneous tissue above the fascia at the periphery of the skin flap is worked into bundles, clamped, transected, and tied with nonabsorbable sutures. This seals superficial lymphatics that drain into the area of dissection. The node-bearing tissue is then freed with a scalpel from the external oblique aponeurosis.

The inferior skin flap is developed using identical techniques. This flap extends to the sartorius muscle laterally, the adductor longus muscle medially, and the apex of the femoral triangle inferiorly. The saphenous vein is encountered above the apex of the femoral triangle and is cross-clamped, transected, and secured with suture ligatures. Most of the lymphatic channels that drain the leg lie superficial to the fascia lata adjacent to the saphenous vein. It is particularly important to work this tissue into several discrete bundles for suture ligation. Some surgeons prefer to approach the distal saphenous vein and surrounding lymphatics after dissection of the femoral triangle.

Unlike the superior portion of the dissection, node-bearing tissue is not freed from the underlying fascia

lata. Rather, the fascia lata is divided over the belly of the sartorius muscle from the anterior superior iliac spine to the apex of the femoral triangle (Figure 17.22). The lateral femoral cutaneous nerve courses beneath the superior portion of this incision and is not disturbed. The edge of the fascia lata is grasped with hemostats and peeled from the sartorius muscle. The femoral nerve is encountered medial to the sartorius, and the fascia lata is carefully dissected from its fibers. Exposure at this juncture is enhanced by dividing the superolateral attachment of the fascia lata and inguinal ligament.

The lateral border of the femoral sheath, which surrounds the proximal femoral artery and vein, is seen

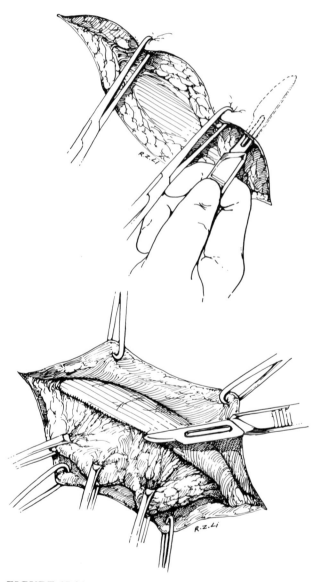

FIGURE 17.21
Development of superior skin flap and dissection of node-bearing tissue from external oblique aponeurosis and inguinal ligament

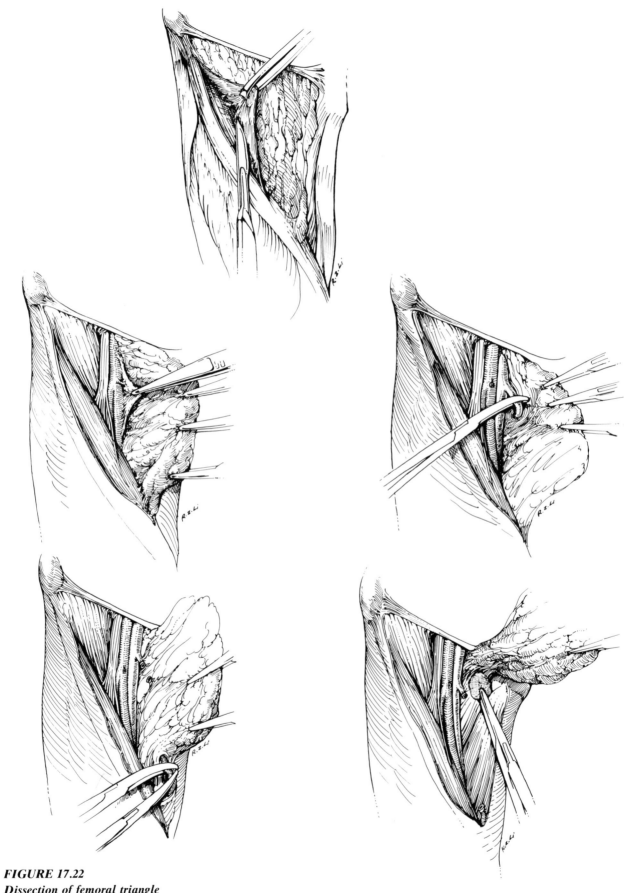

FIGURE 17.22
Dissection of femoral triangle

next and is incised. The anterior component of the sheath and the more distal fascia lata are then freed from the adventitia of the femoral artery and vein. Care is taken to preserve the superior external pudendal artery and the inferior epigastric artery. The saphenous vein is identified beneath the fascia lata as it enters the fossa ovalis. It is clamped flush with the femoral vein, divided, and secured with nonabsorbable ligatures. There is no significant lymphatic tissue behind the femoral artery and vein, and dissection posterior to the vessels is not warranted. The femoral sheath is then divided medial to the vein, and the fascia lata is detached from the medial inguinal ligament.

Fascia lata overlying the lateral border of the adductor longus muscle is incised from the inguinal ligament to the apex of the femoral triangle. If not already done, the saphenous vein and superficial lymphatics surrounding the vessel are transected and secured at this time. Lymphatic tissue at the apex of the femoral triangle beneath the fascia lata is isolated, cross-clamped, transected, and secured with a nonabsorbable suture. Tissue in the groove between the femoral vein and the adductor longus muscle is then mobilized to the femoral canal. The lymphatic trunks coursing under the inguinal ligament medial to the femoral vein are divided and ligated and the specimen is removed. This creates a potential site of herniation if a pelvic lymphadenectomy is also performed. The defect is closed by approximating the inguinal ligament to Cooper's ligament with one or two nonabsorbable sutures.

The origin of the sartorius muscle at the anterior superior iliac spine is divided, and the muscle is mobilized from its sheath for approximately 8 cm. Care must be taken to avoid injury to the neurovascular pedicle that penetrates the posterolateral muscle 10 cm below the spine. The muscle is either shifted or rotated medially to cover the femoral nerve and vessels and is sutured to the inguinal ligament and adductor longus muscle (Figure 17.23).

The wound is liberally irrigated with sterile water and residual bleeders are secured. Two Hemovac drains are positioned over the external oblique and the transposed sartorius muscle and brought out through puncture wounds in the inferior aspects of the lower flap. The flaps are fixed to underlying muscle and fascia with multiple absorbable sutures. Entrapment of the Hemovac drains should be avoided. The edges of the flaps are trimmed if redundant, and the opposing subcutaneous tissue is approximated with interrupted absorbable sutures. The skin is closed without tension using nonabsorbable mattress sutures.

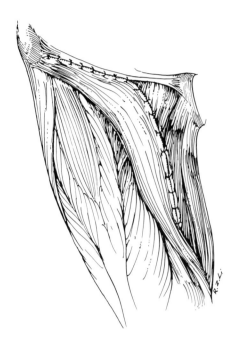

FIGURE 17.23
Transposition of sartorius muscle over femoral nerve, artery, and vein

The incision and flaps are covered with fluff dressings, and the groin and hips are wrapped with an Ace bandage. The legs are also wrapped with an Ace bandage or full-length support stockings.

POSTOPERATIVE CARE AND COMPLICATIONS The patient is kept at bedrest with the legs elevated 30° for 5 to 7 days. Minidose heparin and prophylactic antibiotics are administered for 1 week. The Hemovac drains can usually be removed 4 to 7 days following surgery. The patient is encouraged to elevate the affected leg above the level of the hip whenever sitting or lying down.

Subcutaneous seromas or hematomas are unusual if care is taken to secure all lymphatic channels and blood vessels. Skin flaps that are too thin or are closed under tension predispose to necrosis of the suture line. Extensive necrosis may lead to infection and large cutaneous defects. This complication is best managed by debridement and secondary coverage with a myocutaneous flap rotated from the lateral thigh.

Mild chronic lymphedema of the leg is not unusual after convalescence, and more severe lymphedema is reported to occur in approximately 25 percent of patients. Lymphedema is inevitable when radiation therapy is administered after surgery. The operation produces a depression in the contour of the groin that is accentuated by obesity.

Transurethral Surgery

Endoscopic visualization of the urethra and bladder was introduced in the nineteenth century. Instrumentation for the procedure has evolved from a hollow tube with an external light source to exceedingly durable and practical systems with outstanding clarity and illumination. Fiberoptic technology has led to the development of flexible instruments for examination of the bladder as well as the ureter and renal pelvis.

With the advent of electrosurgery, operative procedures of the prostate and bladder using endoscopic equipment was popularized in the early twentieth century. Most operations for the relief of obstructive voiding symptoms due to benign prostatic hyperplasia (BPH) and for excision of noninvasive malignant tumors of the bladder are now performed by transurethral electrosurgery. Endoscopic laser treatments for inflammatory and neoplastic disorders of the lower urinary tract are also possible with the availability of flexible conductive fiberoptic materials.

Transurethral procedures are a major component of the urologist's day-to-day activities. From a historical perspective their development has helped to define urology as a true surgical subspecialty. For students and non-urologists, full appreciation of the illustrations and discussions in this chapter requires personal observation of the operative procedures. However, we have never encountered a urologist who was unwilling to allow the inquisitive to look through the cystoscope, or to demonstrate the ins and outs of transurethral surgery.

Cystourethroscopy

INSTRUMENTATION

The rigid cystoscope is composed of a sheath, a bridge, and a telescope (Figure 18.1). The sheath is of varying caliber and has inlet and outlet ports for irrigation. The bridge fits on the end of the sheath with a watertight lock and may have one or two ports for the introduction of catheters, electrodes, or forceps into the sheath. A movable deflector that extends to the end of the sheath is incorporated into some bridges. The deflector is used to guide catheters within the bladder lumen.

The telescope is introduced into the sheath through the bridge and is fixed with a watertight lock. Contemporary telescopes are composed of a hollow metal cylinder that contains a series of solid-rod lenses. The image created with solid-rod lenses is superior to that produced by thin lenses separated by air, which were used in telescopes manufactured a decade ago. The eyepiece of the telescope has an ocular lens that magnifies the image. In front of the eyepiece is a light pillar that contains a fiberoptic bundle and connects to a fiberoptic light source. The pillar is continuous with a fiberoptic bundle contained within the telescope, which transmits light to the visual field. The viewing angles of the telescopes are 0° (straight ahead), 30° (foreoblique), and 70° or 90° (right angle). Retroview lenses with viewing angles of 120° are also available.

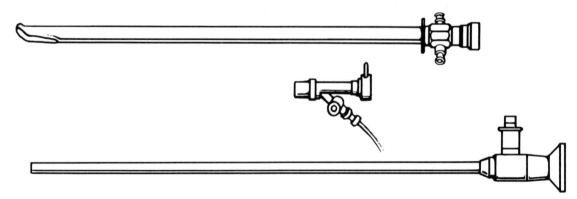

FIGURE 18.1
Sheath, bridge, and telescope of rigid cystoscope

ENDOSCOPIC ANATOMY

The configuration of the male urethra is shown in Figure 18.2. During urethroscopy, the lumen of the urethra expands because retrograde flow of irrigant into the bladder is restricted by the membranous urethra. This facilitates inspection of the entire mucosal surface. One enters the slightly dilated fossa navicularis immediately after introducing the cystoscope through the meatus. After the pendulous and bulbous urethra are traversed, the opposed pleated mucosa of the membranous urethra is seen. The prostatic urethra, which is the widest component of the male urethra, is then entered. When the bladder is distended with irrigant, the outlet expands and the interior of the bladder can be viewed with the end of the cystoscope positioned in the midprostatic urethra.

The mucosa of the prostatic urethra is anchored to the parenchyma and is less pliable than that of the distal urethra. With BPH there are varying degrees of symmetrical protrusion of prostatic tissue from the lateral aspect of the prostatic urethra, as well as elevation of the posterior bladder outlet. The length of the prostatic urethra is about 3 cm but increases with BPH.

The protruding verumontanum is situated at the 6 o'clock position just proximal to the membranous urethra. In the center is the 1- to 2-mm depression of the prostatic utricle, which gives the verumontanum the appearance of a volcano. The orifices of the paired ejaculatory ducts are situated on each side of the utri-

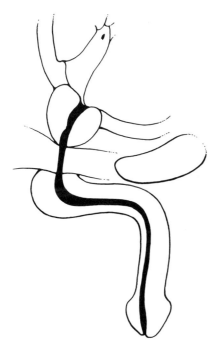

FIGURE 18.2
Male urethra

cle but are often difficult to visualize. A medial longitudinal ridge, the crista urethralis, extends proximal from the verumontanum. The prostatic ducts open lateral to the crista urethralis.

The female urethra is adherent to the anterior vaginal wall, has a relatively uniform caliber from the meatus to the bladder outlet, and is approximately 4 cm long. Distention of the urethra during urethroscopy is less in females than in males because irrigant flows freely into the bladder. This produces a pleated appearance of the entire urethral mucosa that is reminiscent of the membranous urethra in men.

The endoscopic appearance of the bladder is similar in males and females. The epithelium of the trigone is fixed and smooth. In women a whitish "pseudomembranous" mucosa with an irregular proximal border may cover the distal trigone. This is squamous epithelium extending from the urethra and is a variation from normal. The ureteral orifices are usually visualized without difficulty at the superolateral corners of the trigone.

With incomplete bladder distention, the vesical mucosa is rugose. As the bladder expands, the mucosa smoothes out and the fibers of the detrusor muscle become prominent to give the appearance of a grid or lattice. With hypertrophy of the detrusor muscle due to chronic bladder outlet obstruction or neurogenic bladder dysfunction, the muscular fibers form discrete ridges. Mucosa may herniate between these hypertrophied muscular bundles, or trabeculations, to produce small outpockets. With advanced detrusor hypertrophy these cellules may enlarge to form diverticula.

OPERATIVE TECHNIQUE Cystourethroscopy is performed with intraurethral analgesia and sedation. However, regional or general anesthesia is advisable if painful manipulations or electrosurgery is contemplated. The examination is performed in the lithotomy position. A thorough bimanual examination of the pelvis is performed before the patient is draped.

After the endoscopic equipment has been assembled, the sheath of the cystoscope is liberally lubricated with a water-soluble gel. Examination of the bladder is always preceded by inspection of the urethra. Blind insertion of the cystoscope into the bladder may lead to urethral injury or rupture if there is an unsuspected stricture; it can also result in failure to identify potentially serious urethral abnormalities such as neoplasms or diverticula. A 30° telescope is required to visualize the entire circumference of the urethra.

In men the prostatic urethra is systematically examined to assess the presence, size, and location of adenomatous enlargement. Palpation of the prostate per rectum with the cystoscope in the bladder provides a better estimate of prostatic size than does a routine rectal examination. The location and configuration of the ureteral orifices and the nature of efflux from the orifices are noted after the instrument is advanced into the bladder. The concave bladder wall is then examined in an orderly fashion to identify mucosal abnormalities. The interior of all diverticula are inspected if possible. The dome of the bladder is well visualized with the 30° telescope but the 70° telescope is required to examine the base. Suprapubic compression facilitates exposure of the anterosuperior bladder wall.

Transurethral Electrosurgery

Transurethral operations generally employ electrocautery for the cutting and coagulation of tissue. High-frequency current flows from an active electrode (the resecting loop or knife) to an indifferent electrode (the patient grounding plate). The concentrated current at the small surface area of the active electrode produces heat for cutting and coagulation. Heat is not generated at the indifferent electrode because the surface area is substantially greater and the current is dispersed. However, electrical burns can occur if the surface area between the grounding plate and the patient is unintentionally reduced. The electrosurgical unit does not discharge when the connection between the grounding plate and the unit is disrupted. This reduces the possibility of electrical burns at sites where the patient is in contact with conductive materials.

Nonconductive irrigant solutions, such as a glycine solution or water, are required for the conduction of current into the tissues and for the generation of heat. When saline is used, the current disperses into the irrigant, and heat sufficient for cutting and coagulation is not developed.

There is some variability in the form of current produced by different electrosurgical units. For practical purposes, however, the current is of two basic types. An uninterrupted current is used for cutting tissue whereas an interrupted current is used for coagulating tissues. Between the two extremes, current is interrupted for shorter intervals so that a blend of cutting and coagulating current is delivered. The urologist should be familiar with the characteristics of the electrosurgical unit in use and the proper settings for optimal cutting and coagulation.

Two foot pedals control the discharge of cutting and coagulating currents. In most units a sound of different tone is produced when one or the other pedal is depressed. This safety feature helps to prevent activation of the wrong pedal during transurethral surgery.

INSTRUMENTATION

Most transurethral electrosurgical procedures are performed with the resectoscope (Figure 18.3). The resectoscope sheaths for operations in adults range from 24 F to 28 F in caliber. They are made from Bakelite, steel covered in part with Bakelite, or fiberglass and will not conduct an electrical current. The tubing for delivery of irrigation fluids attaches to an inlet port at the hub of the sheath.

The working element comes in a variety of designs and attaches to the end of the sheath with a watertight lock. The telescope is introduced through a lumen in the working element and is secured with a locking mechanism. The cutting loop or other forms of electrodes attach to the working element, and circuits within the element conduct current from an electrical cord to the loop. Back-and-forth movement of the working element produces an identical movement of the loop.

The basic technique of tissue resection is shown in Figure 18.4. The loop is extended beyond the end of the sheath, tissue is engaged, and the cutting current is applied. The loop is then drawn through the tissue and into the sheath. The tissue is sheared off as the loop enters the sheath and is propelled away from the field

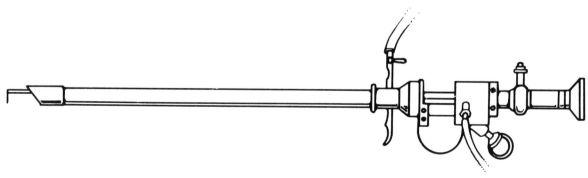

FIGURE 18.3
Resectoscope

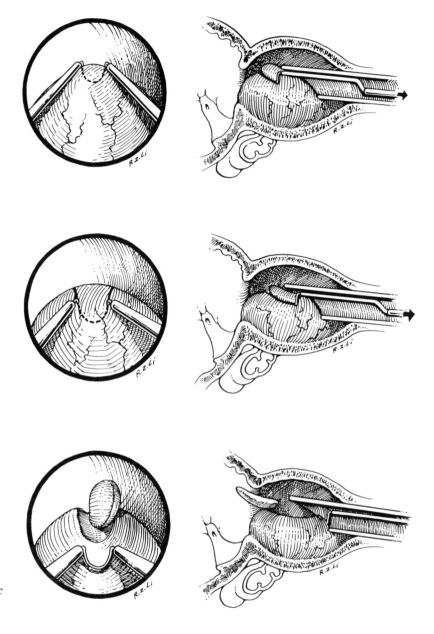

FIGURE 18.4
Resection of prostatic tissue (left, endoscopic view; right, side view)

of vision by the inflowing irrigating solution. Resection of tissue by advancing rather than retracting the loop is dangerous and rarely necessary. One coagulates bleeding vessels by touching the loop to the lumen of the vessel and applying the coagulating current. Fluid and resected tissue that accumulate in the bladder are evacuated passively by removing the working element and attached telescope from the sheath. Continuous-flow resectoscopes—in which the irrigant is delivered through an inner lumen of the sheath and actively evacuated by suction through an outer lumen—are also available.

It is the responsibility of the operating urologist to be certain that all endoscopic and electrosurgical instruments are in good condition and proper working order. Sterile duplicates of all components of the equipment that are planned for use, as well as equipment that might possibly be required if unsuspected conditions are encountered, must be available at the time of surgery. Malfunction of equipment that cannot be replaced immediately may lead to intraoperative disaster.

TRANSURETHRAL RESECTION OF THE PROSTATE

The indications for surgical intervention in the management of BPH are summarized in Chapter 11. Bladder outlet obstruction due to prostate cancer should not be treated by open prostatectomy, but is amenable to transurethral resection.

The anatomy of the upper urinary tract is delineated before surgery with an intravenous pyelogram, and renal function is estimated with a serum creatinine determination. A urine culture is obtained the day before surgery, and the operation is cancelled if there is bacteriuria. We routinely administer a parenteral antibiotic on the morning of surgery as prophylaxis against infection.

OPERATIVE TECHNIQUE Transurethral resection of the prostate (TURP) is performed with the patient in the lithotomy position. Regional anesthesia to the level of the ninth thoracic innervation is preferable to general anesthesia. The degree of relaxation is usually superior and the patient remains alert. Confusion and nausea or vomiting are early symptoms of excessive fluid absorption, and abdominal pain is an early symptom of bladder or prostate perforation. These findings are not manifested by the patient who is asleep.

The genitalia, perineum, lower abdomen, and upper thighs are prepared, and a sterile O'Connor sheath is inserted into the rectum to permit digital manipulation of the prostate during surgery. After preliminary cystourethroscopy the lubricated resectoscope is introduced under direct vision. Dilation or a meatotomy is necessary if the meatus does not accept the sheath. Similarly, if the sheath cannot be moved to and fro in the urethra with complete ease, the urethra is dilated with metal sounds or a smaller sheath is used.

The following considerations and maneuvers apply to all routines of prostatic resection. The resection is always undertaken in a systematic manner by removing a defined portion of the adenomatous tissue before proceeding to another area of resection. Important surgical landmarks include the ureteral orifices, the verumontanum, the circular fibers of the bladder outlet, and the true prostate. Unintentional resection of an orifice rarely leads to stricture and obstruction unless the orifice has been fulgurated also. However, when the resection involves a ureteral orifice, the more distal trigone is almost always resected also and perforation of the bladder outlet is a common complication. The verumontanum lies just proximal to the membranous urethra, and the risks of postoperative incontinence are almost nonexistent if the resection is not carried beyond this landmark. The circular fibers of the bladder outlet and the true prostate are identified after the resection begins. The circular fibers are not thick and demarcate the appropriate depth of resection. Deeper cuts invariably result in perforation and should be avoided. The true prostate is the peripheral constraint of the resection within the prostatic fossa; it has a white, fibrous appearance that is easily

differentiated from the fluffy, dirty snow look of resected adenoma (Figure 18.5).

The stroke of the cutting loop during most of the resection is not flat. Rather, the adenomatous tissue is scooped out by initial engagement, depression of the loop by elevation of the eyepiece, and elevation of the loop as it enters the sheath. This maneuver permits a uniform depth of resection relative to the concave boundary of the true prostate. Rapid retraction of the loop through the prostatic tissue is not necessary, but tissue will adhere to the loop if the stroke is excessively slow. During the procedure the loop becomes coated with proteinaceous material that reduces the efficacy of cutting and coagulation and should be intermittently cleansed with a sterile scrub brush.

Bleeding arteries appear as pulsatile spurts, and bleeding veins resemble clouds of dark blood (Figure 18.5). The vessels are not coagulated during the resection of one portion of the gland unless the field of vision is obscured. Subsequent strokes will only transect the vessels again. However, all bleeders are coagulated before commencing the resection at a different site. This reduces blood loss and improves visibility. In addition, should unexpected complications arise, the procedure can be aborted without concern about hemostasis at previous areas of resection. The identification of large arterial bleeders is facilitated by posi-

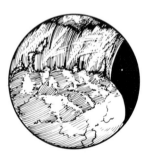

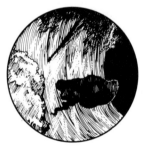

FIGURE 18.5
Endoscopic appearance of resected prostatic adenoma and true prostate (top) and bleeding artery and vein (bottom)

tioning the end of the resectoscope next to the prostatic capsule and advancing the instrument toward the bladder outlet until the lumen of the vessel is visualized. Conversely, the rate of irrigant inflow is reduced to permit localization of the site of venous bleeding.

Tissue fragments within the bladder are cleared with an Ellik evacuator when the resection is completed. Several fragments are often seen lying above the trigone when the process is completed and can be engaged with the loop and pulled through the resectoscope sheath. The integrity of the ureteral orifices is then documented. This is important because oliguria in the postoperative period cannot result from ureteral obstruction if the orifices have not been disturbed.

The prostatic fossa is inspected for bleeding vessels for the final time, the bladder is partially distended with irrigant, and the resectoscope is removed. A lubricated 22-24 F Foley catheter with a 30-ml balloon is introduced and the balloon inflated with 30 to 40 ml of saline. The return of irrigant documents appropriate positioning of the catheter in the bladder lumen. The following maneuvers are then performed to assess the adequacy of hemostasis. The bladder is drained, modest traction is applied to the catheter, the bladder is refilled with 100 to 200 ml of saline, and the catheter is clamped for 2 to 3 minutes. Subsequent drainage from the catheter will be clear or slightly pink if hemostasis is satisfactory. A grossly bloody return suggests active

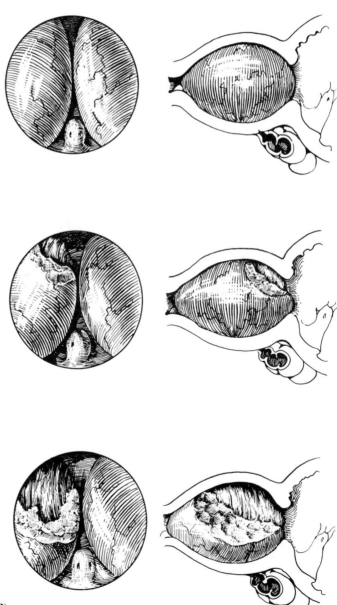

FIGURE 18.6
Technique for transurethral resection of the prostate (TURP)

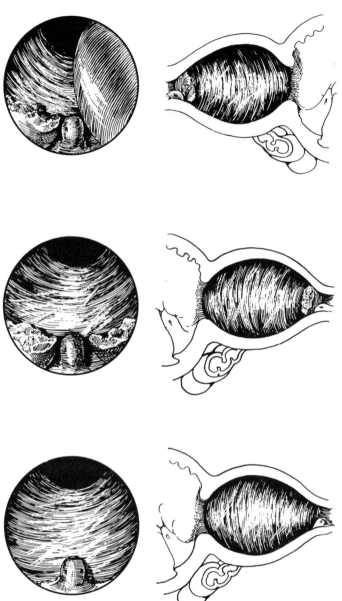

FIGURE 18.7
Transurethral resection of the prostate

arterial bleeding. In this situation the catheter is removed, and the bleeders are identified and fulgurated with the resectoscope. The catheter is then taped to the patient's inner thigh or suprapubic area with modest traction and attached to a sterile drainage bag.

On occasion there is no return of irrigant from the catheter despite seemingly appropriate advancement into the bladder. This is caused usually by introduction of the catheter tip into a defect created by deep resection of the posterior bladder outlet. Perforation of the prostatic capsule and passage of the catheter behind the trigone are inevitable if continued force is applied. The catheter must be removed and reinserted with the aid of a metal stylet curved dorsally.

There is no optimal routine for TURP, and variability in the size and location of adenomatous tissue may necessitate divergence from the general pattern of re-

section that is personally most satisfactory. An approach to TURP employed commonly for the resection of adenomatous tissue that is situated primarily in the lateral aspects of the prostatic urethra is shown in Figures 18.6 and 18.7. With the bladder partially filled to displace the detrusor from the bladder outlet, the resectoscope is rotated clockwise, and the resection is begun at the 9 to 11 o'clock position at the bladder outlet. After circular fibers are exposed, the adenoma is resected to a point adjacent to the verumontanum at the 9 to 11 o'clock position. The resected surface of the lateral lobe is now oriented transversely and can be engaged without rotating the resectoscope. The inferior lateral lobe and posterior adenoma between the 4 and 8 o'clock positions are removed by repetitive strokes that level the surface of the resection to the true prostate. Sculpturing of the posterior fossa can be accomplished without excessive torquing of the resectoscope by elevating the prostate with the index finger in the O'Connor sheath. Adenoma just lateral to the verumontanum is left undisturbed.

Resection of tissue on the left side is performed in a manner identical to that described for the right. When this is completed, attention is turned to the posterior bladder outlet and the remaining anterior and apical tissue. A thin, fibrous ridge at the 3 to 9 o'clock position of the bladder outlet is often developed as the lateral and posterior prostatic fossa is sculptured. This ridge is flattened to make a smooth transition from the trigone to the prostatic fossa. The anterior tissue, which is usually of minimal thickness, is then resected by rotating the resectoscope 180°. As the verumontanum is not visualized during resection of this tissue, care is taken to position the beak of the resectoscope proximal to the verumontanum before rotation. Finally, residual tissue lying just lateral to the verumontanum is carefully resected with short strokes. Elevation of the prostatic apex with a finger in the O'Connor sheath also facilitates this process.

The prostatic fossa is then systematically reexamined. Residual tags or bulging nodules of adenomatous tissue should be removed, but efforts to produce a meticulously smooth prostatic fossa by the resection of small bits of uneven tissue should be avoided. All remaining bleeders are coagulated, paying strict attention to the resected bladder outlet. Arterial bleed-ing at this site may be directed into the bladder and escape identification during cursory inspection.

Several alterations in the routine of resection described above are necessary when the prostatic urethra is longer than 4 or 5 cm. If feasible, the length of the stroke during resection of lateral and posterior tissue is increased by withdrawal of the sheath during retraction of the loop. This technique may permit a pattern of resection as described for smaller adenomas. Alternatively, tissue between the circular fibers of the bladder outlet and the verumontanum may be divided into proximal and distal segments of equal length. The proximal segment is resected at the 9 to 11 o'clock position to expose the true prostate. The distal segment is then resected at the same position. The remaining lateral, posterior, and anterior adenomatous tissues are also removed in a two-step manner.

If the adenoma is large enough to be removed by open prostatectomy but the patient is unsuitable for the procedure, a TURP may be staged. Resection of the right and the posterior adenoma is accomplished at the first sitting. Resection of tissue on the contralateral side is performed at a later date. On occasion the symptoms of bladder outlet obstruction resolve after the initial procedure and further intervention is not necessary.

At times a "median lobe" arising from the posterior bladder outlet protrudes far into the bladder lumen (Figure 18.8). This mass of tissue may obscure the

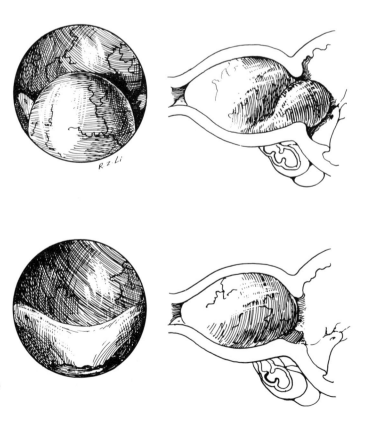

FIGURE 18.8
Transurethral resection of "median lobe" protruding into the bladder lumen

ureteral orifices and interfere with the advancement of the resectoscope and the propulsion of resected tissue into the bladder. It is advantageous to resect this tissue before approaching the lateral and posterior adenoma.

The base of the median lobe is often less thick than the intravesical extension. Complications that may arise during resection include pedunculation and increased mobility, which make engagement by the loop difficult, detachment of a large fragment that cannot be evacuated through the resectoscope sheath, and perforation at the posterior bladder outlet. Injury to unidentified ureteral orifices is also possible. To avoid these problems, the lobe is engaged at its apex, and the loop is retracted to a point just proximal to the bladder outlet. The stroke is made so that the distal portion of the fragment is thicker than the proximal portion. The lobe is approached initially in the midline and then from a lateral perspective. During the last step, it is usually possible to visualize the ipsilateral ureteral orifice. In addition, deliberate resection of the lateral margins helps to prevent the creation of a thin, broad sheet of tissue, which is difficult to engage with the loop. When the intravesical portion of the lobe has been removed, the base is resected flush with the bladder outlet to the level of the circular fibers. Resection of adenomatous tissue within the prostatic urethra is then begun as described previously.

The techniques for resection of prostatic carcinoma, particularly when the tumor is locally extensive, deviates substantially from those described for BPH. The contour of the prostatic urethra is often asymmetric and irregular, and rigidity may restrict the movement of the resectoscope. Most important, however, the appropriate depth of resection is difficult to assess because the appearance of the tissue is generally the same throughout the prostate. Therefore, a "channeling" procedure rather than the customary hollowing out of the prostatic fossa is recommended. The strokes of the loop are flat to create a straight rather than concave contour to the prostatic urethra. Resection of the bladder outlet and prostatic urethra proceeds in a circumferential manner, making no attempt to level the lateral lobes. Resection close to the membranous urethra is avoided because tumor infiltration may limit the functional integrity of the sphincteric mechanism. The complete excision of obstructing tissue, therefore, may lead to incontinence. Tumor regrowth and recurrent symptoms of bladder outlet obstruction are not uncommon. Androgen deprivation therapy may be advisable to reduce the volume of local tumor either in lieu of operative intervention or if symptoms recur following TURP.

INTRAOPERATIVE COMPLICATIONS A number of intraoperative complications are unique to transurethral surgery in general and specifically to TURP.

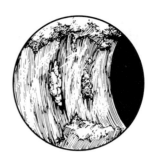

FIGURE 18.9
Endoscopic appearance of perforated prostatic capsule with periprostatic fat visible between capsular fibers

Priapism, urethral stricture disease, or the creation of false passages may make negotiation of the urethra impossible. The former is usually short-lived or responds to the direct injection of alpha-adrenergic agents into the corpus cavernosa. When conservative measures fail, a perineal urethrostomy is performed for introduction of the resectoscope. Extensive strictures or iatrogenic injury may also be circumvented with this procedure.

Uncontrollable bleeding that obscures the field of vision is uncommon if major bleeding arteries are promptly fulgurated. Venous bleeding rarely causes problems with visibility because the pressure of the irrigant exceeds the venous pressure. At the end of the resection, however, excessive bleeding may develop if large venous sinuses have been entered. Traction on the drainage catheter is usually sufficient to tamponade the hemorrhage.

Perforation of the prostatic capsule leads to extravasation of irrigant into the periprostatic space. A perforation characteristically appears as a deep hole with fat protruding through residual capsular fibers (Figure 18.9). Flecks of coagulated blood may be observed disappearing into the cavity. Elongation of the prostatic urethra and elevation and compression of the bladder base are observed when the volume of extravasated fluid is great. Patients managed by regional anesthesia experience restlessness, nausea and vomiting, diaphoresis, and lower abdominal pain as the volume of extravasation increases. Rigidity of the lower abdominal wall and a suprapubic mass may be palpable. The symptoms of excessive systemic fluid absorption may also be manifested.

The operation is aborted when the symptoms and signs of perforation are appreciated. Bleeding vessels are fulgurated, and prostatic fragments are evacuated from the bladder before the resectoscope is removed. A cystogram is then obtained to document the perforation. If a mass is palpable, it is advisable to make a small suprapubic incision for placement of Penrose drains in the retropubic space. Prostatic perforations heal spontaneously, but the duration of postoperative catheter drainage should be extended.

Excessive systemic absorption of irrigating fluid results from perforation of the prostatic capsule or from incision of large venous sinuses. Irrigating fluid enters the venous circulation because the pressure of the irrigant exceeds the venous pressure. Frequently referred to as the TURP syndrome, absorption of irrigant results in dilutional hyponatremia and circulatory overload. When hypotonic solutions (e.g., water) were routinely used for irrigation, intravascular hemolysis and acute renal failure were also components of the syndrome.

Early clinical manifestations of excessive fluid absorption include restlessness, confusion, and nausea and vomiting due to cerebral edema. Expansion of the intravascular volume results in increases of the systolic and diastolic blood pressure, bradycardia, and an elevated central venous pressure. Late central nervous system manifestations include seizures, coma, and transient blindness; pulmonary edema and congestive heart failure are late cardiovascular manifestations.

The procedure is terminated when excessive absorption is suspected; the serum sodium level, osmolality, blood gases, and central venous pressure are monitored closely. The intravenous administration of 10 to 20 mg of furosemide helps to reverse the intravascular overload. Severe hyponatremia is treated with the infusion of 250 to 500 ml of a 3 to 5 percent sodium chloride solution. Sodium chloride, however, must be given cautiously if there is cardiac failure.

Electrical stimulation of the obturator nerve during resection of the lateral prostate results in the forceful and sudden adduction of the ipsilateral leg. Perforation of the prostatic capsule by the relatively fixed resectoscope loop is a complication of the jerking movement. With experience, the urologist learns to immediately remove the foot from the current pedal and loosen his grip on the resectoscope when this startling event occurs. These responses limit the risks of perforation. Reduction in the intensity of the current and resection with the bladder only partially distended to increase the distance between the loop and the nerve help to prevent stimulation during subsequent strokes.

Instrument malfunction may result from such easily correctable problems as a broken loop or the use of saline rather than a nonconductive irrigant. Malfunction of the light source, electrosurgical unit, or endoscopic equipment can be rectified by replacement with duplicate apparatus.

POSTOPERATIVE CARE AND COMPLICATIONS Prophylactic antibiotics are continued throughout the hospitalization and for 1 week after hospital discharge. The catheter is removed 24 hours after the urine is grossly free of blood, and the patient is discharged 1 day later if the urine remains clear and voiding is satisfactory. Most patients experience some degree of urgency and frequency for several weeks after surgery. Urgency incontinence and intermittent gross hematuria of 1 or 2 days' duration are not uncommon but are unsettling for a patient who has not been forewarned.

The patient is seen at 1 week and at 1 to 2 months after surgery for routine follow-up and urine culture. Urethral dilatation is performed only if recurrent obstructive symptoms suggest postoperative stricture formation. The histology of the resected tissue is reviewed with the patient and documented in the chart. Strict attention to this matter is critical so that unsuspected carcinoma identified by the pathologist does not go unrecognized.

Excessive bleeding from the prostatic fossa is the most common postoperative complication. Life-threatening hemorrhage is infrequent, but the accumulation of clot within the bladder and obstruction of the drainage catheter cause painful overdistention of the bladder. Continuous irrigation of the bladder with a three-way catheter system, which is used routinely by some urologists, or intermittent manual irrigation, is required until the bleeding subsides spontaneously. The systemic or intravesical administration of epsilon-aminocaproic acid, an antifibrinolytic agent that may promote hemostasis, is advocated by some authorities. These treatments, however, have been decidedly ineffective in the author's hands. Cystoscopy and fulguration of bleeding sites is always indicated if troublesome hemorrhage persists for 12 to 24 hours or the magnitude of blood loss as determined by serial hematocrit determinations constitutes a threat to the patient's well-being. Not infrequently a bleeding vessel that could account for the hemorrhage is not identified, but the bleeding ceases after clot is evacuated from the bladder.

Other complications that may develop in the early postoperative period include a sterile or bacterial epididymitis and delayed hemorrhage. The latter usually occurs 10 to 14 days after surgery when clots adherent to the prostatic fossa dissolve or break off. In most cases the bleeding resolves with catheterization and evacuation of clot from the bladder.

Urethral stricture and bladder neck contracture are late complications of TURP and are manifested by recurrent obstructive voiding symptoms. Urinary incontinence is remarkably infrequent unless the membranous urethra was damaged at surgery or there is unsuspected neurogenic bladder dysfunction. The bladder outlet and proximal prostatic urethra are rendered incompetent by TURP, and retrograde ejaculation is an anticipated consequence of the operation.

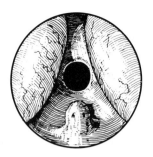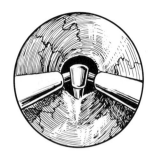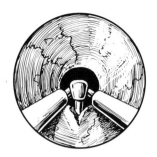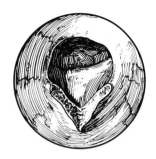

FIGURE 18.10
Transurethral incision of bladder neck contracture using Collings knife

All patients should be appraised of this phenomenon before surgery.

TRANSURETHRAL INCISION OF THE BLADDER OUTLET

Contracture of the bladder outlet usually results from circumferential scarring after TURP or open prostatectomy. Transurethral incision of the outlet with the Collings knife is the treatment of choice because recurrent scar formation is less commonly seen than with transurethral resection of the outlet. The bladder outlet is incised at one to three sites using the cutting current (Figure 18.10). Usually the contracted outlet "springs" open after one or two incisions. We make the first incision at the 6 o'clock position and a second or third incision as needed at the 10 and 2 o'clock positions. Bleeding is minimal but fulguration of several arteries and veins is often necessary. The bladder is drained with a 22 F to 24 F Foley catheter for 1 to 2 days after surgery. Y-V-plasty of the bladder outlet is occasionally necessary when a contracture is refractory to endoscopic management.

Transurethral incision of the prostate has been popularized recently as an alternative to TURP. This approach is most effective when there is symptomatic bladder outlet obstruction but minimal obstructive adenomatous tissue. Incisions at the 4 and 8 o'clock positions extending from the bladder outlet to a point adjacent to the verumontanum are made with a Collings knife. The incisions are preferentially carried into but not through the true prostate. However, extension into periprostatic fat is not uncommon because the appropriate depth of incision is difficult to estimate. Bleeding vessels are fulgurated, and the bladder is drained with a 22 F to 24 F Foley catheter with a 30-ml balloon. A small transurethral biopsy of the prostate using the resecting loop is recommended by some authorities to rule out unsuspected prostatic cancer.

The catheter is removed after 2 to 3 days. Although bleeding during the procedure is usually minimal, delayed hemorrhage several days after surgery has been reported.

TRANSURETHRAL RESECTION OF BLADDER TUMORS

Transurethral resection of the bladder is performed to procure tissue for the histologic diagnosis of urothelial abnormalities, or for the definitive treatment of noninvasive transitional cell carcinomas. Transurethral resection may also be applicable to the management of carcinoma in situ and superficially invasive transitional cell tumors, as well as for the treatment of invasive tumors in patients who are not candidates for radiation therapy or extirpative surgery.

Preoperative management parallels that described for transurethral resection of the prostate. An intravenous pyelogram is always obtained in patients with suspected carcinoma to identify coexisting tumors of the ureter or renal pelvis, or ureteral obstruction caused by the bladder tumor.

OPERATIVE TECHNIQUE Before instrumentation, a bimanual examination with the bladder decompressed is performed to detect palpable induration or masses. Both findings are usually associated with deeply invasive carcinomas. A bimanual examination after resection is often misleading because extravasation of irrigant may produce abnormalities identical to those associated with invasive tumors.

The resectoscope is used in the same manner as described for prostatic resections. However, the margin of error with respect to the depth of resection is not as great. The bladder wall, particularly in women, is not thick and perforation is not unusual. It is advisable to resect the bladder when it is only partially distended to prevent attenuation of the detrusor muscle. Fulguration of bleeding vessels must also be meticulous. Unlike the prostatic capsule, the detrusor muscle does not contract after resection to occlude transected vessels. It may be difficult to position the resectoscope loop adjacent to lesions on the anterosuperior aspect

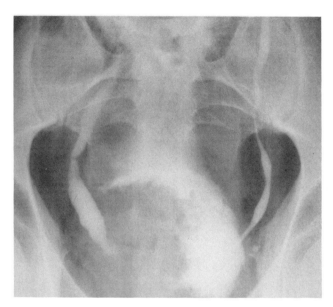 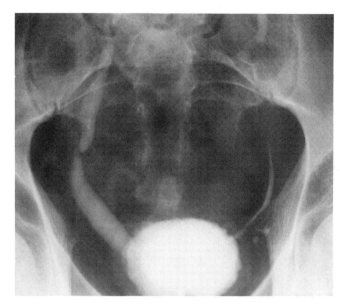

FIGURE 18.11
Intravenous pyelograms demonstrating large noninvasive papillary bladder tumor before (left) and after (right) transurethral resection

of the bladder unless suprapubic pressure is applied. Visualization and resection of tumors situated just inside the lateral and anterior bladder outlet of men is also difficult and may necessitate deliberate resection of the bladder outlet.

Exophytic tumors are frequently multiple and may occupy a large portion of the bladder lumen (Figure 18.11). Most are frondlike in appearance and arise

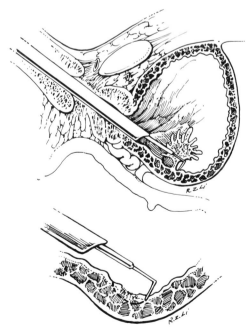

FIGURE 18.12
Transurethral resection of noninvasive papillary bladder tumor

from a small pedicle (Figure 18.12). The papillary component is resected first and evacuated from the bladder. The base or pedicle is then resected and sent for pathologic examination as a separate specimen. This orients the pathologist to the tissue of principal interest for identification of muscle invasion. When there are multiple small exophytic tumors, resection of every lesion and deliberate biopsy of the underlying detrusor is ill-advised. Repetitive removal of tumors using this technique may lead to fibrosis and noncompliance of the bladder. Fulguration alone is preferable for the destruction of these lesions.

Sessile or nodular tumors are usually of a high grade and stage. If the patient is a candidate for cystectomy, complete resection is ill advised. Extravasation of irrigant, which is common during deep resections, results in perivesical inflammation, which makes removal of the bladder more difficult. In addition, deeply resected areas are susceptible to perforation during cystectomy, leading to contamination of the operative field with malignant cells.

If complete removal rather than biopsy of a sessile tumor is undertaken, the lesion is resected to a depth midway into the detrusor muscle (Figure 18.13). The strokes of the loop progress sytematically across the surface of the tumor and correspond to the contour of the bladder wall. Bleeding vessels are carefully fulgurated, and the denuded bladder is liberally cauterized with the ball electrode.

The risks of bladder perforation are substantially less when a biopsy is performed with a cup forceps. The specimens obtained with this technique include epithelium, submucosa, and superficial detrusor and

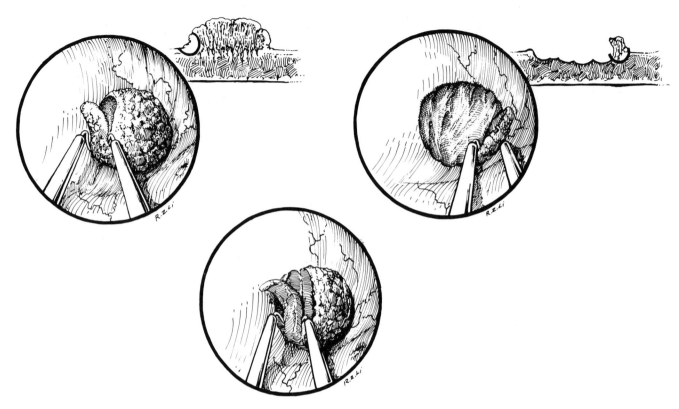

FIGURE 18.13
Transurethral resection of sessile, superficially invasive bladder tumor

are generally adequate for meaningful histologic evaluation. The cup forceps is extremely useful for random biopsy to identify carcinoma in situ among patients with transitional cell carcinoma, or to rule out carcinoma in situ among patients with irritative voiding symptoms of uncertain cause.

INTRAOPERATIVE COMPLICATIONS Perforation is the most common complication during transurethral resection of the bladder or bladder tumors. Defects in the fundus of the bladder may penetrate the overlying peritoneum and produce intraperitoneal extravasation of irrigant. The symptoms and signs of bladder perforation parallel those produced by perforation of the prostatic capsule. The procedure is terminated when a perforation is suspected, and the complication is documented with a cystogram. With intraperitoneal extravasation, contrast is seen between intestinal loops. Extraperitoneal perforations can be managed usually by urethral catheter drainage alone if recognized early and of small size. Intraperitoneal ruptures may also be amenable to this treatment. Open debridement and closure of all intraperitoneal perforations, however, is recommended by some urologists.

Obturator nerve stimulation is not infrequent during resection of the inferolateral bladder. The risks of perforation during this event are substantially greater dur-

ing transurethral resection of the bladder than during prostatic resection. Measures to eliminate obturator nerve stimulation are similar to those described previously.

POSTOPERATIVE CARE AND COMPLICATIONS Hematuria following transurethral resection of the bladder is usually minimal. The urethral catheter is removed after 1 to 2 days if the depth of the resection was not great. When perforation is suspected or documented, the duration of catheter drainage is extended, and a cystogram is obtained before removal of the catheter to be certain that the defect has sealed.

ABLATION OF POSTERIOR URETHRAL VALVES

Posterior urethral valves are the most common cause of congenital urethral obstruction in newborn males. The valves usually consist of two filmy membranous leaflets distal to the verumontanum (Figure 18.14). With voiding the leaflets balloon out and obstruct the flow of urine.

Most patients present with a distended bladder and a weak or dribbling urinary stream. Bacteriuria, sepsis, and renal insufficiency are common. The diagnosis is

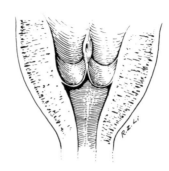 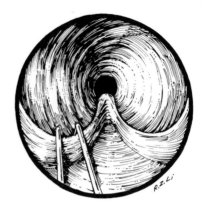

FIGURE 18.14
Side view of prostatic urethra and posterior urethral valves (left) and endoscopic appearance of valves during ablation (right)

made with a voiding cystourethrogram. The prostatic fossa is characteristically dilated, the bladder outlet and detrusor muscle are hypertrophic, and the valvular leaflets are usually identifiable. The degree of hydroureteronephrosis is established with ultrasonography.

Initial management includes decompression of the bladder with a pediatric feeding tube; correction of fluid, electrolyte, and acid-base imbalances; and antimicrobial therapy. The valves are identified and ablated with pediatric endoscopic equipment. If the urethra is too small to accommodate the instrument, a perineal urethrostomy should be performed. A cutaneous vesicostomy is created as a temporary diversion if ablation of the valves is not technically feasible or if pediatric endoscopic equipment is not available. In some cases functional ureteral obstruction necessitates temporary supravesical urinary diversion.

OPERATIVE TECHNIQUE Instrumentation of the delicate neonatal urethra must be gentle to prevent iatrogenic injury and the formation of strictures. The valves are best visualized with the resectoscope positioned distal to the verumontanum, with irrigant draining in an antegrade direction through the sheath. Resection of the valves is not required. Rather, the ballooning valve is engaged with an electrode or bent resectoscope loop at the 7 or 12 o'clock position and current is applied briefly. Most valves disintegrate completely with this maneuver. Regardless, management should err on the conservative side to avoid injury to the adjacent membranous urethra.

The completeness of ablation is assessed in the operating room by comparison of the urinary stream produced with suprapubic pressure before and after the procedure. With satisfactory ablation, the force and caliber of the urinary stream increases dramatically. Bleeding is usually minimal to nonexistent, and postoperative catheter drainage is generally not required.

TRANSURETHRAL INTRAURETERAL MANIPULATIONS

Until recently, transurethral intraureteral manipulations have been limited to retrograde pyelography, the extraction of small distal ureteral calculi with stone baskets, and the advancement of ureteral catheters into the renal pelvis to bypass obstructions. Instruments and techniques developed during the past decade, however, have revolutionized the field. Semirigid and flexible viewing instruments capable of negotiating and visualizing the ureter and renal pelvis are available. Many of these ureterorenoscopes have channels for the introduction of apparatus for biopsy or fulguration of mucosal lesions, or for extracting ureteral calculi. In addition, electrohydraulic, ultrasonic, and laser lithotripters have been adapted for pulverization of ureter calculi. The net result of these advancements is the ability to perform procedures in the upper urinary tract that heretofore could be done only for disorders of the bladder and urethra. The variety of instruments and techniques for these procedures is extensive, and the interested reader should refer to texts and manuals devoted to these topics.

TRANSURETHRAL LITHOLAPAXY AND LITHOTRIPSY

Bladder calculi may be fragmented with stone forceps or by a lithotrite adapted for use with a standard resectoscope sheath and telescope. All but the largest or most dense stones are usually managed with these instruments. Electrohydraulic and ultrasonic lithotrites designed for percutaneous nephrostolithotomy have also been adapted for pulverization of bladder stones.

CHAPTER 19

Extracorporeal Shock-Wave Lithotripsy

Extracorporeal shock-wave lithotripsy (ESWL) is a treatment that pulverizes urinary calculi in vivo and has revolutionized the management of renal and upper ureteral stones. The HM-3 lithotripter developed and manufactured by Dornier of West Germany was the first unit to be approved for use in the United States. Other machines introduced during the past 2 years employ ultrasonography rather than fluoroscopy for targeting the calculus, or generate shock-wave energy with piezoelectric crystals rather than an electric discharge. The following description of ESWL relates to the HM-3 lithotripter, but the general principles of treatment are applicable to all available units.

ESWL pulverizes calculi with shock waves that are generated underwater by an electrical discharge across a spark gap. The spark gap is located in a hemiellipsoidal reflector that focuses the energy at a second focal point within a tub of degassed and deionized water. The patient is submerged in the water, and the shock waves pass through the water and soft tissues with minimal impedance. When the shock wave encounters a calculus with inherent differences in acoustic impedance as compared with water, a portion is reflected (Figure 19.1). Shock waves that pass through the stone are reflected in part at the second acoustical interface between the stone and the surrounding fluid. Reflection of the shock waves results in tensile forces that shear off stone material.

The stone is centered in the second focal point under fluoroscopic control. Radiopaque calculi greater than 3 to 4 mm in diameter are usually visualized without difficulty. Radiolucent stones are identified by the intravenous injection of contrast medium, or by the introduction of contrast into the collecting system through a percutaneous nephrostomy or ureteral catheter. Because expansion during treatment is restricted, upper ureteral stones are more difficult to disrupt than renal pelvic stones and should therefore be pushed into the renal pelvis with a ureteral catheter before treatment. If the push-back is not successful, the catheter is passed beyond the stone to facilitate fluoroscopic localization and to create an "expansion chamber" by dilatation of the ureter.

ESWL is not approved for treatment of lower ureteral or bladder stones. Pregnancy is a contraindication because of the unavoidable radiation exposure. Cardiac pacemakers, distal ureteral obstruction, renal artery calcification, and bleeding diatheses are relative contraindications. Proper positioning of a stone in the second focal point is difficult in obese patients. Individuals taller than 6 ft 6 in or shorter than 4 ft 4 in are difficult to secure in the standard chair. Modifications of the chair, however, permit treatment of short adults or children.

METHODS OF TREATMENT

ESWL is painful and is almost always performed with a general or regional anesthetic. We prefer general an-

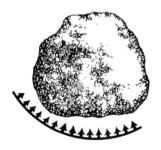 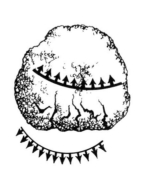 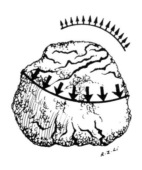

FIGURE 19.1
Reflection of shock waves at the first and second acoustical interfaces of stone and surrounding fluid with fracture of stone

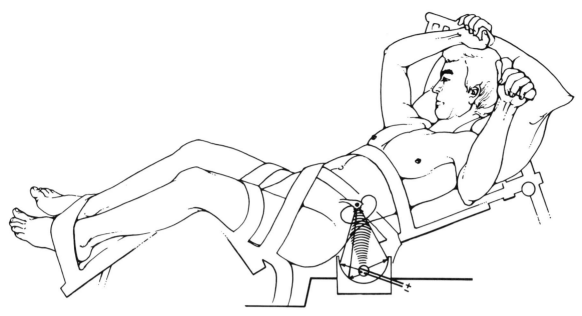

FIGURE 19.2
Patient strapped in chair and stone positioned in fixed second focal point of shock wave

esthetic because excursion of the kidney and stone during respiration is more easily controlled. Antibiotics are administered before treatment if the urine is infected or an infected stone is to be pulverized.

The patient is strapped into the chair, anesthetized, and lowered into the tub (Figure 19.2). The water must cover the anterior abdominal wall so that shock waves leaving the body do not encounter an acoustical interface between the soft tissue and air. This leads to the formation of subcutaneous hematomas. One centers the stone at the stationary second focal point by moving the chair and the patient. Two almost perpendicular x-ray beams cross at the second focal point, and a stone is properly positioned when it is localized at designated sites on each of the two fluoroscopic monitors (Figure 19.3).

The electrical discharges are triggered by the R wave of an electrocardiogram. After every 200 shocks the stone is examined with fluoroscopy to assess fragmentation and to ensure a continued proper location. The number of shocks required for pulverization of a stone is related primarily to its volume. With the exception of cystine stones, most calculi fragment without difficulty. About 1000 to 2000 shocks are usually sufficient, and 2400 shocks are generally thought to be the maximum allowable during one treatment.

POSTOPERATIVE CARE AND COMPLICATIONS Hematuria for 12 to 24 hours is the rule, but most patients with stones measuring less than 2 cm in diameter do not require hospitalization or can be discharged on the first posttreatment day. With larger stones, however, the size and multiplicity of the fragments are increased,

and parenteral analgesics are generally required for the management of ureteral colic. Stones that are not completely pulverized, either unexpectedly or by plan, are retreated. The second treatment may be performed the day after the first.

Ureteral obstruction caused by large fragments or by large volumes of finely pulverized stone material is the primary complication of ESWL. Large

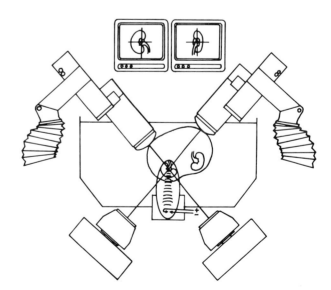

FIGURE 19.3
Two x-ray beams crossing at second focal point for proper positioning of stone

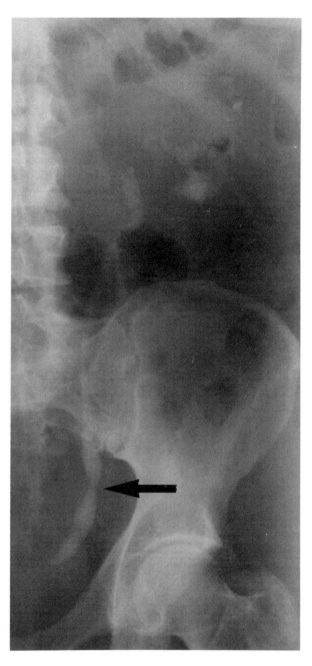

FIGURE 19.4
Column of pulverized stone material in ureter after ESWL

obstructive fragments are extracted with traditional endoscopic techniques or pushed back into the renal pelvis and retreated. Endoscopic manipulations are of little value in the management of large collections of finely pulverized stone material (Figure 19.4), but transurethral incision of the ureteral orifice usually facilitates its passage. A percutaneous nephrostomy or ureteral stent eliminates the obstruction and may also promote clearance of the particles.

Struvite calculi that are caused by infection with urea-splitting bacteria are generally quite large. Bacteria within the stone are liberated by ESWL and partial ureteral obstruction is inevitable. Decompression of the kidney with a percutaneous nephrostomy or ureteral stent before or after treatment is advisable to prevent acute bacterial nephritis.

Unusual but documented complications of ESWL include perinephric or subcapsular hematoma, mild pancreatitis, and fragmentation of coexisting gallstones. Pulmonary contusions may develop if the air-fluid acoustical interfaces of the lung are exposed to shock waves. This complication is seen primarily in children and is prevented by shielding the lower thorax with a sheet of polystyrene foam.

Index